Bradycardias, Complex Tachycardias and Clinical Arrhythmias: the Role of Electrocardiography: Part II

Editors

GIUSEPPE BAGLIANI
ROBERTO DE PONTI
LUIGI PADELETTI

CARDIAC ELECTROPHYSIOLOGY CLINICS

www.cardiacEP.theclinics.com

Consulting Editors
RANJAN K. THAKUR
ANDREA NATALE

June 2018 • Volume 10 • Number 2

ELSEVIER

1600 John F. Kennedy Boulevard • Suite 1800 • Philadelphia, Pennsylvania, 19103-2899

http://www.theclinics.com

CARDIAC ELECTROPHYSIOLOGY CLINICS Volume 10, Number 2
June 2018 ISSN 1877-9182, ISBN-13: 978-0-323-61052-0

Editor: Stacy Eastman
Developmental Editor: Donald Mumford

Cardiac Electrophysiology Clinics (ISSN 1877-9182) is published quarterly by Elsevier Inc., 360 Park Avenue South, New York, NY 10010-1710. Months of issue are March, June, September, and December. Subscription prices are $215.00 per year for US individuals, $344.00 per year for US institutions, $236.00 per year for Canadian individuals, $415.00 per year for Canadian institutions, $299.00 per year for international individuals, $415.00 per year for international institutions and $100.00 per year for US, Canadian and international students/residents. To receive student/resident rate, orders must be accompanied by name of affilliated institution, date of term, and the signature of program/residency coordinator on institution letterhead. Orders will be billed at individual rate until proof of status is received. Foreign air speed delivery is included in all Clinics subscription prices. All prices are subject to change without notice. **POSTMASTER:** Send address changes to Cardiac Electrophysiology Clinics, Elsevier Health Sciences Division, Subscription Customer Service, 3251 Riverport Lane, Maryland Heights, MO 63043. **Customer Service: 1-800-654-2452 (US and Canada). From outside of the US and Canada, call 314-477-8871. Fax: 314-447-8029. E-mail: JournalsCustomerService-usa@elsevier.com (for print support); JournalsOnlineSupport-usa@elsevier.com (for online support).**

Reprints. For copies of 100 or more of articles in this publication, please contact the Commercial Reprints Department, Elsevier Inc., 360 Park Avenue South, New York, NY 10010-1710. Tel.: 212-633-3874; Fax: 212-633-3820; E-mail: reprints@elsevier.com.

Cardiac Electrophysiology Clinics is covered in *MEDLINE/PubMed (Index Medicus)*.

Contributors

CONSULTING EDITORS

RANJAN K. THAKUR, MD, MPH, MBA, FHRS
Professor of Medicine and Director, Arrhythmia
Service, Thoracic and Cardiovascular Institute,
Sparrow Health System, Michigan State
University, Lansing, Michigan, USA

ANDREA NATALE, MD, FACC, FHRS
Executive Medical Director, Texas Cardiac
Arrhythmia Institute, St. David's Medical
Center, Austin, Texas, USA; Consulting
Professor, Division of Cardiology, Stanford
University, Palo Alto, California, USA; Adjunct
Professor of Medicine, Heart and Vascular
Center, Case Western Reserve University,
Cleveland, Ohio, USA; Director, Interventional
Electrophysiology, Scripps Clinic, San Diego,
California, USA; Senior Clinical Director,
EP Services, California Pacific Medical
Center, San Francisco, California, USA

EDITORS

GIUSEPPE BAGLIANI, MD
Arrhythmology Unit, Cardiology Department,
Foligno General Hospital, Foligno, Perugia,
Italy; Cardiovascular Disease Department,
University of Perugia, Perugia, Italy

ROBERTO DE PONTI, MD, FHRS
Department of Cardiology, School of Medicine,
University of Insubria, Varese, Italy

LUIGI PADELETTI, MD
Professor, Heart and Vessels Department,
University of Florence, Florence, Italy; IRCCS
Multimedica, Cardiology Department, Sesto
San Giovanni, Milan, Italy

AUTHORS

GIUSEPPE BAGLIANI, MD
Arrhythmology Unit, Cardiology Department,
Foligno General Hospital, Foligno, Perugia,
Italy; Cardiovascular Disease Department,
University of Perugia, Perugia, Italy

IRMA BATTIPAGLIA, MD
Paediatric Cardiology and Cardiac Arrhythmias
Unit, Department of Paediatric Cardiology and
Cardiac Surgery, Bambino Gesù Children's
Hospital and Research Institute, Rome, Italy

ALESSANDRO CAPUCCI, MD
Cardiology and Arrhythmology Clinic, Marche
Polytechnic University, University Hospital
"Ospedali Riuniti," Ancona, Italy

LAURA CIPOLLETTA, MD
Cardiology and Arrhythmology Clinic, Marche
Polytechnic University, University Hospital
"Ospedali Riuniti," Ancona, Italy

FEDERICO CRUSCO, MD
Radiology, Foligno Hospital, Foligno, Italy

ROBERTO DE PONTI, MD, FHRS
Department of Cardiology, School of Medicine,
University of Insubria, Varese, Italy

DOMENICO GIOVANNI DELLA ROCCA, MD
Texas Cardiac Arrhythmia Institute, St. David's
Medical Center, Austin, Texas, USA

LUIGI DI BIASE, MD, PhD
Texas Cardiac Arrhythmia Institute, St. David's
Medical Center, Department of Biomedical
Engineering, University of Texas, Austin,
Texas, USA; Montefiore Medical Center,
Albert Einstein College of Medicine, Bronx,
New York, USA; Department of Clinical and
Experimental Medicine, University of Foggia,
Foggia, Italy

CORRADO DI MAMBRO, MD
Paediatric Cardiology and Cardiac Arrhythmias
Unit, Department of Paediatric Cardiology and
Cardiac Surgery, Bambino Gesù Children's
Hospital and Research Institute, Rome, Italy

STEFANO DONZELLI, MD
Arrhythmology Unit, Cardiology Department,
Terni Hospital, Terni, Italy

FABRIZIO DRAGO, MD
Head, Paediatric Cardiology and Cardiac
Arrhythmias Unit, Department of Paediatric
Cardiology and Cardiac Surgery, Bambino
Gesù Children's Hospital and Research
Institute, Rome, Italy

FRANCO GIADA, MD
Director, Sports Medicine and Cardiovascular
Rehabilitation Unit, Cardiovascular
Department, PF Calvi Hospital, Venice, Italy

CAROLA GIANNI, MD, PhD
Texas Cardiac Arrhythmia Institute, St. David's
Medical Center, Austin, Texas, USA

FABIO M. LEONELLI, MD
Cardiology Department, James A. Haley
Veterans' Hospital, University South Florida,
Tampa, Florida, USA

DONATELLA LIPPI, PhD
Professor of History of Medicine, Department
of Clinical and Experimental Medicine, School
of Sciences of Human Health, University of
Florence, Florence, Italy

EMANUELA T. LOCATI, MD, PhD
Electrophysiology Unit, Cardiovascular
Department, Niguarda Hospital, Milan, Italy

MASSIMO LOMBARDI, MD, FESC
Multimodality Cardiac Imaging Section,
Policlinico San Donato, San Donato Milanese,
Italy

MAURIZIO LUNATI, MD
Electrophysiology Unit, Cardiovascular
Department, Niguarda Hospital, Milan,
Italy

JACOPO MARAZZATO, MD
Department of Cardiology, School of
Medicine, University of Insubria, Varese,
Varese, Italy

EZIO MESOLELLA, MD
Cardiovascular Diseases Department,
University of Perugia, Perugia, Italy

SANGHAMITRA MOHANTY, MD
Texas Cardiac Arrhythmia Institute, St. David's
Medical Center, Austin, Texas, USA

CARLO NAPOLITANO, MD, PhD
Senior Scientist, Molecular Cardiology, ICS
Maugeri, IRCCS, Pavia, Italy

ANDREA NATALE, MD, FACC, FHRS
Executive Medical Director, Texas Cardiac
Arrhythmia Institute, St. David's Medical
Center, Austin, Texas, USA; Consulting
Professor, Division of Cardiology, Stanford
University, Palo Alto, California, USA; Adjunct
Professor of Medicine, Heart and Vascular
Center, Case Western Reserve University,
Cleveland, Ohio, USA; Director, Interventional
Electrophysiology, Scripps Clinic, San Diego,
California, USA; Senior Clinical Director, EP
Services, California Pacific Medical Center,
San Francisco, California, USA

LUIGI PADELETTI, MD
Professor, Heart and Vessels Department,
University of Florence, Florence, Italy; IRCCS
Multimedica, Cardiology Department, Sesto
San Giovanni, Milan, Italy

MARGHERITA PADELETTI, MD
Cardiology Department, Mugello Hospital,
Florence, Italy

SILVIA G. PRIORI, MD, PhD
Professor of Cardiology, Molecular Cardiology,
ICS Maugeri, IRCCS, Department of Molecular
Medicine, University of Pavia, Pavia, Italy

MARTINA RAFANELLI, MD
Syncope Unit, Department of Geriatrics,
University of Florence, Azienda Ospedaliero
Universitaria Careggi, Florence, Italy

ANTONIO RAVIELE, MD, FEHRA, FESC, FHRS
President of ALFA Alliance to Fight Atrial Fibrillation, Former Director of Cardiovascular Department, Dell'Angelo Hospital, Venice, Italy

KETTY SAVINO, MD
Cardiology and Cardiovascular Physiopathology, University of Perugia, Perugia, Italy

ALESSIO TESTONI, MS
Electrophysiology Unit, Cardiovascular Department, Niguarda Hospital, Milan, Italy

ALESSANDRA TONDINI, MD
Arrhythmology Unit, Cardiology Department, Terni Hospital, Terni, Italy

CHINTAN TRIVEDI, MD, MPH
Texas Cardiac Arrhythmia Institute, St. David's Medical Center, Austin, Texas, USA

ANDREA UNGAR, MD, PhD, FESC
Associate Professor of Internal Medicine - Geriatrics, Geriatrics and Intensive Care Unit, University of Florence, Azienda Ospedaliero Universitaria Careggi, Florence, Italy

Contents

> This article reconstructs the steps leading to the identification of the atrioventricular block, from its first descriptions to current studies, highlighting the roles of Arthur Keith (1866–1955) and Martin Flack (1882–1931), who contributed to establish the theoretic basis for electrocardiography.

> The sick sinus syndrome includes symptoms and signs related to sinus node dysfunction. This can be caused by intrinsic abnormal impulse formation and/or propagation from the sinus node or, in some cases, by extrinsic reversible causes. Careful evaluation of symptoms and of the electrocardiogram is of crucial importance, because diagnosis is mainly based on these 2 elements. In some cases, the pathophysiologic mechanism that induces sinus node dysfunction also favors the onset of atrial arrhythmias, which results in a more complex clinical condition, known as "bradycardia-tachycardia syndrome."

> This article describes the different anatomic structures involved in normal atrioventricular conduction and their pathologic states. It defines their effects on the electrocardiogram and describes how to localize the level and evaluate the severity of conduction disease by electrocardiographic analysis. It illustrates the relevance of intracavitary recordings in the diagnosis of level of block.

> From the atrioventricular node, electrical activation is propagated to both ventricles by a system of specialized conducting fibers, His-Purkinje system (HPS), guaranteeing a fast, synchronous depolarization of both ventricles. From the predivisional common stem, a right and left branch separate, subdividing further in a fairly predictable fashion. Synchronous ventricular activation results in a QRS with specific characteristics and duration of less than 110 milliseconds. Block or delay in any part of

the HPS changes the electrocardiographic (ECG) morphology. This article discusses the use and limitations of standard ECG in detecting abnormal ventricular propagation in specific areas of the HPS.

Surface electrocardiograms, both resting 12-lead electrocardiographs and ambulatory electrocardiograph monitoring, play an essential role in establishing indications for cardiac implantable electronic devices (pacemakers, cardiac implantable defibrillators, and cardiac resynchronization therapies) and in the evaluation of patients who have already undergone implantation. Current devices have prolonged memory capabilities (defined as Holter functions) and remote monitoring functions, to evaluate the electrical properties and for the automatic detection of arrhythmias. Nonetheless, surface electrocardiography remains the critical tool to detect device malfunction, evaluate programming and function, verify the automatic arrhythmia analysis and the delivered electric therapy, and prevent inappropriate intervention.

Premature complexes are electrical impulses arising from atrial, junctional, or ventricular tissue, leading to premature heart beats. Premature atrial beats are much more frequent than those arising in the atrioventricular junction but less frequent than premature beats from the ventricles. Although they are usually benign and highly prevalent in the general population, they could trigger sustained supraventricular and ventricular arrhythmias and cause cardiomyopathies. This article reviews the main electrocardiology features of premature complexes and discusses their implications in clinical practice.

Atrioventricular node reentrant tachycardia (AVNRT) is a supraventricular arrhythmia easily diagnosed by 12-lead electrocardiogram. What is far more challenging is the understanding of the reentrant circuit in its typical and atypical presentations. The function of the atrioventricular node is still incomplete, and this knowledge gap is reflected in the reconstruction of the pathways used by AVNRT in its multiform presentations. This article illustrates the heterogeneous electrocardiographic manifestations of AVNRT. The authors reconstruct the reentrant circuits involved using more recent understanding of the anatomic and electrophysiologic characteristics of the atrioventricular node.

The common arrhythmia atrial fibrillation (AF) is incompletely understood. The mechanism of initiation and the perpetuation of AF remain speculative. This article summarizes current knowledge of the complex relationship between arrhythmias triggering AF and their long-term effects on atrial tissue leading to perpetuation of tachycardia. It focuses on the role of the electrocardiogram (ECG) from AF diagnosis in the identification of sinus P wave abnormalities predicting future occurrences. The role of ambulatory ECG recordings in managing AF and the use of frequency analysis to determine the degree of organization and the identification of AF triggers are discussed.

Wide complex tachycardia may represent a challenge for correct interpretation of standard electrocardiogram, which is crucial for proper patient management. For this reason, algorithms based on electrocardiographic criteria have been developed to guide interpretation in a step-by-step approach. Despite their greater accuracy, some cases of wide QRS complex tachycardia are a challenge. Some peculiar forms of ventricular tachycardia, and complex supraventricular substrate or particular clinical condition, may originate a challenging electrocardiographic pattern. In this article, a series of peculiar cases of wide QRS complex tachycardia is presented as paradigm of how important a comprehensive clinical approach is in these patients.

The surface electrocardiogram (ECG) is a valuable mapping tool in patients with idiopathic and scar-related ventricular arrhythmias (VAs). A detailed analysis of the 12-lead ECG can provide useful information in localizing the VA site of origin; this might help tailoring the ablation strategy to optimize procedural duration, increase the probability of success, and prevent complications. This article reviews the ECG features of both idiopathic and scar-related VAs and discusses their potential implications for optimizing the ablation strategy.

Early repolarization, Brugada syndrome, and pathologic J waves have been described for decades, but only recently experimental and clinical data have allowed reconciliation of Brugada and early repolarization under the common definition of J-wave syndromes. The concept was derived from studies showing, in both conditions, the presence of transmural dispersion of repolarization, localized conduction abnormalities, and abnormal transition between QRS and ST segment on electrocardiogram. Although several clinical studies have addressed the clinical presentation and epidemiology of J-wave syndromes, relevant knowledge gaps exist. Incomplete pathophysiologic understanding and uncertain electrocardiographic definitions limit effective risk stratification. Here, the authors review the current knowledge and recommendations for diagnosis and clinical management of these arrhythmogenic disorders.

Syncope is a frequent condition caused by a transient global cerebral hypoperfusion, which may depend on a reduction of vascular total peripheral resistance and/or cardiac output. Cardiac syncope doubled the risk of death from any cause and increased the risk of nonfatal and fatal cardiovascular events. Arrhythmias are the most common cardiac causes of syncope. Both bradyarrhythmias and tachyar-rhythmias may predispose one to syncope. The first-line evaluation relies on clinical history, physical examination, active standing test, and 12-lead echocardiogram. The diagnostic yield of electrophysiologic study in detecting the cause of syncope depends highly on the pretest probability.

CARDIAC ELECTROPHYSIOLOGY CLINICS

FORTHCOMING ISSUES

September 2018
Lead Management for Electrophysiologists
Noel G. Boyle and Bruce Wilkoff, *Editors*

December 2018
His Bundle Pacing
Pramod Deshmukh and Kenneth A. Ellenbogen,
Editors

March 2019
Cardiac Resynchronization : A Reappraisal
Jagmeet P. Singh and Gopi Dandamudi, *Editors*

RECENT ISSUES

March 2018
**Contemporary Issues in Patients with
Implantable Devices**
Amin Al-ahmad, Raymond Yee, and
Mark S. Link, *Editors*

December 2017
**Contemporary Challenges in Sudden Cardiac
Death**
Mohammad Shenasa, N.A. Mark Estes III, and
Gordon F. Tomaselli, *Editors*

September 2017
**Normal Electrophysiology, Substrates, and
the Electrocardiographic Diagnosis of
Cardiac Arrhythmias: Part I**
Luigi Padeletti and Giuseppe Bagliani, *Editors*

ISSUE OF RELATED INTEREST

Cardiac Electrophysiology Clinics, September 2017 (Vol. 9, No. 3)
**Normal Electrophysiology, Substrates, and the Electrocardiographic Diagnosis of
Cardiac Arrhythmias: Part I**
Luigi Padeletti, Giuseppe Bagliani, *Editors*

THE CLINICS ARE AVAILABLE ONLINE!
Access your subscription at:
www.theclinics.com

Foreword
Remembering Luigi Padeletti

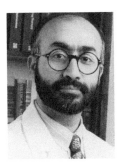

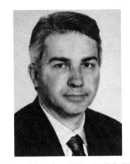

Ranjan K. Thakur, MD, MPH, MBA, FHRS   Andrea Natale, MD, FACC, FHRS

Consulting Editors

We introduce this issue of *Cardiac Electrophysiology Clinics* by expressing our sorrow and paying tribute to an editor, Dr Luigi Padeletti. Dr Padeletti was in the process of editing the current issue when he passed away unexpectedly. We are grateful to his coeditors, Drs Bagliani and De Ponti, who completed what Dr Padeletti could not. Dr Padeletti had been an ardent supporter of the *Cardiac Electrophysiology Clinics*, having contributed several articles and having edited multiple issues over the years.

Dr Padeletti inspired and edited two recent issues of *Cardiac Electrophysiology Clinics*; the first issue focused on basic electrocardiography in normal and diseased hearts. That issue took a unique approach to discussing electrocardiography of arrhythmias. It first detailed what can be learned about physiology, pathology, and neural control from each wave and interval of the electrocardiogram and then built on that to discuss arrhythmias originating in each cardiac structure. This companion issue of the *Cardiac Electrophysiology Clinics* focuses on electrocardiography of various arrhythmias:

bradycardias, tachycardias, and some specific arrhythmias.

We and the coeditors of this issue are grateful to have known and worked with Dr Padeletti and draw inspiration from his example of dedication to scholarship. We hope the readers will enjoy reading and learning from this issue, because that will be the most fitting tribute to his memory.

Ranjan K. Thakur, MD, MPH, MBA, FHRS
Sparrow Thoracic and Cardiovascular Institute
Michigan State University
1440 East Michigan Avenue, Suite 400
Lansing, MI 48912, USA

Andrea Natale, MD, FACC, FHRS
Texas Cardiac Arrhythmia Institute
Center for Atrial Fibrillation at
St. David's Medical Center
1015 East 32nd Street, Suite 516
Austin, TX 78705, USA

E-mail addresses:
thakur@msu.edu (R.K. Thakur)
andrea.natale@stdavids.com (A. Natale)

Card Electrophysiol Clin 10 (2018) xiii
https://doi.org/10.1016/j.ccep.2018.03.002
1877-9182/18/© 2018 Published by Elsevier Inc.

Preface
On the Shoulder of Giants and Luigi Padeletti Is One of Them

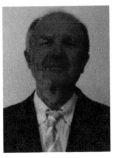

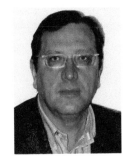

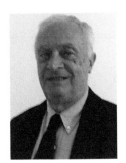

Giuseppe Bagliani, MD   Roberto De Ponti, MD, FHRS   Luigi Padeletti, MD
Editors

When, after completing the first issue inspired by the work of the big names in the field of cardiac arrhythmias, we moved on to the second issue, we were so satisfied with the work that we felt as we were "on the shoulders of giants."

The first issue was focused on basic electrocardiography in normal and diseased heart, apparently a very simple topic, but very frequently neglected by the hypertechnologic young generations. Along with Luigi Padeletti, it was decided that a second issue was necessary to complete the body of knowledge on electrocardiographic interpretation in bradycardias, complex tachycardias, and peculiar clinical conditions. This was to remind the readership of the information necessary to use the surface electrocardiogram as a fundamental instrument to orient diagnosis in the universe of cardiac arrhythmias. To this aim, we invited Roberto De Ponti, a friend for ages, to join the editors.

At that time, we would have never expected that the person who inspired these issues, our mentor and friend Luigi, would have left us by the time the second issue was completed. He passed away on a sad December evening and, as in a nightmare, we are still unable to cope with this. Although he is no longer with us in our professional and personal life, his culture, experience, equilibrium, and savoir faire remain.

Looking at the hard work done and the long years of fruitful cooperation with Luigi, we realize that we have been so lucky to have known a giant like him and to have been on his shoulders. The strength of his example spurs us on to continue the study of and the rational approach to cardiac arrhythmias, both based on the surface electrocardiogram.

On behalf of all the contributors, who have been willing to participate in this venture and support the hard work with their scientific and practical experience, we dedicate this issue to Luigi.

Thank you, Luigi. We will never forget you.

Giuseppe Bagliani, MD
Arrhythmology Unit
Cardiology Department
Foligno General Hospital
Via Massimo Arcamone
Foligno, Perugia 06034, Italy

Cardiovascular Disease Department
University of Perugia
Piazza Menghini 1
Perugia 06129, Italy

Roberto De Ponti, MD, FHRS
Department of Cardiology
School of Medicine
University of Insubria
Viale Borri, 57
Varese 21100, Italy

Luigi Padeletti, MD
Heart and Vessels
University of Florence
viale Morgagni, 85
Florence, Italy

E-mail addresses:
giuseppe.bagliani@tim.it (G. Bagliani)
roberto.deponti@uninsubria.it (R. De Ponti)
lpadeletti@interfree.it (L. Padeletti)

cardiacEP.theclinics.com

Card Electrophysiol Clin 10 (2018) xv
https://doi.org/10.1016/j.ccep.2018.03.001
1877-9182/18/© 2018 Elsevier Inc. All rights reserved.

In Memoriam

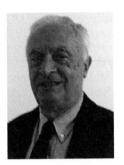

Luigi Padeletti

Luigi Padeletti was born July 15, 1947 in Gubbio, Italy. He spent all his life in Florence, Tuscany, where he lived with his family and worked at the University of Medicine. He graduated in 1972 from medical school and gained two fellowships, one in cardiology and cardiovascular diseases and the other in anesthesiology and critical care, at the University of Florence. In 1992, he became an Assistant Professor in Cardiology, and, finally, in 2006 a Full Professor of Cardiology at the University of Florence, School of Medicine, Careggi Medical Center. For eighteen years he was the Director of the Fellowship Cardiology Program at the University of Florence. He ended his academic career in November 2017 at the age of 70, when he retired. He moved from Florence to Milan and, from 2015 until 2017, he was the Director of the Cardiovascular Department IRCCS Multimedica. From 2012 to 2014, he was President of the Italian Association of Arrhythmology and Cardiac Pacing.

Dr Padeletti dedicated most of his life to studying medicine and cardiology and to transferring his knowledge to a new generation of medical doctors. He was always surrounded by students, residents, and fellows that were involved in his multiple areas of research. He trained and mentored innumerable electrophysiology cardiologists from all over Italy and abroad. His electrophysiology cardiology lab and his office were always open to anyone who wanted to be trained in this field and follow his research.

Dr Padeletti's area of expertise covered many fields of cardiology and electrophysiology. He started to pace the Koch triangle in order to prevent atrial fibrillation burden in patients implanted with pacemakers. In addition, he dedicated a lot of his research to optimization for cardiac resynchronization therapy in congestive heart failure. In his late years, he dedicated his attention to hemodynamic changes in failing hearts by His bundle stimulation. Based on all his studies and his ability to guide research, he headed several randomized controlled trials that were presented and published at European Heart Rhythm Association, European Society of Cardiology (ESC), and American College of Cardiology, at American Heart Association's annual meetings, and in various journals (MASCOT, PACMAN, WHERE,

Card Electrophysiol Clin 10 (2018) xvii–xviii
https://doi.org/10.1016/j.ccep.2018.04.001
1877-9182/18/© 2018 Published by Elsevier Inc.

DASAP, INSYNC, and so on). He also wrote more than 350 peer-reviewed research papers.

Along with this innovative research, he joined and led many national and international steering committees, as, for example, the 2013 ESC guidelines for cardiac pacing and resynchronization therapy. In addition, he guided an Expert Consensus Statement on the management of cardiovascular implantable electronic devices in patients nearing end of life or requesting withdrawal of therapy in Europe, the composition of which required not only expertise in medicine but also an understanding of the connection of medicine with other fields, such as philosophy, religion, and ethics.

His leadership was associated with a friendly relationship with all his colleagues, and with a sense of humor and a propensity to help young researchers, medical doctors, and his patients.

Giuseppe Bagliani, MD
Arrhythmology Unit
Cardiology Department
Foligno General Hospital
Via Massimo Arcamone
Foligno, Perugia 06034, Italy

Cardiovascular Disease Department
University of Perugia
Piazza Menghini 1
Perugia 06129, Italy

E-mail address:
giuseppe.bagliani@tim.it

Gerbezius' Pulsus Mira Inconstantia and the First Descriptions of the Atrioventricular Block

Donatella Lippi, PhD

KEYWORDS

- Atrioventricular block • Maladie de Stokes-Adams • Morgagni • History of medicine

KEY POINTS

- The atrioventricular block, known also as cardiovascular syncope, is a pathologic condition that has many appellations.
- The first description of the cardiovascular syncope was recorded in 1692.
- Observations and studies of this syndrome led to the birth of electrocardiography.

The atrioventricular block, known also as cardiovascular syncope, is a pathologic condition that has many appellations. In 1899, Henry Huchard[1] named the condition of slow pulse with apoplectic seizures after Stokes and Adams. In modern practice, the names are ordered chronologically and the names of Spens and Morgagni have often been added. Roberts Adams (1791–1875) and William Stokes (1804–1878) were Irish physicians (Stokes is also famous for the Cheyne-Stokes respiration, a pattern of breathing characteristically seen in coma). Thomas Spens (1764–1842) was a Scottish physician. Giovan Battista Morgagni (1682–1771) can be considered the founder of pathologic anatomy.

Although Adams, Stokes, and Spens described the syndrome independently in the early nineteenth century, the first descriptions were recorded in 1692 and 1717 by Marcus Gerbezius (1658–1718), a notable Slovenian physician and scientist.

In 1692 Gerbezius[2] published *Pulsus Mira Inconstantia*, which was a case of temporary cardiac arrest with syncopal attacks.

In 1731, the Swiss pathologist Jean Jacques Manget[3] (1652–1742), in his work *Bibliotheca Scriptorum Medicorum Veterum et Recentorium*, quoted this case.

In 1717, Gerbezius described 2 very important cases, providing the description of an extremely slow pulse rate of his patients, who also suffered from seizures. He observed these patients very carefully, recognizing unusual bradyarrhythmia with epileptic seizures, and writing down every detail.

Both patients had a slow but regular pulses, dizziness, syncope, and occasional epileptic seizures: "*Rarius tamen quid observaveram in duobus subjectis circa pulsum: nimirum quod unus eorum melancholico-hypochondriacus qua sanus communiter habuerit pulsum adeo tardum, ut priusquam subsequens pulsus consequebatur antecedentem, facile apud alium sanum tres pulsationes praeterierint… Vir alias erat robustus, et in actionibus accuratus; sed tardissimus, saepius vertiginosus, et subinde leviter insultibus epilepticis obnoxious…*"[2]

Disclosure Statement: The author has nothing she wishes to disclose.
Department of Clinical and Experimental Medicine, School of Sciences of Human Health, University of Florence, Largo Brambilla 3, Florence 50134, Italy
E-mail address: donatella.lippi@unifi.it

According to this description, the first patient "…had such a slow pulse that the pulse of a healthy person would beat three times before his pulse would beat for a second time…" The second patient was a strong and Meticulous man "…very sluggish, frequently dizzy, and from time to time subject to mild epileptic attacks."[4,5]

These cases, considered the first descriptions in medical literature of a complete atrioventricular block,[5] were followed by the account of the Italian pathologist Giovanni Battista Morgagni (1682–1771) some years later. Morgagni, in the anatomymedical letter LXIV, reported the case of a 64-year-old merchant from Padua, a full-bodied man, who had already suffered from rheumatic and nervous diseases.[6]

He had recovered from these ailments, but he was overwhelmed by ordinary problems, which caused him sadness, fear, and rage ("vehementissimis animi affectibus terrore, timore, iraque, deinde et moestitia corriperetur").[6]

Then, he collapsed following vertigo ("ingruente quasi vertigine cecidit") and, in the following days, he had frequent epileptic attacks.[6] His pulse was vigorous but hard and rare ("Erant pulsus eo tempore validi quidem, sed duri et rari…").[6] Doctors had used bleedings and purges, as was usual in epilepsy. After a short recovery, the attacks started again, with lack of appetite and difficulty of breathing. The symptoms reappeared after only 4 months of remission.

In this phase, Morgagni was asked for a consultation. The pulse rate, about two-thirds less than normal ("Raritas praecipue pulsuum illa tanta, ut eorum numerus duabus circiter tertiis partibus minor esset quam oporteret, tum inculcabatur, tum a me quoque reperiebatur") was evaluated as the most dangerous symptom.[6] Moreover, the variation in beating was considered the first premonitory sign of an attack ("Medici si instantem praedicerent insultum: quo durante, pulsus non modo ex raro frequens, fed ita frequens fiebat, ut in aegris frequentem vocamus").[6] After 15 months from the onset of the disease, death occurred. At autopsy, Morgagni observed that "the heart was dilated because of the enlargement of ventricles (Cor vero amplum valde ob dilatatos ventriculos, non ob parietes factos crassiores) and the aorta was dilated in the same way from the beginning of its curve (Magna etiam arteria ad curvatura; usque initium aequo latior)."[6]

Morgagni remarked that the slow pulse rate could not be connected to aneurisms of the heart and aorta ("Sed neque ad ejusmodi causas aut solum, aut praecipue, pulsuum tantam raritatem esse referendam, vel hinc intelligere proclive fore, quod in tot aliis quorum cordis, et arteriae Aortae aneurysmata, multo etiam istis majora, deprehendimus, ejuscemodi pulsus non fuere; ut nisi aliud aliquod accedat, eos non inde fieri satis constet")[6] and that the disease had been produced by a disorder of the nerves ("spirituum et nervorum vitium").[6,7]

After Morgagni, another very important description of a heart block, dating back to 1792, was reported by Thomas Spens[8]:

On the 16th of May, 1792, about 9 o'clock in the evening, I was sent for to see T. R., a man in the 54th year of his age, a common labouring mechanic…I was much surprised, upon examining the state of his pulse, to find that it beat only twenty-four strokes to the minute. These strokes, however, as far as I could judge, were at perfectly equal intervals, and of the natural strength of the pulse of a man in good health. He informed me, that about 3 o'clock in the afternoon, he had been suddenly taken ill while standing in the street; that he had fallen to the ground senseless; and that, according to the accounts given him, by those who were present, he had continued in that state for about 5 minutes…From the time of his first attack till I saw him, he had been affected with three other fits, mainly of a similar nature. These, however, were attended with some convulsive movements of his limbs, and with screaming during the fit…nor had he, at any time, any other complaint…Upon visiting him on the morning of the 17th, I found that he had been attacked with several fits during the night…Upon examining his pulse I found that it beat only twenty-three beats in the minute…an hour after, I found it in precisely the same state as before. He was now directed to take some spirits of hartshorn; but, by mistake, it was given him very little diluted, and produced much uneasiness in his throat and mouth. From this cause I found him in great distress at one o'clock; but it seemed to' have produced no change in the state of his pulse, which at this time beat twenty-four strokes in a minute and was of the same strength and regularity as before-…In the morning of the 18th I was informed that…he had been frequently faint… his pulse beat only twenty-six strokes in in the minute. About 8 in the evening he had no sooner smelt it (newly toasted bread) than he felt some of the sensations of a beginning fit; and, as soon as he had tasted it he almost instantly cried out, and fell back senseless, with smart convulsions of all his muscles. He *apparently recovered in a few seconds; but hardly any pulse could be felt for a good many seconds. On the morning of the 19th I learnt that...he had been attacked with frequent fits, attended with violent convulsions...at three in the afternoon, I found that it (the pulse) beat only ten strokes a minute, though it still continued equally strong and regular as before...he expired on the 20th. The day after his death the body was opened by Mr. Fyfe, and, upon the most careful examination, no morbid appearance of any consequence could be discovered either in the thorax or abdomen.*[8]

All the elements of the case indicate its being an absolute example of heart-block: the slow, regular pulse; the random faints; losses of consciousness; and convulsions, during which, if prolonged, hardly any pulse could be felt, are distinctive signs. Particularly important is the state of the pulse, even following the dosage of the too strong hartshorn; this stationary character of the pulse under variable circumstances could be another striking feature of heart-block.[9]

Despite other descriptions of heart block that followed, the eponyms of heart block are bound to 2 Irish physicians: Robert Adams (1791–1875) and William Stokes (1804–1877). Adams' description of syncope associated with bradycardia dates back to 1827 and Stokes described the same association in 1846.[10]

Robert Adams described a 15-year-old youth with severe mitral obstruction and pulsatile neck veins. At autopsy, the severe mitral obstruction appeared accompanied by massive right ventricular enlargement concealing the small left ventricle. Adams reflected on the pulsations seen in the jugular veins which "demand our consideration...the cause of this symptom has been much disputed," and established that the jugular venous distention and pulsation "results from the regurgitation of blood from the right ventricle into the auricle, by which the current descending from the jugular veins is repelled back into these vessels during the systole of the ventricle. The pulsations in the jugular veins I have always observed to be synchronous with the action of the heart, even with the pulsations which were not perceptible in the arteries!"[11]

Another case reported by Adams regarded "an officer in the revenue, aged 68 years...just recovering from the effects of an apoplectic attack...and remarkable slowness of the pulse, which general, ranged at the rate of 30 in a minute." The patient had suffered from recurrent attacks for 7 years, and died suddenly following an attack. Adams commented on the circumstances: "where the heart is slow in transmitting the blood it receives ... a means of accounting for the lethargy, loss of memory, and vertigo, which attends these cases." He concluded that "apoplexy must be considered less a disease in itself than symptomatic of one, the organic seat of which was the heart."[12] Adams' contribution was very important in connecting the heart rate with problems in consciousness.

In fact, slow pulse with epileptic paroxysms had been described earlier but William Stokes published his *Observations* in 1846 and extended the clinical field because he clarified how a slow heart could inhibit consciousness and he recovered Adams' earlier case presentation. Restoring to life Adams' earlier report provided the link that contributed to the Stokes-Adams eponym.

Huchard[1] named the condition *"maladie de Stokes-Adams"* in his text in 1889 and it is still quoted in this way. However, the comprehensive identification of the cardiac conduction system was reached between the end of the nineteenth and the beginning of the twentieth century, with the findings by Wilhem His[13] (1831–1934), who discovered the bundle that now bears his name: a collection of specialized cardiac muscle cells in the heart that transmits the electrical impulses and helps synchronize contraction of the cardiac muscles. Sunao Tawara[14] (1873–1952) revealed the atrioventricular node and bundle. Tawara's monograph confirmed the existence of the atrioventricular node and the function of Purkinje cells. Before him, it was supposed that electrical conduction through the bundle of His was slow because of the long interval between atrial and ventricular contractions. Tawara managed to demonstrate that the ventricular contraction occurs with the apex contracting earlier than the base; he believed that the heart's electrical conduction was not slow but rapid. He worked under the guidance of his mentor, Ludwig Aschoff, carrying out the histologic examination of 150 hearts with myocarditis. He started by examining the atrioventricular bundle before conducting an inclusive study of the anatomy and histology of the heart's conduction system.

His observations started a great debate, paving the way to the discovery of the sinoatrial node by Arthur Keith (1866–1955) and Martin Flack (1882–1931). Keith and Flack[15] contributed to establishing the theoretic basis for electrocardiography.

REFERENCES

1. Huchard H. Traité des maladies du Coeur et des vaisseaux. Paris Octave Doin 1899;262:309.

2. Gerbezius M. Pulsus mira inconstantia. Miscellanea curiosa, sive Ephemeridum medico-physicarum Germanicum Academiae Caesareo-Leopoldinae Naturae. Norimbergae 1692;10:115–8.

3. Joannis Jacobi Mangeti, medicinae doctoris, et serenissimi ac potentissimi regis Prussiae archiatri, Bibliotheca scriptorum medicorum, veterum et recentiorum in qua sub eorum omnium qui a mundi primordiis ad hunc usque annum vixerunt, nominibus, ordine alphabetico adscriptis, vitae compendiô enarrantur, opiniones, & scripta, modestâ subinde adjectâ [epikrisei] recensentur, ac sectae praecipuae, sub quârumque propriâ appellatione explicantur sicque historia medica vere universalis exhibetur opus doctis omnibus, maximeque medicis utile, ac perjucundum pro quô concinnandô, necessaria undique, sive ex ipsis scriptoribus medicis antiquis, quorum opera ad nostra usque tempora pervenerunt, aut aliis, tùm iisdem contemporaneis, tùm etiam subsequentibus, qui de illis verba fecerunt, sive variis dictionariorum compilatoribus, & scriptorum medicorum catalogis, miscellaneis, praeterea, Germanor. curiosis, Actis Bartholinianis, Actis Lipsiensib. ephemerid. per totam Europam jam à multis annis, variis linguis emissis, &c. non mediocri labore ac curâ, sunt exquisita/Genevæ: sumptibus Perachon & Cramer, M. DCCXXXI [1731]: 458.

4. Gerbezius M. Constitutio anni 1717 a Dn. D. Marco Gerbezio Labaco 10 Decemb. descripta (Constitution of the year 1717 by D. D. Marco Gerbezio Labaco). Academiae Caesareo-Leopoldinae Carloninae Naturae Curiosorum…centuria VII. Et VIII. Cum Appendice…Norimbergae, Sumptibus Academiae. Litteris M.G.Heinii, Anno 1719. [Appendix: 22–24].

5. Slavec ZZ, Neudauer U. Marcus Gerbezius (1658–1718) and his first description. Block Zdrav Vestn 2015;84:855–60.

6. Morgagni GB. De sedibus, et causis morborum per anatomen indagatis libri quinque, Tomus primus: 420. Venetis: typ. Remondiniana; 1761 (The seats, and the causes of diseases investigated by anatomy …. 2 volumes in 1 Reprinted in English translation in Willius & Keys, Cardiac Classics, 1941:177–182).

7. Zampieri F, Zanatta A, Basso C, et al. Cardiovascular medicine in Morgagni's De sedibus: dawn of cardiovascular pathology. Cardiovasc Pathol 2016;25: 443–52.

8. History of a case in which there took place a remarkable Slowness of the Pulse. Communicated to Dr. Duncan by Dr. Thomas Spens, physician in Edinburgh. Medical commentaries, for the years 1792, 1793. Exhibiting a concise view of the latest and most important discoveries in medicine and medical philosophy Printed by Thomas Dobson, at the stonehouse, no 41, South Second-Street.[1795]: 458.

9. Lea CE. Dr. Thomas Spens: the first describer of the Stokes-Adams syndrome. Proc R Soc Med 1914; 7(Sect Hist Med):243–6.

10. Stokes W. Observations on some cases of permanently slow pulse. Dublin Q J Med Sci 1846;2:73–85.

11. Adams R. Cases of diseases of the heart, accompanied with pathological observations. Dublin Hosp Rep 1827;4:353–453.

12. Wooley CF. Robert Adams-a Dublin master of clinical expression. Clin Cardiol 1996;19:523–4.

13. His W. The activity of the embryonic human heart and its significance for the understanding of the heart movement in the adult. Arb Med Klin Leipzig 1893;2:14–49.

14. Tawara S. Das Reizleitungssystem des Säugetierhezens. Verlag von Gustav Fischer, Jena 1906.

15. Keith A, Flack M. The form and nature of the muscular connection between the primary divisions of the vertebrate heart. J Anat Physiol 1907;41: 172–89.

Sick Sinus Syndrome

Roberto De Ponti, MD, FHRS[a],*, Jacopo Marazzato, MD[a],
Giuseppe Bagliani, MD[b,c], Fabio M. Leonelli, MD[d], Luigi Padeletti, MD[e,f]

KEYWORDS

- Sinus node • Bradycardia • Sick sinus syndrome • Bradycardia-tachycardia syndrome
- Sinus node dysfunction • Sinus arrest • Sinoatrial block

KEY POINTS

- The sick sinus syndrome includes a spectrum of symptoms and heart rhythm disturbances related to abnormal sinus impulse formation and/or propagation.
- This disease has different electrocardiographic presentations, such as bradycardia, sinus arrest, sinoatrial block, and alternant episodes of bradycardia and tachycardia.
- Symptoms related to these heart rhythm disturbances are generally fatigue, effort dyspnea, dizziness, syncope or presyncope, and palpitations, although patients can be asymptomatic in the early phase of the disease.
- When symptoms are related to intrinsic dysfunction of the sinus node, pacemaker implantation is required, whereas when a reversible cause is present, identification and correction of this extrinsic cause are necessary.
- Diagnosis is mainly based on clinical and electrocardiographic evaluation, but in some cases, further noninvasive and invasive diagnostic workup may be required.

INTRODUCTION

The sinus node (SN) is located in the superior right atrium and is the natural pacemaker of the human heart.[1] The electrical activity of the SN is under a precise regulation of the autonomous nervous system that allows it to adjust the heart rate according to the body's needs.[2] The sick sinus syndrome includes symptoms and signs related to abnormal sinus impulse formation and/or propagation caused by intrinsic sinus node dysfunction (SND). This heterogeneous clinical entity includes rhythm disturbances, which may lead to major cardiovascular events,[3] thromboembolism,[4] inadequate heart rate response to exercise/stress known as chronotropic incompetence, or any other symptom requiring pacemaker implantation. The annual number of new cases with sick sinus syndrome in the United States is expected to increase from 78,000 in 2012 to 172,000 in 2060.[5]

ETIOLOGY AND PATHOPHYSIOLOGY

The different forms of primary and secondary SND are listed in **Table 1**. SND is better conceptualized as a spectrum of disorders, rather than a single entity, where different pathophysiologic mechanisms lead to a very similar disease phenotype.

Disclosure: The authors have nothing to disclose.
[a] Department of Cardiology, School of Medicine, University of Insubria, Viale Borri, 57, Varese, Varese 21100, Italy; [b] Arrhythmology Unit, Cardiology Department, Foligno General Hospital, Via Massimo Arcamone, Foligno, Perugia 06034, Italy; [c] Cardiovascular Disease Department, University of Perugia, Piazza Menghini 1, Perugia, Perugia 06129, Italy; [d] Cardiology Department, James A. Haley Veterans' Hospital, University of South Florida, 13000 Bruce B Down Boulevard, Tampa, FL 33612, USA; [e] Heart and Vessels Department, University of Florence, Largo Brambilla, 3, Florence, Florence 50134, Italy; [f] Cardiology Department, IRCCS Multimedica, Via Milanese, 300, Sesto San Giovanni, Milan 20099, Italy
* Corresponding author.
E-mail address: roberto.deponti@uninsubria.it

Card Electrophysiol Clin 10 (2018) 183–195
https://doi.org/10.1016/j.ccep.2018.02.002
1877-9182/18/© 2018 Elsevier Inc. All rights reserved.

cardiacEP.theclinics.com

Table 1
Different forms of primary and secondary sinus node dysfunction

Primary SND	SND Secondary to Reversible Causes
Degenerative fibrosis	Metabolic disorders
• Aging	• Hyperkalemia
• Atrial tachyarrhythmias	• Hypocalcemia
• Chronic ischemia (?)	• Hypothermia
Genetic	• Hypoxia
• Inherited primary arrhythmia syndromes with mutations for SCN5A, HCN4, calsequestrin, ryanodine	• Acute ischemia
	Pharmacologic agents
	• Antiarrhythmic medication (class I and III)
	• β-Blockers
	• Calcium channel blockers (nondihydropyridine)
Associated with atrial myopathy:	• Digoxin
• Amyloidosis	• Cimetidine
• Connective tissue diseases	• Clonidine, methyldopa, reserpine
• Hemochromatosis	
• Sarcoidosis	• Lithium, phenothiazine, amitriptyline
• Hereditary muscle dystrophies	Extracardiac diseases
• Myocarditis	• Hypothyroidism
• Valvular heart disease	• Intracranial hypertension
• Heart failure	
• Hypertension	
• Diabetes	
• Obesity	
• Obstructive sleep apnea	
Infective	
• Rheumatic fever	
• Chagas disease	
• Diphtheria	

Degenerative Fibrosis

Aging causes both a decrease in the intrinsic heart rate and an increase in SN conduction time.[6] The latter could be well explained by atrial remodeling, more evident in the region around the crista terminalis, leading to conduction slowing and voltage loss and evidence of a decrease in SN reserve.[7] Indeed, previous experimental[8] and clinical studies[7] showed that aging was associated with a significant increase in the atrial effective refractory period and prolonged conduction time associated with areas of low voltage and double potentials consistent with age-related development of interstitial fibrosis. Furthermore, in patients with normal heart and no previous history of atrial fibrillation (AF), electroanatomic mapping of the right and left atrium[9] showed an inverse correlation between age and left atrial wavelength, which may explain the age-related modifications of the atrial substrate and the increase in the prevalence of AF. Hence, the association between SND and atrial tachyarrhythmias observed during aging favors the hypothesis that these 2 entities share several pathophysiologic aspects and interstitial atrial fibrosis is a possible link. Earlier in 1954, aging was first noted to be associated with fibrosis of the SN.[10] However, fibrosis cannot explain all cases of SND. Although morphologic studies in the 1970s[11,12] revealed that most cases of patients with SND were associated with SN fibrosis, the same studies showed that other patients with the same clinical presentation had normal SN histology. In experimental studies, widespread electrical remodeling with loss of connexin 43,[13] age-related changes in the expression of ion channels and clock genes in the SN,[14] and downregulation of genes responsible for collagen and elastin[15] have been advocated as possible causes of SND. Therefore, aging is associated with both structural and molecular remodeling, and the cause of SND in the elderly is likely to be complex and heterogeneous.

As mentioned earlier, atrial structural alterations leading to SND predispose also to the development of atrial arrhythmias. However, AF per se could also cause SND. In dogs, pacing-induced chronic AF causes SND and a reversible electrical remodeling with atrial conduction time prolongation and shortening of atrial refractoriness, which favors perpetuation of AF.[16] In patients undergoing electrical cardioversion of long-standing persistent AF, a depressed SN function is observed, which is independent from the autonomic tone and recovers after sinus rhythm restoration, suggesting that AF remodels the SN.[17] More recently, in a canine model,[18] it has been demonstrated that atrial tachyarrhythmias downregulate ion channel expression in the SN, particularly the pacemaker subunit I(f), which may contribute to worsening SND when AF is concomitantly present. These data highlight the pathophysiologic bi-univocal relationship between SND and atrial arrhythmias.

Although acute myocardial ischemia is listed (see **Table 1**) among the causes of reversible SND,[19] whether chronic ischemia is a cause of SND is controversial. In fact, data from morphologic studies that in the past investigated the role of chronic ischemia of SN function showed mixed results,[20] and a definite conclusion cannot be reached.

Sinus Node Dysfunction in Young Patients

SND can be also observed in the first decades of life. These "early-onset" cases are associated either with direct SN injury from previous cardiac surgery for congenital heart disease performed early in life or without any clear structural heart disease.[21,22] In the latter group of patients, the presence of a genetic disease should be suspected. Multiple gene mutations for the cardiac sodium channel SCN5A have been described with a suggested autosomal recessive pattern of inheritance and are associated with isolated SND, AF in the context of the Brugada syndrome, long QT3 syndrome, and syndromes associated with cardiac conduction disease.[23–25] Mutations in the HCN4 gene have also been identified in patients with idiopathic SND[26] and in individuals with a combination of mild sinus bradycardia, AF, and acquired long QT syndrome in the absence of any detectable structural heart disease.[27] Finally, mutations in both the calsequestrin (CASQ 2) and the ryanodine (RYR2) genes could lead to forms of catecholaminergic polymorphic ventricular tachycardia associated with a significantly lower resting heart rate and bradycardia, mainly because of sarcoplasmic reticulum dysfunction within the SN.[28,29] These genetic disorders are associated with an increased risk of sudden cardiac death related to the occurrence of malignant ventricular arrhythmias.

Atrial Cardiomyopathies

In some patients, several cardiovascular and non-cardiovascular conditions can affect the atria more than the ventricular myocardium, leading to an atrial cardiomyopathy associated with SND.[30] Many diseases (see **Table 1**) can cause alterations in the atria, which can be evident as primarily cardiomyocyte changes, primarily fibrotic changes, a combination of both, or noncollagen infiltration.[30] Fibrotic atrial cardiomyopathy and muscular dystrophies are worth considering from the heterogeneous spectrum of atrial cardiomyopathies. The former has been recently recognized as a distinct entity in patients with normal-sized atria, without AF and any detectable structural heart disease,[31] and it is thought to be responsible for atrial arrhythmias associated with SND because of progressive atrial fibrosis. Genetics as well as inflammatory processes may play a role in the pathophysiology of this entity. Muscular dystrophies include a group of inherited disorders involving both the skeletal muscles and the myocardium. In myotonic dystrophy type 1, Emery-Dreifuss and Limb-Girdle type IB muscular dystrophy, specific atrial involvement can be present, leading to SND or atrial arrhythmias.[32–34]

Infective Diseases

About 15% of the patients presenting with diphtheric myocarditis develop sinus bradycardia, which is one of the heart rhythm disturbances that can be associated with this disease and seems to be associated with a more benign prognosis compared with atrioventricular conduction disturbances or ventricular arrhythmias.[35] Chagas cardiomyopathy is associated with SND, often requiring permanent pacing, and new AF during follow-up has a higher incidence in these patients.[36]

ELECTROCARDIOGRAPHIC PRESENTATIONS OF SINUS NODE DYSFUNCTION
Bradyarrhythmias

Severe and symptomatic sinus bradycardia can be the initial manifestation on standard electrocardiogram (ECG) of an intrinsic dysfunction of the SN, as shown in **Fig. 1**. Opposite to what could be observed overnight in normal subjects exhibiting an increased parasympathetic tone (juveniles, athletes, and so forth), bradycardia due to SND is typically observed also during the day, even in the absence of any drug that may affect the sinus rate, with minimal or no variation during physical activities. Consequently, patients usually complain of fatigue, dizziness, and poor effort tolerance.

In these patients, slowing of sinus rate allows the emergence of low-frequency atrial ectopic rhythms with similar or slightly higher rate. As a result, the "wandering pacemaker" phenomenon may appear, which can be observed also in normal subjects during vagal hypertonia.[1] **Fig. 2** shows a typical example of this phenomenon with 4 different morphologies of the P wave cyclically alternating and resulting in a heart rate ranging from 43 to 50 beats per minute.

In some cases, SND presents suddenly with SN arrest and prolonged asystole, causing syncope and even worse consequences if a significant structural heart disease is associated and a junctional or idioventricular escape rhythm does not promptly emerge. An example of a sinus arrest is reported in **Fig. 3**. Because it is caused by the loss of automaticity of the SN, this term should be strictly used when the value of the sinus pause is not a multiple of the basic PP interval. If so, a prolonged pause could be due to the occurrence of a third-degree sinoatrial block, which is an expression of an altered conduction between the SN and the surrounding atrial myocardium, not

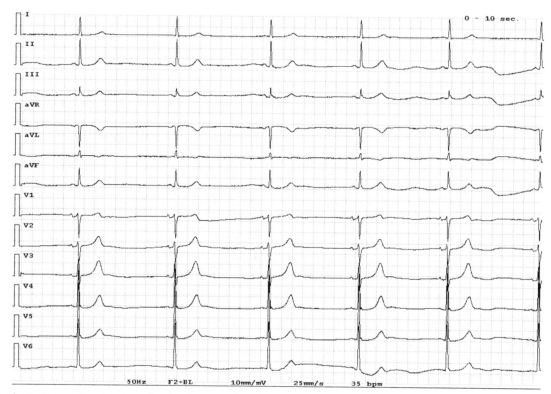

Fig. 1. Severe sinus bradycardia: the sinus rate is 35 beats per minute; QRS complex is normal.

necessarily associated with a marked depression of the SN automaticity: (see next paragraph). A prolonged absence of SN activity favors the emergence of a junctional escape rhythm with an acceptable rate (**Fig. 4**), which can be what is observed at the presenting ECG of patients coming to medical attention for a recent syncope, worsening fatigue, or heart failure.

The tissue in the periphery of the SN has peculiar characteristics with intermingling of nodal and atrial muscular cells. This complex structure may include areas of conduction block or delay, which can be the expression of both anatomic structures and functional phenomena.[20] The surface ECG of sinoatrial conduction blocks can be a sequence of irregular and longer PP cycles with the same P-wave morphology and of sinus pauses, which may be of difficult interpretation. Notably, careful evaluation of the P-wave morphology is needed to discriminate between sinoatrial block and the presence of atrial premature beats with a longer coupling interval, mimicking sinoatrial block (**Fig. 5**). As for the atrioventricular block three degrees of sinoatrial conduction block are reported. The first degree is merely a conduction delay between the area of sinus impulse formation and the atrial tissue, which originates the P wave: when this delay

results in a fixed time interval, this phenomenon cannot be detected on surface ECG, showing only sinus bradycardia. During second-degree sinoatrial block in a sequence of sinus impulses, one remains blocked within the SN and does not originate a P wave. The modality of sinoatrial conduction delay before the block results in different peculiar electrocardiographic aspects that may require prolonged recording for correct interpretation. If, before the block, sinoatrial conduction occurs with a periodic conduction delay (type 1), the tracing shows sinus bradycardia, typically with a progressive minimal decrease in the PP cycle length before a pause with an interval definitely longer than the preceding PP cycle, but not matching its double (**Fig. 6**). If, conversely, the blocked impulse is not preceded by progressive delay of the sinoatrial conduction (type 2), the PP cycles before the pause have a relatively constant value and the pause originated by the blocked impulse measures the double of the preceding PP cycle (**Fig. 7**). When this type of block occurs with a 2:1 periodicity, an alternant sequence of shorter and longer PP cycles is observed, with the longer measuring the double of the shorter cycles. Finally, in third-degree sinoatrial block, multiple sinus impulses are blocked, and this originates a sudden and

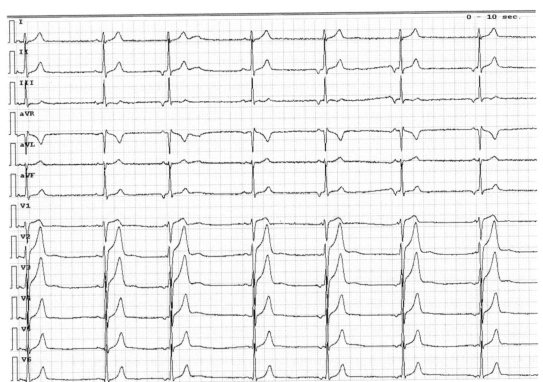

Fig. 2. Wandering pacemaker phenomenon in a patient with sinus bradycardia: beats originating in the SN (first and second) or close to the SN (fourth) alternate with beats (third, fifth, and last) originated by the lower right atrium, possibly the coronary sinus os, as suggested by the negative P-wave morphology in the inferior leads. A fourth P-wave morphology is also present (sixth beat), possibly originated by a septal focus. Of note, the PQ interval may be slightly different, depending on the location of the focus: it is usually shorter when the distance between the focus and the atrioventricular node is shorter compared with the one between the sinus and the atrioventricular node. Interestingly, sinus beats exhibit a very low voltage, suggesting the presence of fibrotic atrial myocardium.

longer pause with an interval multiple of the basic sinus cycle. This condition can be diagnosed only when the sinus rate is relatively regular before and after the pause (**Fig. 8**).

Bradycardia-Tachycardia Syndrome

As mentioned earlier, the pathophysiologic mechanism determining SND also modifies the atrial

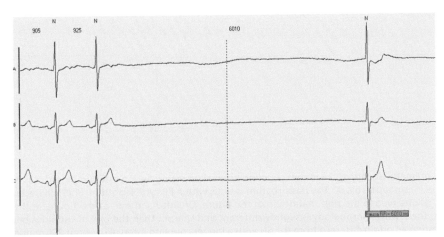

Fig. 3. SND resulting in asystole: after a sequence of sinus beats at 65 beats per minute, sinus activity suddenly interrupts with a 6.2-second pause with subsequent emergence of junctional escape rhythm.

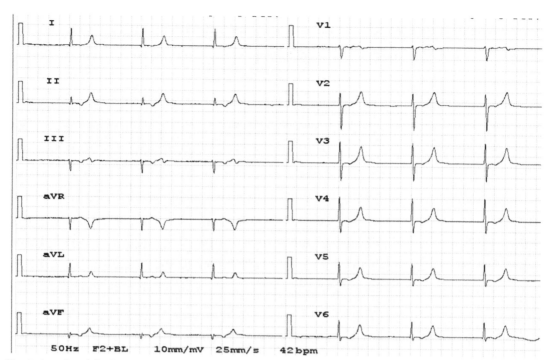

Fig. 4. Junctional rhythm at 42 beats per minute: the narrow QRS morphology not preceded by P waves suggests origin from the atrioventricular node or His bundle region. Every QRS complex is followed by a retrogradely conducted P wave (negative morphology in the inferior leads), which rules out the concomitant presence of complete atrioventricular block.

myocardium to generate arrhythmogenic substrate leading to development of atrial arrhythmias. Among supraventricular arrhythmias, AF is the most frequently encountered, affecting up to 68% of the patients undergoing DDDR pacemaker implantation for SND.[37] This datum confirms that the association between SND and atrial arrhythmias is not casual and, on the other hand, mutually

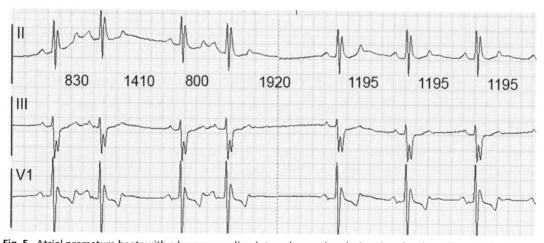

Fig. 5. Atrial premature beats with a longer coupling interval occurring during sinus bradycardia and mimicking a certain degree of sinoatrial block. The basic rhythm is sinus with a PP cycle length of 1195 milliseconds (50 beats per minute), as observed in the right-hand side of the figure. On left-hand side of the figure, in the second and fourth beats, the P-wave morphology is slightly different and sharper than the one of the sinus beats (first and third), suggesting an origin different from the SN with a longer coupling interval of about 800 milliseconds. After the second atrial premature beat and a longer pause, sinus rhythm with a stable PP interval resumes. In this and in the following figures, numbers refer to PP intervals in milliseconds.

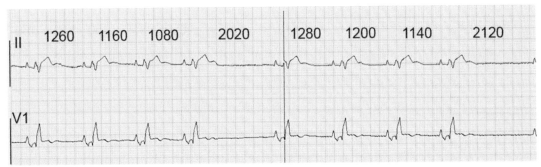

Fig. 6. Second-degree type 1 sinoatrial block: sinus bradycardia shows minimal decrease in the PP cycle length, before a sinus pause, which measures less than the double of the preceding PP cycle. The second sequence before the second pause shows a very similar phenomenon. In this type of sinoatrial block, the PP interval decreases as the delay in sinoatrial conduction decreases over the sinus beats preceding the missing P wave. The sinus pause does not match the double of the preceding PP interval, because of the variable delay in sinoatrial conduction.

noxious with a strong clinical impact. As shown in **Fig. 9**, onset of AF may be favored by marked sinus bradycardia, during which a greater dispersion of atrial refractoriness and increased ectopic activity from the pulmonary veins are present.[38] If sudden onset of AF with fast ventricular response may be poorly tolerated by patients, the symptoms can be even worse when the arrhythmia terminates **(Fig. 10)**, because the preautomatic pause can be particularly long for several reasons. In fact, short-lasting fast atrial rates can alter the SN function even in humans without sick sinus syndrome,[39] and they may have a stronger influence in patients with preexisting SND. Moreover, concomitant use of antiarrhythmic drugs in the attempt to prevent paroxysmal AF episodes or to control their ventricular rate worsens the SND. Of note, in up to 70% of the patients affected by bradycardia-tachycardia syndrome, paroxysmal AF does not progress to a persistent or permanent form,[40] and this, in the absence of an adequate treatment and although the SND progresses with age, exposes the patients to more frequently recurrent episodes of postarrhythmia sinus arrests or marked bradycardia with syncope or disabling symptoms related to low cardiac output.

In some patients with prior cardiac surgery for congenital[41] or acquired structural heart disease,

SND is associated with postsurgical atriotomy, scars, or areas of slow atrial conduction. In these cases, tachycardias associated with bradycardia can be different from AF, and the presenting arrhythmia could be typical or atypical atrial flutter, or macro-reentrant or focal atrial tachycardia. Peculiarly, the control of the ventricular rate during these arrhythmias is generally more difficult, and higher dose of drugs used in these cases to slow the ventricular rate can worsen bradycardia when sinus rhythm resumes.

DIFFERENTIAL DIAGNOSIS
Pseudobradycardia

In some cases, what appears as sinus bradycardia with an extremely low heart rate is not necessarily due to an overt SND requiring permanent pacing **(Fig. 11A)**. In fact, in these cases, the presence of a blocked bigeminal premature atrial beat hidden in the T wave of the sinus beat prolongs the PP interval, which is the sum of the coupling interval of the premature atrial beat and the compensatory pause before the next sinus beat. The blocked P wave, superimposed to the T wave, may not be easy to detect, because it modifies only slightly the morphology of the T wave, and a comparison with an electrogram recorded when this phenomenon

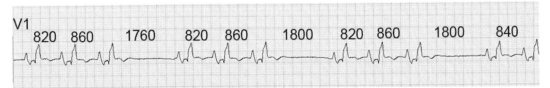

Fig. 7. Second-degree type 2 sinoatrial block: the sinus rate is rather stable with only 40-millisecond cycle variations. After the third beat, the pause is roughly the double of the last PP cycle. The same phenomenon is cyclically observed in the following beats.

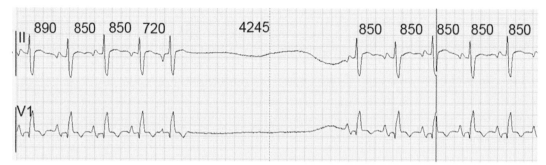

Fig. 8. Third-degree sinoatrial block: the pause is quintuple of the basic sinus cycle length. The 2 beats before the pause show a slightly different (second last) or different (last) P-wave morphology, suggesting a different exit of the impulse from the SN or a different origin, which combines with a shorter cycle length.

is absent may be of help in identifying the presence of the blocked P wave (**Fig. 11**B). The more premature the atrial beat is, the greater is the chance of not being conducted to the ventricle. Very premature atrial beats with the characteristic "P on T" aspect have been described to originate from the pulmonary veins,[42] and they can be more frequently seen in patients with paroxysmal AF.

Respiratory Sinus Arrhythmia

Respiratory sinus arrhythmia is a physiologic change in heart rate synchronized with respiration, so that the heart rate increases with inspiration and decreases with expiration. Vagal influence and respiratory-circulatory interaction determine this phenomenon, which is thought to have a positive influence on gas exchange for optimization of the ventilation/perfusion matching.[43] Because this arrhythmia occurs in asymptomatic healthy young subjects and it is clearly related to the respiratory rhythm, it is easily distinguished from sinus rate variations due to SND.

Neuromediated Bradycardia

Severe sinus bradycardia and sinus arrest could be due to an abnormally increased vagal influence in dysautonomic syndromes (**Fig. 12**). Although this clinical presentation is more frequently observed in younger people, it is currently being diagnosed with an increasing frequency in patients older than 70 years of age,[44] and it may have more severe consequences in this age group because of the lack of prodromal symptoms. In these cases,

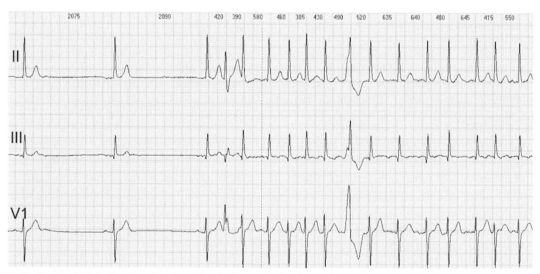

Fig. 9. Onset of AF during sinus bradycardia: the heart rhythm is regular and very slow (29 beats per minute) with a biphasic P-wave morphology in the inferior leads, suggesting an origin for the lower part of the SN or the crista terminalis. An early atrial ectopy superimposed to the previous T wave ("P on T" phenomenon) and conducted with aberrancy initiates AF with fast ventricular response.

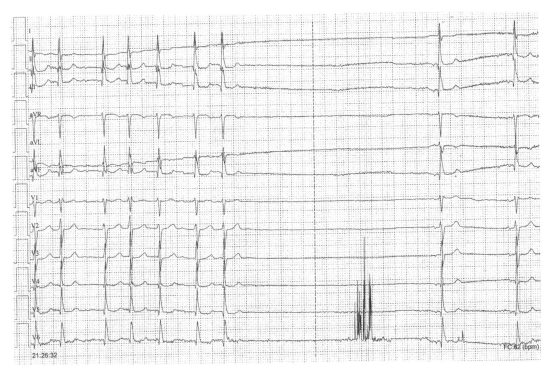

Fig. 10. Termination of AF followed by a pause of 3.7 seconds with subsequent emergence of a rhythm originating from the low right atrium (negative P waves in the inferior leads), consistent with SND.

accurate clinical evaluation and proper diagnostic workup are required to discriminate this condition from intrinsic SND.

BRADYCARDIA DUE TO REVERSIBLE CAUSES

The second column of **Table 1** reports different forms of SND related to reversible causes, such as metabolic disorders, drugs, and extracardiac diseases. In these cases, the electrocardiographic presentation of the bradyarrhythmias may be similar to one of the intrinsic forms. Therefore, in a correct diagnostic workup, the presence of a reversible cause of SND should be excluded before a pacemaker is implanted. **Fig. 13** shows a case of sinus arrest related to acute hypoxia in a patient with acute respiratory insufficiency.

METHODOLOGIES TO DIAGNOSE SINUS NODE DYSFUNCTION

Diagnosis of SND can be straightforward if a clear association between ECG abnormalities and symptoms, such as dizziness, syncope, heart failure, fatigue, and exercise intolerance, is found. Nevertheless, when SND presents intermittently and the relationship between electrocardiographic abnormalities and the clinical presentation are

difficult to evaluate, further investigation may be required.

Holter monitoring can be useful when SND occurs transiently, but with an expected recurrence frequent enough to allow documentation during monitoring. Usually, a 24- or a 72-hour ECG monitoring can be used to evaluate the association between ECG abnormalities and symptoms, and it may be helpful also in detecting other clinical arrhythmia, such as AF in bradycardia-tachycardia syndrome. When Holter monitoring is insufficient and SND is highly suspected based on the clinical presentation, an implantable loop recorder can be considered for a more prolonged monitoring (up to 24 months) in selected cases, especially when patients come to medical attention for syncope.

Exercise stress test is useful to discriminate an intrinsic form of SND from bradycardia due to a vagal hypertonia, which may be responsible for electrocardiographic aspects similar to the ones due to SND. In the former condition, chronotropic incompetence with inadequate increase of the heart rate during exercise is evident, resulting in functional limitation, whereas in the latter, a regular and progressive increase of sinus rate is observed with the ability to perform a maximal exercise stress test. Such a discrimination is critical to guide appropriate therapeutic choices.

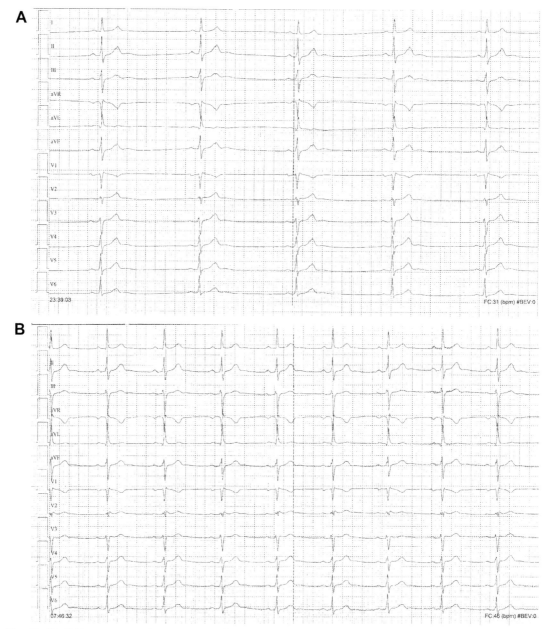

Fig. 11. (A, B) The presence of extreme sinus bradycardia at 31 beats per minute (A) is due to blocked atrial bigeminism in which the ectopic P wave with a very short coupling interval is superimposed to the T wave of the sinus beat. In this patient with paroxysmal AF, the short coupling interval and the P-wave morphology (positive in the inferior and precordial leads) suggest origin from the pulmonary veins. As soon as the bigeminism terminates (B), sinus rhythm at 52 beats per minute resumes.

Head-up tilt test is used to diagnose conditions in which bradycardia is due to abnormal influences of the autonomic nervous system, possibly responsible for neuromediated syncope.

Finally, in selected cases when other diagnostic tools have been inconclusive in the diagnosis of SND, an electrophysiologic study can be performed, and the SN recovery time as well as the

sinoatrial conduction time can be calculated using specific pacing maneuvers.

THERAPEUTIC OPTIONS

In the sick sinus syndrome, symptoms related to SND can be prevented by pacemaker implantation. The management of the bradycardia-tachycardia

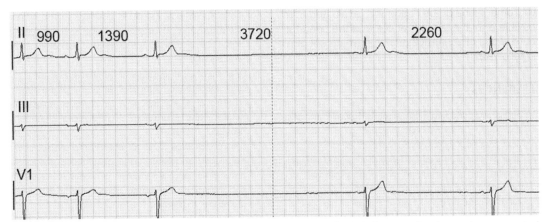

Fig. 12. Example of neuromediated bradycardia: under parasympathetic influence, the sinus rate progressively slows until sinus pause and severe sinus bradycardia (26 beats per minute) appear.

syndrome could be more challenging, because antiarrhythmic drugs administered to control atrial arrhythmias worsen the SND, and, therefore, a combined therapy is often required. In this specific clinical setting, when a pacemaker is implanted, the modality of pacing has to be carefully considered, because it can have an impact on the progression of the coexisting atrial arrhythmias. Dual-chamber pacing with specific algorithms to minimize ventricular pacing and prevent and treat atrial tachyarrhythmias is superior to standard dual-chamber pacing in the reduction of death and hospitalization for cardiovascular causes,[45,46] and this benefit is driven by the reduction in the progression to long-standing or permanent AF due to the use of the specific algorithms. As an alternative to pacemaker implantation in patients with bradycardia-tachycardia syndrome, catheter ablation of AF is considered reasonable (class IIa, level of evidence B, non-randomized) by a recently published expert consensus document.[47] However, although catheter ablation can be curative of more organized atrial arrhythmias, even if complex (such as atypical atrial flutter or atrial tachycardias in congenital heart disease patients[48]), its benefit to prevent recurrences of AF in bradycardia-tachycardia

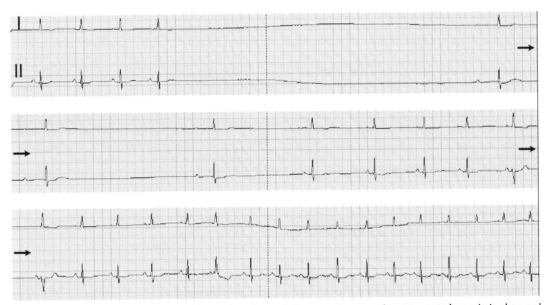

Fig. 13. After normal sinus rhythm, sudden and prolonged sinus arrest concomitant to acute hypoxia is observed. Sinus rhythm promptly resumes upon correction of hypoxia with progressive increase in sinus rate and some premature ventricular complexes. Interestingly, during hypoxia also atrioventricular conduction is delayed with first-degree atrioventricular block. *Arrows* indicate that the sequence of tracings is uninterrupted.

syndrome should be carefully evaluated for possible arrhythmia recurrences and the need for continuation of antiarrhythmic drug treatment during follow-up.

REFERENCES

1. Bagliani G, Leonelli F, Padeletti L. P wave and the substrates of arrhythmias originating in the atria. Card Electrophysiol Clin 2017;9:365–82.
2. Chandler NJ, Greener ID, Tellez JO, et al. Molecular architecture of the human sinus node insights into the function of the cardiac pacemaker. Circulation 2009;119:1562–75.
3. Brubaker PH, Kitzman DW. Chronotropic incompetence: causes, consequences, and management. Circulation 2011;123:1010–20.
4. Sutton R, Kenny RA. The natural history of sick sinus syndrome. Pacing Clin Electrophysiol 1986;9:1110–4.
5. Jensen PN, Gronroos NN, Chen LY, et al. Incidence of and risk factors for sick sinus syndrome in the general population. J Am Coll Cardiol 2014;64: 531–8.
6. Dobrzynski H, Boyett MR, Anderson RH. New insights into pacemaker activity: promoting understanding of sick sinus syndrome. Circulation 2007; 115:1921–32.
7. Kistler PM, Sanders P, Fynn SP, et al. Electrophysiologic and electroanatomic changes in the human atrium associated with age. J Am Coll Cardiol 2004;44:109–16.
8. Anyukhovsky EP, Sosunov EA, Plotnikov A, et al. Cellular electrophysiologic properties of old canine atria provide a substrate for arrhythmogenesis. Cardiovasc Res 2002;54:462–9.
9. Kojodjojo P, Kanagaratnam P, Markides V, et al. Age-related changes in human left and right atrial conduction. J Cardiovasc Electrophysiol 2006;17:120–7.
10. Lev M. Aging changes in the human sinoatrial node. J Gerontol 1954;9:1–9.
11. Thery C, Gosselin B, Lekieffre J, et al. Pathology of sinoatrial node. Correlations with electrocardiographic findings in 111 patients. Am Heart J 1977; 93:735–40.
12. Evans R, Shaw D. Pathological studies in sinoatrial disorder (sick sinus syndrome). Br Heart J 1977; 39:778–86.
13. Jones SA, Lancaster MK, Boyett MR. Ageing-related changes of connexins and conduction within the sinoatrial node. J Physiol 2004;560:429–37.
14. Tellez JO, Mczewski M, Yanni J, et al. Ageing-dependent remodelling of ion channel and Ca2+ clock genes underlying sino-atrial node pacemaking. Exp Physiol 2011;96:1163–78.
15. Yanni J, Tellez JO, Sutyagin PV, et al. Structural remodelling of the sinoatrial node in obese old rats. J Mol Cell Cardiol 2010;48:653–62.
16. Elvan A, Wylie K, Zipes DP. Pacing-induced chronic atrial fibrillation impairs sinus node function in dogs: electrophysiological remodeling. Circulation 1996; 94:2953–60.
17. Manios EG, Kanoupakis EM, Mavrakis HE, et al. Sinus pacemaker function after cardioversion of chronic atrial fibrillation: is sinus node remodelling related with recurrence? J Cardiovasc Electrophysiol 2001;12:800–6.
18. Yeh YH, Burstein B, Qi XY, et al. Funny current down-regulation and sinus node dysfunction associated with atrial tachyarrhythmia: a molecular basis for tachycardia-bradycardia syndrome. Circulation 2009;119:1576–85.
19. Rokseth R, Hatle L. Sinus arrest in acute myocardial infarction. Br Heart J 1971;33:639–42.
20. Choudhury M, Boyett MR, Morris GM. Biology of the sinus node and its disease. Arrhythm Electrophysiol Rev 2015;4:28–34.
21. Ector H, Van Der Hauwaert LG. Sick sinus syndrome in childhood. Br Heart J 1980;44:684–91.
22. Beder SD, Gillette PC, Garson A Jr, et al. Symptomatic sick sinus syndrome in children and adolescents as the only manifestation of cardiac abnormality or associated with unoperated congenital heart disease. Am J Cardiol 1983;51:1133–6.
23. Benson DW, Wang DW, Dyment M, et al. Congenital sick sinus syndrome caused by recessive mutations in the cardiac sodium channel gene (SCN5A). J Clin Invest 2003;112:1019–28.
24. Zimmer T, Surber R. SCN5A channelopathies. An update on mutations and mechanism. Prog Byophys Mol Biol 2008;98:120–36.
25. Ruan Y, Liu N, Priori SG. Sodium channel mutations and arrhythmias. Nat Rev Cardiol 2009;6:337–48.
26. Schulze-Bahr E, Neu A, Friederich P, et al. Pacemaker channel dysfunction in a patient with sinus node disease. J Clin Invest 2003;111:1537–45.
27. Duhme N, Schweizer PA, Thomas D, et al. Altered HCN4 channel C-linker interaction is associated with familial tachycardia-bradycardia syndrome and atrial fibrillation. Eur Heart J 2013;34:2768–75.
28. Postma AV, Denjoy I, Hoorntje TM, et al. Absence of calsequestrin 2 causes severe forms of catecholaminergic polymorphic ventricular tachycardia. Circ Res 2002;91:e21–26.
29. Postma AV, Denjoy I, Kamblock J, et al. Catecholaminergic polymorphic ventricular tachycardia: RYR2 mutations, bradycardia, and follow up of the patients. J Med Genet 2005;42:863–70.
30. Goette A, Kalman JM, Aquinaga L, et al. EHRA/HRS/APHRS/SOLAECE expert consensus on atrial cardiomyopathies: definition, characterization, and clinical implication. Europace 2016;18:1455–90.
31. Kottkamp H. Fibrotic atrial cardiomyopathy: a specific disease/syndrome supplying substrates for atrial fibrillation, atrial tachycardia, sinus node

disease, AV nodal disease, and thrombotic complications. J Cardiovasc Electrophysiol 2012;23:797–9.

32. Boriani G, Gallina M, Merlini L, et al. Clinical relevance of atrial fibrillation/flutter, stroke, pacemaker implant, and heart failure in Emery-Dreifuss muscular dystrophy: a long-term longitudinal study. Stroke 2003;34:901–8.

33. Dello Russo A, Pelargonio G, Parisi Q, et al. Widespread electroanatomic alterations of right cardiac chambers in patients with myotonic dystrophy type 1. J Cardiovasc Electrophysiol 2006;17:34–40.

34. Hsu DT. Cardiac manifestations of neuromuscular disorders in children. Paediatr Respir Rev 2010;11: 35–8.

35. Stockins BA, Lanas FT, Saavedra JG, et al. Prognosis in patients with diphtheric myocarditis and bradyarrhythmias: assessment of results of ventricular pacing. Br Heart J 1994;72:190–1.

36. Arce M, Van Grieken J, Femenia F, et al. Permanent pacing in patients with Chagas' disease. Pacing Clin Electrophysiol 2012;35:1494–7.

37. Gillis AM, Morck M. Atrial fibrillation after DDDR pacemaker implantation. J Cardiovasc Electrophysiol 2002;13:542–7.

38. Chen YC, Lu YY, Cheng CC, et al. Sinoatrial node electrical activity modulates pulmonary vein arrhythmogenesis. Int J Cardiol 2014;174:378–80.

39. Hadian D, Zipes DP, Olgin JE, et al. Short-term rapid atrial pacing produces electrical remodeling of sinus node function in humans. J Cardiovasc Electrophysiol 2002;13:584–6.

40. Nielsen JC, Themsen PEB, Hojberg S, et al. A comparison of single-lead atrial pacing with a dual chamber pacing in sick sinus syndrome. Eur Heart J 2011;32:686–96.

41. Drago F, Silvetti MS, Grutter G, et al. Long term management of atrial arrhythmias in young patients with sick sinus syndrome undergoing early operation to correct congenital heart diseases. Europace 2006; 8:488–94.

42. Haissaguerre M, Jais P, Shah DC, et al. Spontaneous initiation of atrial fibrillation by ectopic beats originating in the pulmonary veins. N Engl J Med 1998;339:659–66.

43. Yasuma F, Hayano J. Respiratory sinus arrhythmia: why does the heartbeat synchronize with the respiratory rhythm? Chest 2004;125:683–90.

44. Tan MP, Pary SW. Vasovagal syncope in the older patient. J Am Coll Cardiol 2008;51:599–606.

45. Boriani G, Tukkie R, Manolis AS, et al. Atrial antitachycardia pacing and managed ventricular pacing in bradycardia patients with paroxysmal or persistent atrial tachyarrhythmias: the MINERVA randomized multicentre international trial. Eur Heart J 2014;35:2352–62.

46. Padeletti L, Puererfellner H, Mont L, et al. New-generation atrial antitachycardia pacing (reactive ATP) is associated with reduced risk of persistent or permanent atrial fibrillation in patients with bradycardia: results from the MINERVA randomized multicenter international trial. Heart Rhythm 2015;12:1717–25.

47. Calkins H, Hindricks G, Cappato R, et al. HRS/ EHRA/ECAS/APHRS/SOLAECE Expert consensus statement on catheter and surgical ablation of atrial fibrillation. Heart Rhythm 2017;14:e275–444.

48. Drago F, Russo MS, Marazzi R, et al. Atrial tachycardias in patients with congenital heart disease: a minimally invasive simplified approach in the use of the three-dimensional electroanatomic mapping. Europace 2011;13:689–95.

Atrioventricular Nodal Conduction Disease

Giuseppe Bagliani, MD[a,b,]*, Fabio M. Leonelli, MD[c], Roberto De Ponti, MD, FHRS[d], Ezio Mesolella, MD[b], Luigi Padeletti, MD[e,f]

KEYWORDS

- Atrioventricular conduction • Atrioventricular conduction anatomy • Conduction disorders
- Atrioventricular blocks

KEY POINTS

- Anatomic description of the atrioventricular components of the conduction system.
- Clinical relevance of a correct diagnosis of level of block.
- Electrocardiographic analysis of conduction disorders.

INTRODUCTION

The term atrioventricular conduction describes the whole mechanism allowing the conduction of an electrical impulse from sinoatrial node to the ventricles. Many structures participate in this task and constitute a complex net that is physiologically and ontologically deputized to optimize and synchronize atrial and ventricular activation. This system is able to regulate the speed of conduction according to specific needs.[1] In fact, in a normal sinus rhythm, atrial contraction substantially contributes to ventricular end-diastolic filling and only a flexible system will guarantee constant atrioventricular synchrony at all sinus rates. Furthermore, some of the components of this net (eg, the atrioventricular junction) may act as an emergency pacemaker in case of sinus arrests.

THE PR INTERVAL AND ITS COMPONENTS

Atrioventricular conduction is analyzed observing the PR interval, defined as the time from onset of atrial depolarization, the beginning of P wave, to onset of ventricular activation, the beginning of QRS. This interval includes the activation of 3 different parts of the conduction systems: the internodal conduction, the atrioventricular junction, and the His bundle branches and Purkinje fibers (**Fig. 1**).

Internodal Conduction

The internodal conduction consists of 3 internodal tracts (anterior, middle, and posterior). These are fibers radially coursing the atrium in an anteroposterior direction to reach the atrioventricular junction. Conduction velocity in the atrial fibers encompassing the atrioventricular node (AVN) progressively decreases in an anteroposterior direction because of different connexins expression and diminished density of sodium (Na) channels. Therefore, the anterior pathway, also referred as transitional tissue, located in the superior and middle part of the triangle of Koch, by expressing connexins of large or medium conductance and having high density Na channels, has the fastest conduction. This area (fast pathway) is responsible for the shortest PR intervals both because of its electrophysiological characteristics and because of its more direct connection to the penetrating bundle of His bypassing the AVN (**Fig. 2**). Moving

---

There are no relevant conflicts to disclose.
[a] Cardiology Department, Arrhythmology Unit, Foligno General Hospital, Foligno, Italy; [b] Cardiovascular Diseases Department, University of Perugia, Perugia, Italy; [c] Cardiology Department, James A. Haley Veterans' Hospital, University South Florida, Tampa, FL, USA; [d] Cardiology Department, University of Insubria, Varese, Italy; [e] Heart and Vessels Department, University of Florence, Florence, Italy; [f] IRCCS Multimedica, Sesto San Giovanni, Italy
* Corresponding author. Via Centrale Umbra 17, Spello, Perugia 06038, Italy.
E-mail address: giuseppe.bagliani@tim.it

cardiacEP.theclinics.com

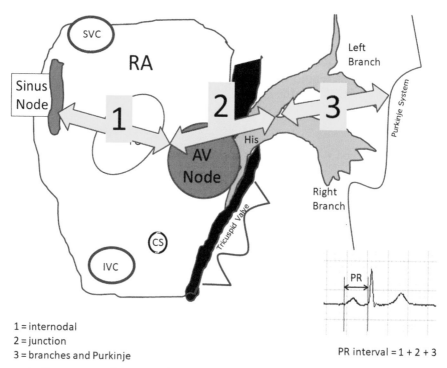

1 = internodal
2 = junction
3 = branches and Purkinje

PR interval = 1 + 2 + 3

Fig. 1. The conduction system and the normal activation of the heart. AV, atrioventricular; CS, coronary sinus; IVC, inferior vena cava; RA, right atrium; SVC, superior vena cava.

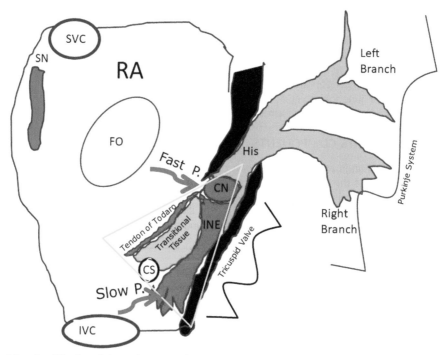

Fig. 2. The triangle of Koch and the atrioventricular junction. Fast and slow pathways of the atrioventricular junction. CN, compact node; FO, fossa ovalis; INE, inferior nodal extension.

toward the posterior bundles, situated in the middle and inferior part of the triangle of Koch, conduction becomes progressively slower owing to expression of low conductance connexins and decreased Na channel content. This region, also called the inferior nodal extension, is associated with longer PR intervals (slow way).

The competition between faster and slower pathways conducting the impulse to the ventricle is based on a delicate balance between their conduction speed and refractory period modulated by phasic influences mediated by the neurovegetative system. In fact, refractoriness is longer in the fast conducting pathway because a prolonged action potential is required to eliminate the increased amount of intracellular Na. Conversely, the slow conducting pathways with decreased expression of Na channels exhibit a shorter action potential duration and refractoriness.

Atrioventricular Junction

The atrioventricular junction is composed of the AVN and the His bundle before branching (see **Fig. 2**). The AVN, placed at the apex of the triangle of Koch, with calcium-dependent fibers, weak electrical coupling, and low conductance connexins, shows the slowest velocity of conduction. The His bundle is the fastest cardiac conducting structure, carrying the impulse from the AVN to the left and right bundle branches. Different connexins expression appears to dissociate longitudinally along this bundle creating 2 parts: the superior, with direct input from the fast pathway, and the inferior, linked to the slow conducting fibers incoming from the inferior nodal extension.[2]

Branches and the Purkinje Network

The His bundle divides into a left branch and a right branch that reach and activate the ventricular myocardium via a specialized cellular arborization called the Purkinje network. Electrical activation proceeding through the AVN, His bundle, and bundle branches cannot be recorded using a standard 12-lead electrocardiogram (ECG). Therefore, the earliest ventricular activation recorded in the surface ECG determines the end of the PR interval.

ANALYZING THE PR INTERVAL AND ITS ANOMALIES

The analysis of the PR interval provides precise information regarding the components of atrioventricular conduction. Localization and severity of conduction abnormalities are necessary to assess their clinical relevance and prognosis.

A block within the His-Purkinje system (HPS) often progresses to compete heart block, whereas AVN block is often either a side effect of commonly used AVN blockers, a benign effect of aging, or a physiologic response to hypervagotonia. Conduction deficits of different severity may present with an apparently similar ECG. In-depth evaluation of all available tracings to assess the PR-interval response to different stressors and consideration of the clinical context are essential to guide correct management of the patient.[3]

His Bundle Recording in the Study of Atrioventricular Conduction

The PR interval contains general information on the atrioventricular conduction but a detailed analysis of the 3 fundamental parts of the conduction system can only be obtained by endocavitary recording. Introducing special catheters in the AVN-His region make it possible to record the His bundle activation potential (**Fig. 3**), which represents the cornerstone of the analysis of the conduction system.[4] In fact, by combining surface and His Bundle recording, it is possible to measure the following intervals representing the activation time of every single part of the conduction system:

- PA interval (from P wave beginning to the His potential recording), corresponding to internodal conduction
- AH interval (from atrial activation at the His level to the His potential), corresponding to atrioventricular node conduction time
- HV interval (from the His potential to the beginning of surface QRS), representing His Purkinje conduction, which includes the His bundle, branches, and the distal Purkinje network.

ATRIOVENTRICULAR CONDUCTION DISORDERS
First-Degree Atrioventricular Block

Electrocardiogram characteristics
First-degree atrioventricular block (I-AVB) is defined as a delay of atrioventricular conduction in which all P waves are followed by QRS complexes with a PR interval constantly longer than 200 ms (**Fig. 4**).

Clinical issues and prognosis
It is possible to identify the site of delay through the analysis of the surface ECG by considering the PR and QRS interval duration, and eventual coexistence of second-degree AVB (II-AVB), as well as reaction to carotid sinus massage (CSM), atropine administration, and/or an ergometric test.

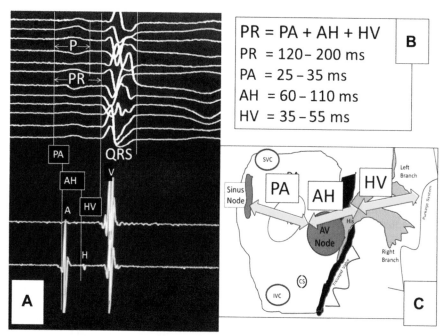

$$PR = PA + AH + HV$$

B

$$PR = 120 - 200 \text{ ms}$$
$$PA = 25 - 35 \text{ ms}$$
$$AH = 60 - 110 \text{ ms}$$
$$HV = 35 - 55 \text{ ms}$$

Fig. 3. Surface and intracavitary study in the analysis of atrioventricular conduction. The endocavitary recordings of a normal conduction system and its genesis. (*A*) The different intervals from the beginning of recorded atrial activity (beginning of P wave) to the arrival of the excitation front in the region of the AVN (PA). The activation of the AVN is not directly recorded but the time of transit through this structure (AH) is inferred from the time of depolarization of the atrial tissue in this region (A deflection) to the time of activation of the His bundle (H). Total time of impulse transit through the HPS, including right and left bundle, is represented by the HV interval recorded from the common His deflection to the first depolarization of ventricular tissue (beginning of QRS). (*B*) The normal values of the different intervals. (*C*) The different wave-fronts of propagation from the sinus node to the ventricles and its corresponding interval at intracardiac recording (PA, AH, HV).

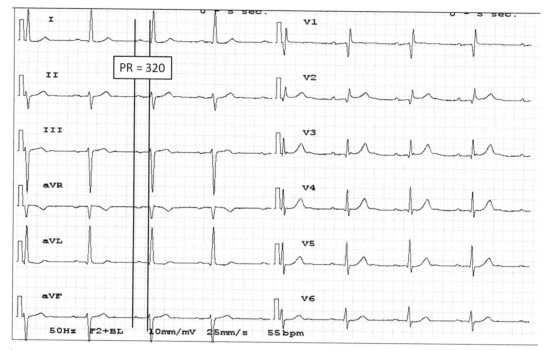

Fig. 4. I-AVB. PR interval is prolonged (320 ms). bpm, beats per minute.

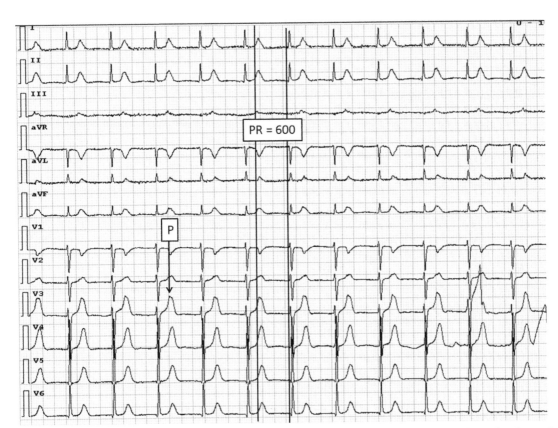

Fig. 5. I-AVB. An important impairment of atrioventricular conduction is evident by a very prolonged PR interval (600 ms). P wave is synchronous and inscripted into the previous T wave.

A marked intraatrial delay could, at times, increase the PR interval to longer than 200 ms; however, the delay is never very pronounced, and it is accompanied by ECG evidence of atrial enlargement. A PR interval longer than 300 ms (**Fig. 5**) almost certainly indicates some degree of AVN delay. Equally, narrow QRS complexes, worsening of the block with CSM, or its improvement with atropine suggests a nodal origin of the delay and thus a better prognosis. On the contrary, a block within the HPS, an infrahisian block manifested by prolonged QRS complexes, and an opposite response to CSM, atropine, or an ergometric test carries a worse prognosis. The clinical setting in which I-AVB is observed is fundamental in determining the level of block.

I-AVB in the young is usually a physiologic expression of increased vagal tone and it disappears as the adrenergic tone increases (eg, during a physical effort). Equally, when diagnosed in an asymptomatic elderly patient with an otherwise normal ECG, it carries a good prognosis due to its intranodal localization. In rare case it is possible to record a sudden prolongation of the PR interval as expression of a jump in a very slow AVN conducting pathway (**Fig. 6**); this double AVN conduction is, in many cases, the substrate of an AVN reentry tachycardia.

Conversely, localization of I-AVB is more complex and it acquires a different prognostic significance when associated with ECG evidence of abnormal intraventricular conduction. In the presence of bifascicular block (eg, Right Bundle Branch Block and Left Anterior Fascicular Block/Left Posterior Fascicular Block), PR interval prolongation could be due to an added AVN delay or represent a severe prolongation of HPS conduction. Twelve-lead ECG cannot distinguish between these 2 possibilities and the precise localization of the site of delay needs an electrophysiological study with the His bundle electrogram recording (see **Fig. 3**). An AH interval prolongation implies an intranodal site of delay and a good prognosis. A delay in delivery of the impulse due to HPS disease delaying the propagation of the impulse to the ventricle is accompanied by a progressive increase in the HV interval. Particularly ominous is the observation of fragmentation of the His electrogram, signifying advanced disease in the common bundle, or an HV delay longer than 100 ms.

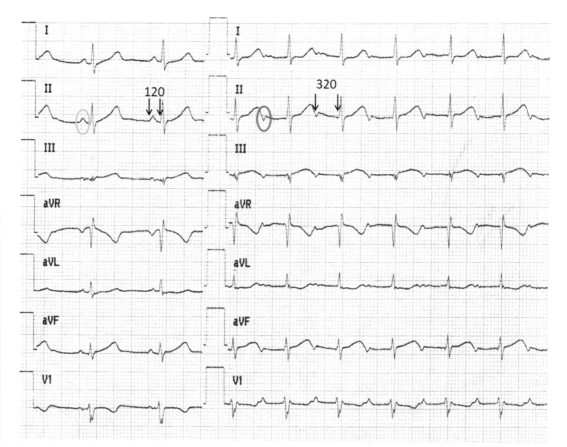

Fig. 6. PR prolongation and double atrioventricular node conduction. The green circle shows normal P wave and AVC (PR = 120 ms, PP = 800 ms). The red circle shows an ectopic activation of the atria that is associated with an abrupt prolongation of the AVC (PR 320 ms, P'-P' = 600 ms).

Either of these findings demand permanent pacemaker implant because the risk of progression to complete heart block is all but assured.

Second-Degree Atrioventricular Block

Electrocardiogram characteristics

II-AVB occurs when at least 1 impulse is not conducted from atria to ventricles. Different manifestations of II-AVB are classified as type 1 (also called Mobitz 1 or Luciani-Wenckebach), type 2 (also called Mobitz 2 or simply Mobitz), fixed 2:1 (ratio) AVB, and paroxysmal AVB (PAVB).

Mobitz type I atrioventricular block (Wenckebach) Wenckebach II-AVB is characterized by a sequence of P waves showing prolongation of the PR interval until a P wave is not followed by a QRS complex (**Fig. 7**). After the block, the atrial impulse conducts normally with a PR interval that is the shortest of the series. Over a longer period of observation, the sequence is repeated multiple times with a cyclicity that is a feature of the Wenckebach periodicity.[5]

In a typical Wenckebach II-AVB, the maximum perceptual increase of the PR interval occurs in the second beat of the sequence.

As the PR intervals of the series continue to prolong, they will do so by a smaller fraction each time. The prolongation of the PR intervals can be inappreciable after a long sequence; therefore, the PR interval shortening after the nonconducted P wave is the typical electrocardiographic sign of the Wenckebach sequence (**Fig. 8**).

As a rule, in a typical Wenckebach sequence, no PR interval should be shorter than the previous and no RR interval should be longer than the previous.[6] If this simple rule is not observed, the Wenckebach periodicity is defined as atypical (**Fig. 9**). Although most type I II-AVBs will demonstrate the typical periodicity previously described, several variations, so-called atypical Wenckebach, have also been described. Atypical manifestations include the last RR interval

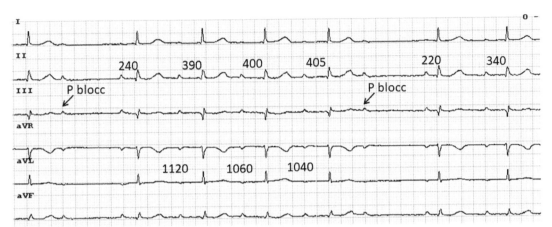

Fig. 7. Typical Mobitz type I-AVB (Wenckebach sequence). During normal sinus rhythm, a progressive prolonga-tion of PR interval is evident until a blocked P wave (not followed by a QRS complex). After the block, the PR interval is the shortest of the series. The prolongation of the PR interval is associated with the shortening of the RR interval.

of the series longer than the previous by 40 ms or more, several PR intervals of the same duration, unexpected decrease of a PR interval or failure of the second PR interval to show maximum increase. To diagnose typical or atypical Wenck-ebach and, therefore, localize the block to the AVN, it is necessary, as previously discussed, to measure the PR interval of the beat before and after the blocked P wave. Equally important is the precise evaluation of the PP interval before and at the time of the blocked P wave. A prema-ture atrial beat, in fact, may not be conducted

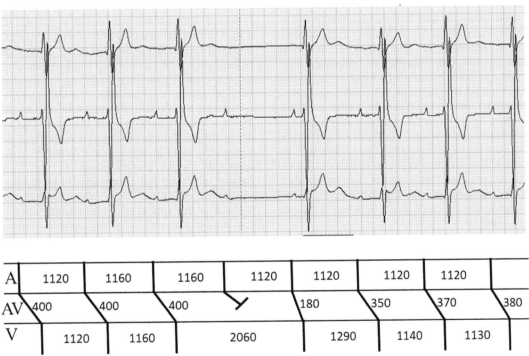

A	1120		1160		1160		1120		1120		1120		1120	
AV	400		400		400				180		350		370		380
V		1120		1160			2060			1290		1140		1130	

Fig. 8. A laddergram of typical Mobitz type I-AVB (Wenckebach sequence) prolongation of the PR interval (and shortening of RR interval) until a P wave is not followed by a QRS complex. After the block, the atrial impulse conducts normally with the shortest PR interval. The prolongation of the PR intervals is inappreciable before the nonconducted P wave and, therefore, the PR interval shortening after the nonconducted P wave is the typical sign of Wenckebach sequence.

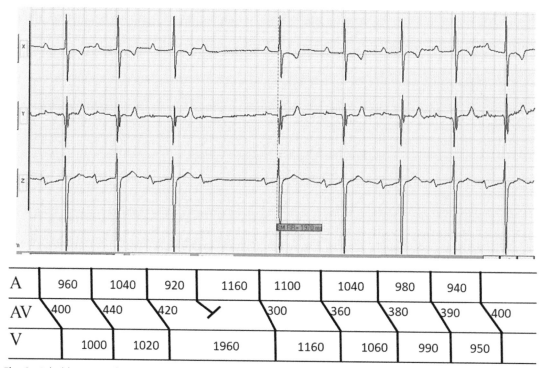

A	960	1040	920	1160	1100	1040	980	940	
AV	400	440	420		300	360	380	390	400
V		1000	1020	1960	1160	1060	990	950	

Fig. 9. A laddergram of atypical Mobitz type I-AVB (Wenckebach sequence). A blocked P wave due to a shortening of the sinus cycle (PP: 960-1040-920 ms).

and be preceded and followed by similar PR intervals, therefore giving, at first sight, the impression of a Mobitz type II phenomenon. The level of block, in this case, cannot be definitely diagnosed. In another scenario, a faster atrial rhythm may conduct with a longer PR interval as normal physiologic response. When the tachycardia terminates, the PR interval shortens in response to increase in cycle length. Furthermore, a blocked P wave may be followed by a junctional escape encroaching on the next P. In this case, the PR interval of this beat cannot be interpreted, limiting observation of the data and making it impossible to distinguish between a Mobitz type I and II.

Mobitz type II-atrioventricular block The observation of a single nonconducted P wave associated with a constant PR interval before and after the blocked P wave is defined as Mobitz type II-AVB (**Fig. 10**). If this observation occurs in the setting of a stable sinus rate, the block occurs in the HPS and, because it carries an ominous prognosis, it will require pacemaker implant.[7]

Atrioventricular block
The electrocardiographic pattern of a II-AVB manifested by a sequence of 2 or more blocked

P waves alternatively conducted in a 2:1 ratio (**Fig. 11**) represents a very challenging diagnostic dilemma because this finding could occur both at the AVN or HPS level with a marked difference in prognosis. To reach a diagnosis, it is necessary to review any available tracing, focusing on some very relevant observations. The finding of Wenckebach periodicity in the same patient, often obtained during prolonged recordings, localizes the level of block to the AVN. The presence of bundle branch block in the same patient, although not diagnostic, is highly suggestive of HPS block.[7] The occurrence of type II block in the setting of a slowing of the sinus rate is suggestive of hypervagotonia and, therefore, most likely localizes the block at the AVN level. The endocavitary recording is able to identify the site of the block (**Fig. 12**).

Paroxysmal or advanced atrioventricular block
PAVB is defined by the loss of conduction of 2 atrial impulses or more (**Fig. 13**). It is characterized by the presence of at least 2 P waves not followed by QRS complexes. The block occurs in the setting of heart rate change, either deceleration or, more often, acceleration. Tachycardia-dependent PAVB is often preceded by multiple episodes of Mobitz type II during a

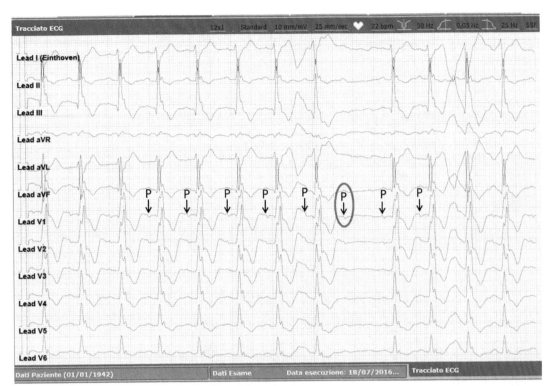

Fig. 10. Mobitz type II. Regular sinus rhythm with PR of 210 ms. The red circle shows a nonconducted P wave. There are no variations in sinus rate and PR duration (the first conducted PR following the block measures 210 ms).

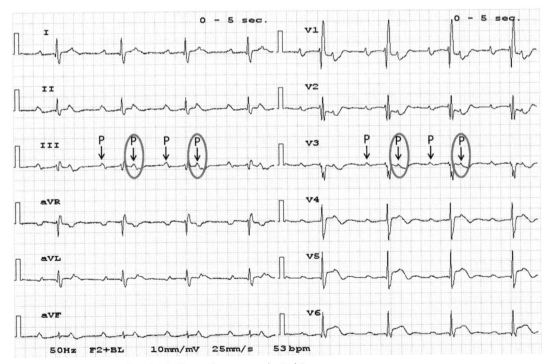

Fig. 11. 2:1 AVB. The red circles indicate the nonconducted P wave.

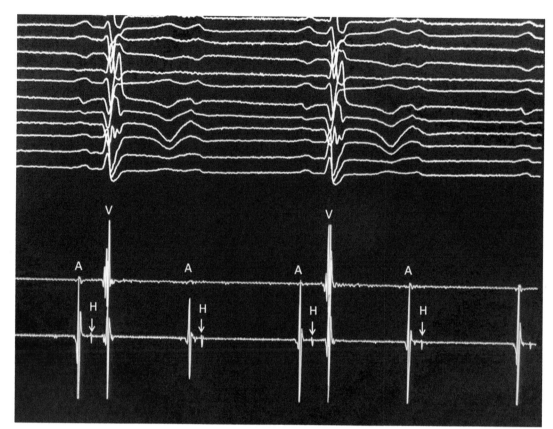

Fig. 12. 2:1 AVB. His bundle recording in the localization the site of the block. Each P wave (A) is followed by an activation of His bundle (H). This is typical of a site of block distal to the His bundle.

spontaneous, often subtle gradual increase of heart rate. Onset of bradycardia-dependent PAVB occurs during spontaneous slowing of sinus rate or is it ushered in by a pause, usually a compensatory pause following a premature atrial or ventricular beat, or it is due to tachycardia-induced overdrive suppression of the sinus node.

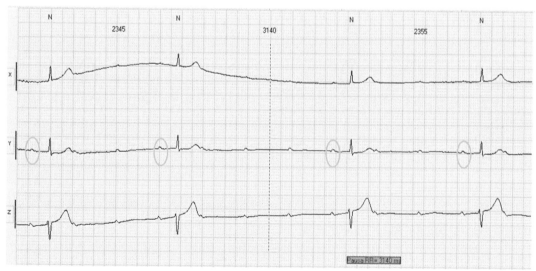

Fig. 13. Advanced AVB or PAVB. P waves not followed by QRS complexes. Only occasionally is a P wave is conducted to the ventricles (*red circles*).

Both can occur in the setting of cardiac ischemia or variations of autonomic sympathetic tone. Both also occur because of severely diseased HPS with its fibers demonstrating major electrophysiological abnormalities, affecting both cellular depolarization and repolarization The site of block in forms of PAVB is frequently the common His, at times accompanied by more extensive bundle branch disease. Therefore, either block can occur in patient with normal or wide QRS. The electrophysiological mechanism of the block is unclear. Concealed conduction within the diseased HPS has been suggested as the mechanism triggering tachycardia-mediated PAVB, whereas bradycardia-dependent block is still missing a satisfactory explanation. Although PAVB is often associated with symptoms of syncope and presyncope, its relationship with sudden cardiac death is unclear.[4]

Third-Degree Atrioventricular Block (Complete Heart Block)

Electrocardiogram characteristics

In third-degree AVB (III-AVB) none of the P waves is linked to a specific QRS complex because of the complete interruption of atrioventricular conduction. Cardiac standstill is avoided by the emergence of a subsidiary pacemaker.

The AVN and HPS, in addition to the sinus-atrial node, are capable of spontaneous automaticity, becoming, in the absence of a faster rhythm, a subsidiary cardiac pacemaker generating an escape rhythm.[7] Emergence of a pacemaker is determined by its intrinsic rate. The sinus node is, in normal circumstances, the usual pacemaker because its higher intrinsic rate will depolarize any other subsidiary pacemaker before they spontaneously discharge. The intrinsic rate of automatic tissue is progressively slower moving down along the conducting system structures. When the rhythm originates from the atrio-ventricular junction, it is characterized by narrow QRS (QRS similar to SR) and a heart rate of 45 to 50 beats per minute (**Fig. 14**). A lower subsidiary pacemaker from 1 of the branches of the HPS, idioventricular rhythm, will have a wide QRS with a morphology resembling a bundle branche block of the opposite chamber. The ECG will, therefore, demonstrate a regular escape rhythm dissociated, without any relationship with sinus P waves (**Fig. 15**). Rarely, a complete heart block can be congenital and asymptomatic. The escape is junctional with narrow QRS and often normal chronotropic response (**Fig. 16**). In this case, life expectancy of patients with and without pacemakers is similar and implanting a device it is not necessary.

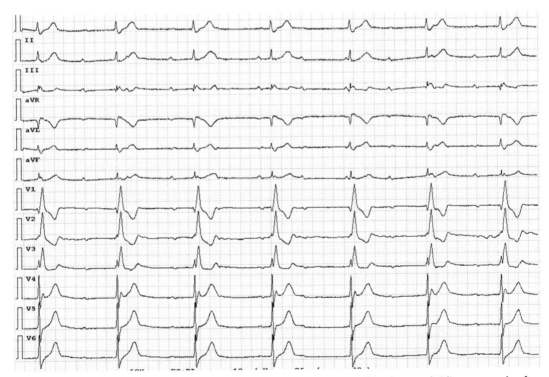

Fig. 14. III-AVB and escape junctional rhythm. A complete AVB is present with a lower subsidiary pacemaker from 1 of the branches of the HPS, with RBBB morphology.

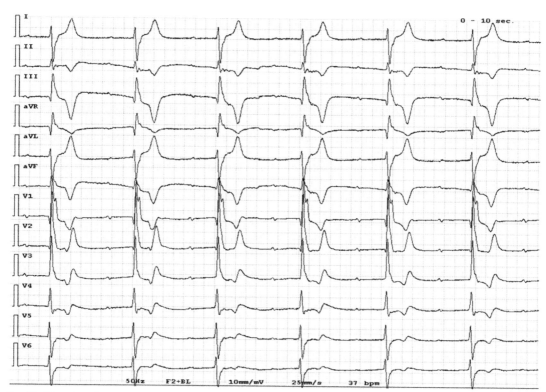

Fig. 15. III-AVB and escape ventricular rhythm. A lower subsidiary pacemaker from 1 of the branches of the HPS generates an idioventricular rhythm with a wide complex RBBB morphology.

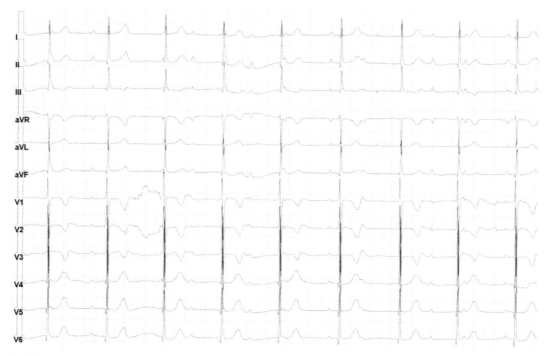

Fig. 16. Congenital III-AVB and junctional escape rhythm. Very narrow QRS in an asymptomatic pediatric patient and normal chronotropic response.

REFERENCES

1. Bagliani G, Della Rocca DG, Di Biase L, et al. PR interval and junctional zone. Card Electrophysiol Clin 2017;9:411–33.
2. Di Biase L, Gianni C, Bagliani G, et al. Arrhythmias involving the atrioventricular junction. Card Electrophysiol Clin 2017;9:435–52.
3. Kurian T, Ambrosi C, Hucker W, et al. Anatomy and electrophysiology of the human AV node. Pacing Clin Electrophysiol 2010;33(6):754–62.
4. Hwang HJ, Ng FS, Efimov IR. Mechanisms of atrioventricular nodal excitability and propagation. In: Zipes DP, Jalife J, editors. Cardiac electrophysiology: from cell to bedside. 6th edition. Philadelphia (PA): Elsevier; 2014. p. 275–85.
5. Kinoshita S, Konishi G. Atrioventricular Wenckebach periodicity in athletes: influence of increased vagal tone on the occurrence of atypical periods. J Electrocardiol 1987;20(3):272–9.
6. Mond HG, Vohra J. The electrocardiographic footprints of Wenckebach block. Heart Lung Circ 2017; 26(12):1252–66.
7. Schamroth L. The disorders of cardiac rhythm. Johannesburg: Blackwell Scientific Publications; 1971.

Intraventricular Delay and Blocks

Fabio M. Leonelli, MD[a],*, Giuseppe Bagliani, MD[b,c], Roberto De Ponti, MD, FHRS[d],
Luigi Padeletti, MD[e,f]

KEYWORDS

- Bundle branch block • Left bundle branch • Right bundle branch block • Hemiblocks
- His Purkinje disease

KEY POINTS

- Diseases affecting the His Purkinje system will alter the propagation of the electrical wave front in left and right bundle.
- Changes in propagation will induce vectorial shifts recorded on the 12-lead electrocardiogram (ECG) with changes often diagnostic of a specific bundle branch block.
- Delays or blocks of conduction can minimally involve a bundle branch or one of its subdivisions or be widespread, affecting different segments of both branches.
- Analysis of the ECG can often assess the severity of the injury but is limited in its ability to predict long-term risk of complete heart block or death.
- ECG limitations also include anatomic localization of some ECG abnormalities and distinction among conduction blocks and delays.

INTRODUCTION

The specialized tissue conducting cardiac impulses from sinus node, to the atria and to the ventricles comprises the 3 following anatomic regions (Fig. 1):

1. The atria
2. The atrioventricular (AV) junctional region (AV node and the nonbranching portion of the His bundle)
3. The branching of the His Purkinje system (HPS) into right and left bundle (LB) with its anterior, posterior subdivision and terminal arborizations.

The significance of conduction block in either bundle was recognized more than 100 years ago by observing electrocardiographic (ECG) tracings following experimental destruction of each branch. Further human and animal studies, including accurate endocardial and epicardial mapping, allowed the identification of changes in electrical wavefront propagation during left and right bundle branch block (LBBB and RBBB). The initial observations of vectorial shifts induced by conduction blocks were confirmed and expanded by these mapping studies.

It was observed that the main consequence of bundle branch block (BBB) is a profound alteration of activation of the ventricle supplied by the affected branch. A normally functioning HPS ensures fast and sequentially optimized wavefront propagation. In BBB, the intact bundle activates the muscle in a physiologic manner, and from

[a] Cardiology Department, James A. Haley Veterans' Hospital, University of South Florida, Tampa, FL, USA; [b] Cardiology Department, Arrhythmology Unit, Foligno General Hospital, Foligno, Italy; [c] Cardiovascular Diseases Department, University of Perugia, Perugia, Italy; [d] Cardiology Department, University of Insubria, Varese, Italy; [e] Heart and Vessels Department, University of Florence, Florence, Italy; [f] IRCCS Multimedica, Sesto San Giovanni, Italy
* Corresponding author. James A Haley Veterans' Hospital, 13000 Bruce B. Downs Boulevard (111A), Tampa, FL 33612.
E-mail address: fabio.leonelli@va.gov

Card Electrophysiol Clin 10 (2018) 211–231
https://doi.org/10.1016/j.ccep.2018.02.003

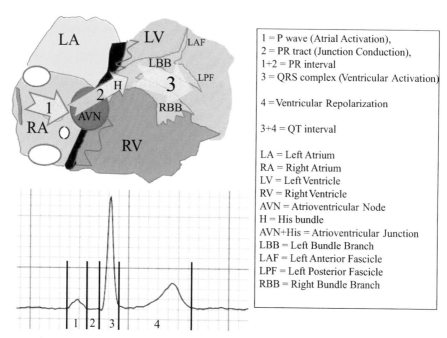

1 = P wave (Atrial Activation),
2 = PR tract (Junction Conduction),
1+2 = PR interval
3 = QRS complex (Ventricular Activation)

4 = Ventricular Repolarization

3+4 = QT interval

LA = Left Atrium
RA = Right Atrium
LV = Left Ventricle
RV = Right Ventricle
AVN = Atrioventricular Node
H = His bundle
AVN+His = Atrioventricular Junction
LBB = Left Bundle Branch
LAF = Left Anterior Fascicle
LPF = Left Posterior Fascicle
RBB = Right Bundle Branch

Fig. 1. The normal conduction system.

there the activation proceeds as a discontinuous wavefront to the affected chamber propagating from myocyte to myocyte. A marked decrease in conduction velocity and alterations in vector direction lead to the changes observed in the 12-lead electrocardiogram (ECG) often diagnostic of a specific BBB. As a result, the ECG is now considered the gold standard in the diagnosis of conduction disorders. Even so, limitations of ECG sensitivity and specificity in the diagnosis of conduction system disease need to be recognized and are discussed in this article.

Notwithstanding these limitations, several electrocardiographic criteria for intraventricular conduction defects were agreed upon and still constitute the most useful tool in the diagnosis of this condition (**Box 1**).

LEFT BUNDLE BRANCH BLOCK

Immediately after crossing the membranous septum, the common bundle of His divides into a right and a left branch coursing down both sides of the intraventricular septum from the base toward the apex. The LB begins below the noncoronary aortic cusp, thickening as it fans out with several unpredictable divisions variably interconnected, extending from the septum to the anterior and posterior wall of the LV (see **Fig. 1**). Variations in the anatomy of this branch are extensive, and there is no full agreement on the nomenclature of the different fascicles.

Nevertheless, an anterior and a posterior division are often identified as distinct fascicles with a variable number of fibers proceeding from the proximal portion of the anterior LB toward the basal third of the anterior left ventricular wall. Equally recognizable, a fan of LB fibers proceeds posteriorly after coursing one-half to two-thirds of the septum from the base to the apex. The existence of a separated third or septal branch of this bundle is still debated. In human and animal studies, a third radiation covering the midseptal surface was observed originating directly from the common LB or from a variable and convoluted plexus of ramifications from either the anterior or the posterior fasciculi.

Following Rosenbaum's observations, the concept of trifascicular left ventricle (LV) activation was enshrined in ECG literature. More than an anatomic observation, the division of LB in left anterior (LA) and left posterior (LP) fascicles conceptualized the fact that there is a clear anterior and a posterior vector in LV activation. During typical conduction, vectors balance each other, producing a QRS lasting up to 110 milliseconds with normal morphology. Any delay or "block" of conduction system ramifications supplying the anterior or posterior wall will lead to the ECG abnormalities defined as hemiblocks, as later discussed.

Conduction can be affected at multiple levels of the HPS, from its predivisional location in the common bundle of His to the terminal arborization.

Box 1
World Health Organization criteria for intraventricular conduction disturbances

Left bundle branch block

1. The QRS duration is 0.12 seconds or more

2. Left-sided precordial leads, Vs and V6, as well as lead 1 and aVL show broad and notched or slurred R waves. Occasionally, an RS pattern may occur in leads Vs and V6 in uncomplicated LBBB associated with posterior displacement of the left ventricle. An R pattern may then be seen if leads V7 and V8 are recorded in these patients.

3. With possible exception of lead aVL, Q waves are absent in the left-sided leads, specifically in leads Vs, V6, and I.

4. The R peak time is prolonged to more than 0.06 second in lead Vs or V6, but is normal in leads VI and V2 when it can be determined.

5. In the right precordial leads VI and V3, there are small initial r waves in most cases, followed by wide and deep S waves. The transition zone in the precordial leads is displaced to the left. Wide QS complexes may be present in leads VI and V2 and rarely in lead V3.

Left anterior fascicular block

1. Frontal plane QRS axis −45° to −80°;

2. QRS duration of 0.11 second or less; and

3. Small Q wave of 0.02 second or less in leads I and aVL.

Left posterior fascicular block

1. A frontal plane QRS axis of +90° to +180°;

2. rS configuration in leads I and aVL, associated with a qR pattern in the inferior leads and obligatory Q waves in leads III and aVF.

Right bundle branch block

1. Prolongation of QRS to 0.12 second or more.

2. An rsr′, rsR′, or rSR′ pattern in lead VI or V2. The R′ is usually greater than the initial R wave.

3. Leads V6 and 1 show a QRS complex with a wide S wave (S duration is longer than the R duration or >40 ms in adults).

4. The R peak time should be greater than 0.05 second in lead VI and should be normal in leads Vs and V6.

Adapted from Willems JL, Robles de Medina EO, Bernard R, et al. Criteria for intraventricular conduction disturbances and pre-excitation. World Health Organizational/International Society and Federation for Cardiology Task Force Ad Hoc. J Am Coll Cardiol 1985;5:1261–75; with permission.

Defects can vary from minor delay to complete block. In general, the more proximal and more severe the block, the more obvious the ECG changes will be, although there is no strict correlation between pathologic condition location and specific ECG alterations. In fact, a small predivisional lesion can produce an ECG similar to that caused by a very extensive pathologic condition affecting multiple LB ramifications. Furthermore, QRS complex prolongation generating ECG morphologies similar to LBBB can be produced by clinical situations not specifically affecting LB conduction, such as antiarrhythmic drugs, electrolytes imbalance, myocardial infarction (MI), left ventricular dilatation, and marked left ventricular hypertrophy. The difference between LBBB proper and the widening of QRS caused by these other conditions lies in the alteration in activation sequence caused by the branch block.

From a large number of animal and human studies, a correlation has been established between LBBB and certain alterations of the ECG, showing major abnormalities of LV activations in the presence of an unchanged RV depolarization.

The most reproducible alteration is the reversal of normal septal activation, not from left to right as expected, but from right to left accompanied by a marked decrease in velocity of propagation. In normal hearts, the earliest endocardial activation is recorded simultaneously at 3 distinct locations. One is the anterobasal wall of the LV near the aortic root, with the impulse probably carried on by a branch of the anterior fascicle. A second wavefront appears in the mid septum, with the impulse possibly propagated by mid-septal branches. Last, the posterior branch depolarizes the lower third of the septum at its the junction with the posterior wall. RV activation, on the other hand, begins at the level of the anterior right papillary muscle approximately 10 milliseconds after the onset of the left ventricular cavity potential.[1]

A delay of LB activation longer than 6 milliseconds is sufficient to alter the sequence of normal septal activation.[2] When LBBB is complete, LV septal activation is reversed and proceeds from the RV across the septal muscle. Instead of 3 specific activation sites, left septal activation appears in single or multiple breakthroughs with a delay of 40 to 80 milliseconds. The abnormal right to left septal activation explains the absence of Q in leads I, V5, and V6 and r in V1 and V2 (**Fig. 2**).

It is conceivable that, in some patients with LBBB, a well-developed septal branch will continue to function while the anterior and posterior fascicles are blocked. In these patients, left to right septal conduction will persist together with abnormal depolarization vectors of the anterior and posterior LV wall. Recently, a study of LBBB[3] reported that an r wave of ≥1 mm in V1 was a sensitive sign of persisting L to R septal conduction. This finding was possibly due to a distal block that spared the distal septal fibers. These patients were observed to develop RBBB during right heart catheterization despite a preprocedural LBBB on ECG and were less likely to progress to complete heart block (CHB) at follow-up.

From the septum, the wavefront propagates with different vectors depending on the presence of concomitant cardiac pathologic conditions. In a patient with LBBB and normal heart or LBBB and dilated cardiomyopathies, endocardial activation proceeds rapidly, with the free wall activation wavefront ahead of the posterior wall. In these patients, LV propagation is fairly uniform with the latest activation found in the posterolateral wall. In LBBB associated with MI, on the contrary, the site and the extent of the scar appear to influence LV endocardial activation. Large anterior MIs profoundly disrupt the endocardial activation time, whereas inferior MIs have a less marked effect on ventricular activation time.[4]

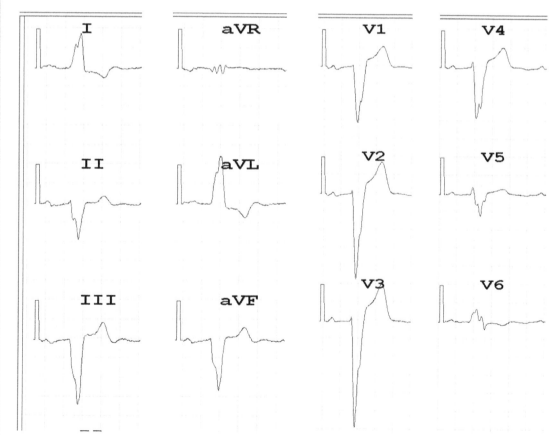

Fig. 2. Typical LBBB: QRS duration of 190 milliseconds, absence of q in I, aVL, V5, and V6 and r in V1, small r in V2-V3. Increased intrinsecoid deflection, broad R with notching in I, aVL, and V6.

This effect on conduction could be due to more extensive destruction of the specialized distal conduction system in anterior MIs; extensive damage prevents late reentry of the depolarizing wavefront into a still intact Purkinje arborization. The lower density of His Purkinje fibers in the basal inferior LV wall explains the minor effect on total endocardial activation.

Regardless of the causing pathologic condition, in LBBB, the slowing of impulse propagation, now conducted from fiber to fiber, generates a large, slow-rising vector directed leftward terminating at the base the heart in patients with normal hearts or cardiomyopathies. On the contrary, in patients with MIs, the last site of endocardial activation is variable and often corresponds to the location of prior infarction.

ECG changes reflect these alterations: slow propagation increases R-wave peak time to more than 60 milliseconds in leads V5 and V6. The dominant leftward vector inscribes a dominant R wave typically broad, notched, or slurred in leads I, aVL, V5, and V6 with occasional RS in leads V5 and/or V6. RV depolarization is completely obscured by the predominant, long-lasting, and high-voltage LV depolarization. The S waves in V5 or V6 are therefore not related to RV activation but simply represent a more posterosuperior direction of a late LV vector possibly because of biventricular enlargement (**Fig. 3**).

In computer simulation of LBBB, the first component of the notch coincides with the beginning of LV endocardial depolarization following R to L septal activation. The second notch corresponds to the arrival of the depolarization wave front at the epicardium of the posterolateral wall. The 2 notches have similar amplitude because they share magnitude and direction of the mean electrical vector.[5]

A preexisting LBBB without overt cardiac disease is associated with minimal mortality risk. On the other hand, the same condition whether newly acquired or in the contest of structural heart disease confers an increased mortality risk.[6] This risk is higher in part because of the LV contraction dyssynchrony induced by LBBB. Because cardiac resynchronization therapy (CRT) reverses in part or totally this hemodynamic complication, the ECG

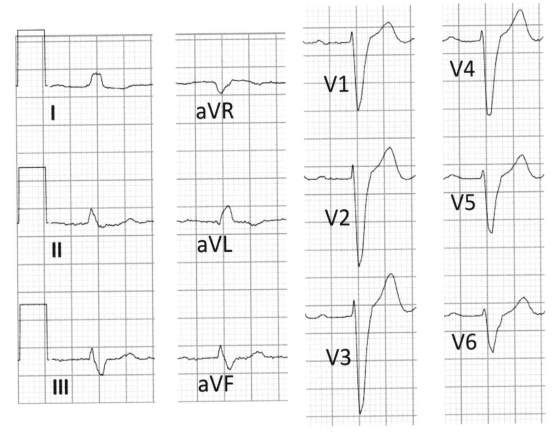

Fig. 3. Effect of RV enlargement on typical LBBB: first-degree AV block with marked S waves in the precordial leads in a patient with normal LV function, paradoxic septal motion, and enlarged RV with RV hypertension.

criteria of this conduction defect have assumed new relevance.

It is not as yet clear whether the level of LB block influences the response to CRT. Because the ECG cannot reliably distinguish between proximal or distal conduction system disease, it is unclear what level of block would respond better to CRT. There is a general consensus, however, that in the presence of LBBB the wider the QRS the more consistent the clinical benefits.

LEFT ANTERIOR FASCICULAR BLOCK

The concept of trifascicular conduction system and therefore of left hemiblocks represents a clear advancement in the understanding of the pathophysiology of the conduction system. Nevertheless, given the extensive arborization of the LB, transferring this schematic approach directly to clinical practice may be difficult. The ECG has limitations in defining the site and extent of the lesions, causing fascicular blocks; multiple studies have in fact identified hemiblocks as manifestations of LBBB disease. The underlying pathologic lesions are generally much more widely distributed than what could be expected from the reductive electrocardiographic terminology of let anterior or posterior hemiblocks.

The LA fascicle fans out from the main LB branch as a thinner branch directed anterosuperiorly to the anterior wall of the LV and anterior papillary muscle. Complete damage to this structure delays depolarization of the anterior LV and shifts the initial vector more posteriorly toward the inferior LV wall supplied by an intact Left Posterior Fascicle (LPF). Thanks probably to the extensive arborization between the 2 fascicles, the wavefront then reaches the anterior wall later and generates an unopposed vector directed anteriorly, superiorly, and toward the left.

The typical ECG findings in pure left anterior fascicular block (LAFB) therefore are (**Fig. 4**) as follows:

- A QRS interval of ≤100 milliseconds with a frontal plane QRS axis to the left of −30°; an initial activation directed to the right and posteriorly with a small q in lead aVL and a small r in III; followed by a leftward superior vector with tall R in lead I and aVL and deep S wave in II, III, and aVF.

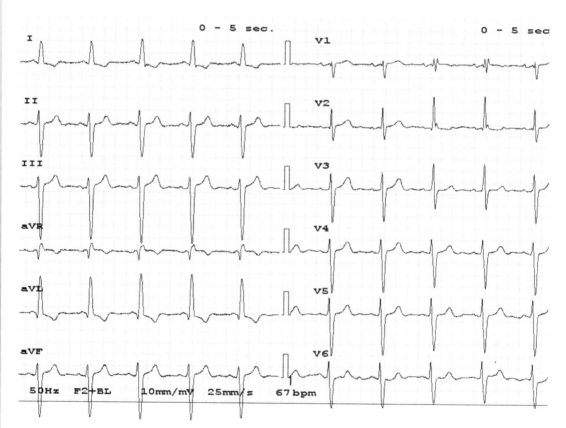

Fig. 4. LAH: QRS interval ≤100 milliseconds with a frontal plane QRS axis to the left of −30°, small q in lead aVL, and a small r in III; tall R in lead I and aVL and deep S wave in II, III, and aVF.

The specificity of these findings is not very high because any pathologic condition leading to left-axis deviation (most often left ventricular hypertrophy [LVH] or inferior MI) will mimic LAFB.

A differential diagnosis must be considered with any condition leading to left-axis deviation, such as, among others:

1. Horizontal heart;
2. Isolated LVH;
3. Inferior MI;
4. Straight back syndrome;
5. Wolff-Parkinson-White syndrome; and
6. Regional anterosuperior right ventricular block

The initial vector shift (small q in lead aVL and a small r in III) can help the interpretation of these different conditions (see **Fig. 4**).

These ECG findings are optimally demonstrated during functional block. In this situation, in fact, there is an alternans of normal and aberrant conduction, and the vector shift is easily observed comparing the 2 QRSs (**Fig. 5**). The dominant anterior forces generated by LAFB can alter the

characteristic features of other pathologic conditions, thus interfering with their diagnosis. In an inferior wall MI, the typical qR or qS morphology of the inferior limb leads may be hampered by LAFB. In a typical LAFB, an r wave is always observed in leads II, III, and aVF because of the early and unopposed activation of the LV inferior wall, caused by the posterior division of the LBB. This r wave will totally or partially disappear whenever the necrotic zone includes the areas of early activation. Conversely, if the infarction spares those areas, an initial r wave will occur in the inferior leads, and the inferior infarction may be concealed. Moreover, the repolarization of secondary changes of LAFB that produce a positive T wave in the inferior limb leads also contributes to mask the signs of a diaphragmatic MI. Accordingly, a negative T wave in II, III, and aVF in the presence of LAFB is a strong sign of the coexistence of significant inferior ischemia or even of a concealed inferior infarction. When a dominant anterolateral wavefront depolarizes the LV, its vector will oppose the late depolarization vector of RBBB. This

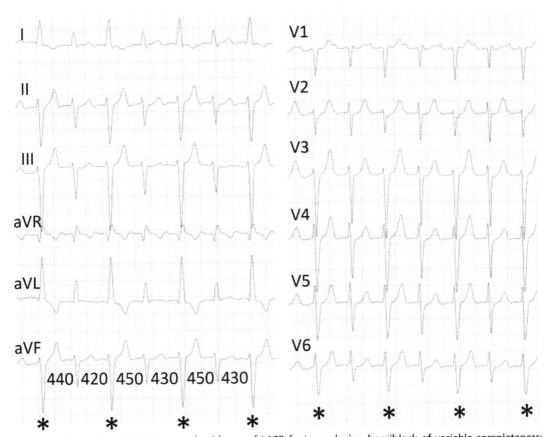

Fig. 5. Rate-dependent LAFB. Increased evidence of LAFB features during hemiblock of variable completeness: The rhythm is atrial tachycardia with variable PR interval. The short RR interval ends with a QRS with more marked evidence of LAFB (*asterisks*). Note deeper q in aVL, deeper S in III and V4 to V6.

discordance can occur in LVH, LV focal conduction blocks due to myocardial fibrosis, and LAFB. All these conditions, and LAFB in particular, may partially conceal the diagnosis of RBBB by causing the S waves of RBBB to disappear from leads I, aVL, and in some cases, the left precordial leads.

LEFT POSTERIOR FASCICULAR BLOCK

This thicker branch of the LB, in most cases, takes off first, at the level of the posterior aortic cusp. In a posteroinferior course, the fascicles reach the lateral and posterior LV wall as well as the posterior papillary muscle. This branch is the least likely division of the intraventricular conduction system to be affected by conduction disturbances. Its resilience is probably due to a combination of factors, including its limited length and wide ramifications, its blood supply from both the anterior and the posterior descending coronary arteries, and its location in the LV inflow tract, a region + n with less turbulent blood flow than the outflow tract. Isolated LPF block is very rare (**Fig. 6**) and when present is frequently associated with RBBB (**Fig. 7**). Extensive lesions are required to alter the conduction in the posterior fascicle; when they occur, it is highly likely that the extent of the disease has already affected both the right bundle (RB) branch and the anterior division of the LBB. The presence of such widespread pathologic condition explains the high incidence of progression to complete AV block when RBBB and left posterior hemiblock (LPH) are present.

Both the ECG and vectorcardiogram (VCG) of LPH are the mirror images of left anterior hemiblock (LAH).

The initial forces oriented superiorly and to the left, responsible for the small r waves in leads I and aVL, and the small q waves of leads II, III, and aVF are caused by early activation of the anterolateral wall of the LV.

The terminal forces of the QRS loop are oriented inferiorly and to the right and are responsible for the S in leads I and aVL and R in leads II, III, and aVF. Other conditions causing right-axis deviation, such as right ventricular hypertrophy (RVH), horizontal heart, need to enter in the differential diagnosis. Differential diagnosis with RVH vertical heart and lateral infarction is at times difficult but, as for LAH, fulfillment of all the ECG criteria and review of the VCG loop should be of great help.

Although more rarely than LAH, the marked axis shift as observed in LPH could interfere with the ECG diagnosis of inferior ischemia or infarct. The QRS force's shift inferiorly and to the right can mask to variable degrees the signs of inferior MI. As previously noted, subtle ST segment changes, such as elevation in lead III and marked ST segment depression in leads I and V5–V6, could be the only sign of evolving ischemia.

PERSISTING CONTROVERSIES IN LEFT BUNDLE BRANCH BLOCK
Incomplete Left Bundle Branch Block and the Existence of a Septal Branch

The concept of incomplete LBBB derives from observations of progressive, rate-dependent, LB conduction abnormalities ranging from normal QRS to complete LB block. Because of the rarity of these reports, however, and the stringent

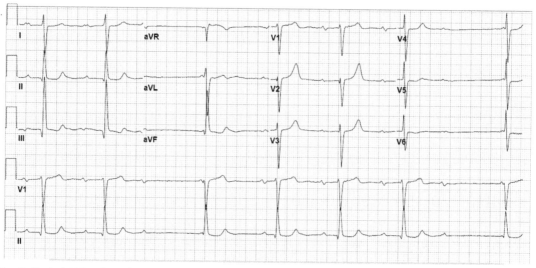

Fig. 6. Typical LPFB: Sinus rhythm, junctional escape, Mobitz type I AV block and LPFB. Note frontal plane QRS axis of +110°; rS configuration in leads I and aVL, associated with a qR pattern in the inferior leads.

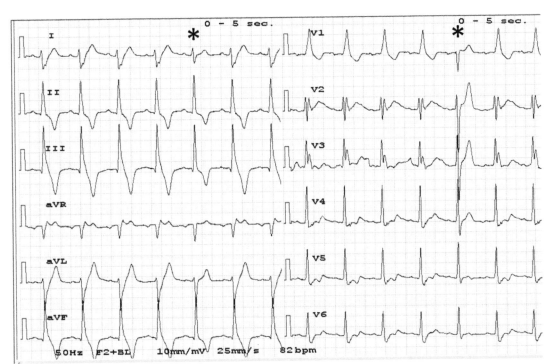

Fig. 7. RBBB and LPFB: The features of both blocks are present. Note beat 5 and 12 (*asterisks*) show a disappearance of the RBBB and clear features of solitary LPFB.

diagnostic criteria, this electrocardiographic entity remains incompletely defined.[7]

The first consequence of LB conduction delay is an alteration of septal activation. Minor degrees of LBBB do not alter the left to right septal activation, and therefore, this condition remains electrocardiographically silent. As the LB delay approaches 10 milliseconds, transseptal activation will be altered with manifested ECG changes.

Once the electrical wavefront has reached the left side of the septum, the remainder of the LV depolarization will proceed unchanged, maintaining the rest of the QRS within normal limits. As the block increases, the normal septal depolarization is progressively reversed with inversion and delay of the septal vector. The first evidence of such incomplete block is loss of the initial q wave in V5 and V6, followed by slurring of the upstroke of the R wave in left-oriented leads (**Fig. 8**).

As the LBB progresses, the T wave will invert, and finally, the QRS will progressively widen, developing a plateau that eventually will become notched.[8]

Some investigators have suggested that incomplete LBB is due to an initial conduction delay limited to septal arborization of the LB.

As more and more LB branches become functionally incapacitated, the activation will progressively depend on muscle to muscle propagation

and will result in an increasingly abnormal ECG. This explanation is supported by some observations describing a third or septal branch of the LB.

However, in the classical understanding of the LB,[9] this branch is anatomically bifascicular with a distinct anterosuperior and posteroinferior division. Interruption of these fascicles results in ECG patterns commonly described as LAH and LPH. In reality, the LB anatomic variations are very large, and, at least in a consistent number of them, a middle or left septal fascicle (LSF) can be recognized.[10] A controversy still exists on the functional and clinical significance of this branch and more importantly whether a block of this branch generates a specific ECG pattern. Some support for trifascicular activation of the LV comes from observations of isolated heart[11] endocardial excitation, where 3 distinct subendocardial breakthroughs were identified in areas corresponding to the arborization of the 3 fascicles. According to this interpretation, LSF would contribute to the initial 10 milliseconds of ventricular depolarization with a septal vector oriented left to right and inferiorly. As the opposite vectors generated by the LAF and LPF will cancel each other, the main direction of septal depolarization is determined by LSF recording a q wave in left facing leads. A block in this branch will cause a delay in septal activation, leading to a predominance of anterior forces,

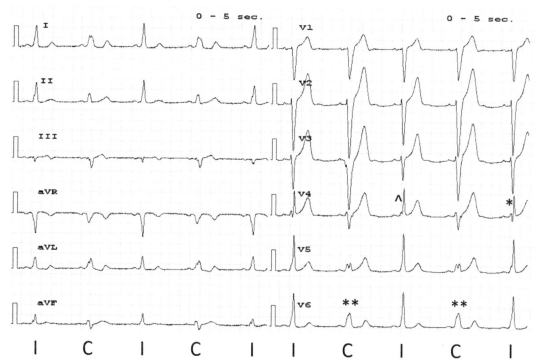

Fig. 8. Variable LBBB severity. The figure shows an alternant LBBB (C complete LBBB, I incomplete LBBB). Note the variation in septal activation manifested with presence (*asterisk*) or absence (*caret*) of q in V4 in the incomplete LBBB. In the complete block (*double asterisks*), the features of LBBB are present, including small or absent r in V1 to V3, wide notched QRS in V6.

because they will be less counterbalanced by the inferoposterior vector associated with LSF depolarization. Most of the literature on the subject therefore associates LSF block with the loss of q waves in leads I, aVL, and more obviously, in leads V5 and V6, and the emergence of prominent anterior forces in V1 and V2 (**Fig. 9**). Block in this fascicle could help explain some ECG findings that defy interpretation if one adopts a strict bifascicular LV activation model. In severe LVH, LAFB, RBBB, and in incomplete rate-related LBBB, LSF block is invoked to explain the loss of septal r in V1, V2 and of septal q in left precordial and limb leads.

Specificity of Electrocardiographic Diagnosis of Left Bundle Branch Block

The specificity of the ECG criteria for LBBB has been under scrutiny for well over 50 years. The correlation between the nature and degree of intraventricular delay occurring in complete LBBB and its ECG manifestations has become more relevant in the era of CRT. More than a third of symptomatic patients, fulfilling LBBB electrocardiographic criteria, do not clinically improve after receiving a CRT device.

Several cardiac pathologic conditions can induce ECG changes suggestive of LBBB mostly by inducing notching of the R wave or increasing the total duration of the QRS. In most of these cases, LV activation is prolonged, but the propagation sequence is not changed. "Pseudo" LBBB has been observed following antiarrhythmic drugs, electrolytes abnormalities, ventricular hypertrophy, or dilatation, or with a localized propagation block from scars or infiltrative disease.

The most important diagnostic criteria defining true LBBB are the presence of a reversal of septal activation with delayed spread of activation from the RV to the LV free wall. These abnormalities are at the core of the ECG diagnostic criteria proposed by the World Health Organization and most widely accepted. Unfortunately, a substantial discrepancy exists between the ECG features of LBBB and the degree of real electrical impairment so that even strict adherence to these criteria does not completely eliminate the limited specificity of ECG diagnosis of LBBB.

Observation of serial ECGs is very useful in differentiating true LBBB from conditions mimicking this abnormality.

Progressive widening of QRS can be documented in LVH or cardiomyopathies, whereas in

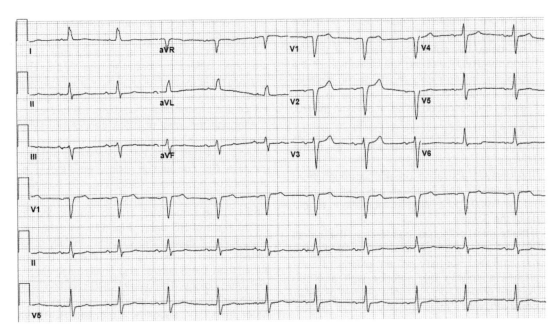

Fig. 9. Electrocardiographic features of LVH: Sinus rhythm in a patient with echocardiographic evidence of mild LVH in an otherwise normal heart. Note the absence of q in V1/V2 and r in V5/V6, suggesting block of the left septal branch.

true LBBB electrocardiographic changes consistent with abnormal and delayed conduction will occur suddenly.

No prospective studies evaluating the accuracy and clinical usefulness of these observations are as yet available, making strict adherence to the previously referred criteria (see **Box 1**) the best tool in the diagnosis and management of LBBB.

RIGHT BUNDLE BRANCH BLOCK
Complete and Incomplete

The RB branches take off from the common His at the anterior-inferior margin of the membranous septum toward the right side of the interventricular (IV) septum, traveling through a layer of collagen a millimeter or less in thickness (see **Fig. 1**). The thin and narrow RB remains superficial and mostly an unbranched structure throughout the IV septum. From the septum, most of the bundle enters the moderator band, which terminates at the foot of the anterior papillary muscle. From here, the RB divides into septal, free wall, and outflow fascicles spreading over the entire right ventricular myocardium.

The characteristics of the RB mostly determine the anatomic location of the block. Predivisional His bundle lesions of the RB are very rare given its thin structure, absence of proximal branches, and lack of collagen septation. Numerous studies, on the other hand, have shown that fibrosis at the

distal branching portion of the bundle of His, where the RB originates, is the most common pathologic condition associated with RBBB. More uncommonly, extensive anterior MI can affect the RB upper third, where this penetrates deeply into the interventricular septum. In other cases, the infarct can destroy the RB ramifications distal to the moderator band. A third type of lesion, observed exclusively following surgical procedures for congenital heart disease,[12] is due to complete transection of the moderator band. Numerous human and animal mapping studies have described the specific alterations of RV depolarization following each of these 3 distinct levels of block: proximal, moderator band, and peripheral ramifications.

- Proximal RBBB, the most common form, results in a total delay of RV activation of the septum, the apex, and the outflow tract. These structures now activate transeptally from the LV, where impulse propagation remains normal. Activation begins in the apical septum approximately 30 milliseconds later than surface QRS onset, and it proceeds inferosuperiorly, ending at the right ventricular outflow tract (RVOT).
- Distal RBBB due to transection of the moderator band results in delayed activation of the RV free wall and RVOT, whereas activation of the septum remains normal.

- A more peripheral pathologic condition affecting the distal ramifications of the RB will delay the anterobasal region of the RV and the RVOT, leaving the activation of the septum, inferior, and much of the anterior wall unchanged. The ECG reflects to some extent the described levels of block in the RB.

The more proximal the RB lesion, the wider the QRS and more marked the alteration in the terminal forces.

The delayed activation breaking through from the LV at the RV apical septum progresses up toward the RVOT, generating an increase in amplitude of the S wave.

If the terminal branches are affected, the overall QRS duration is within normal limits, as most of the RV is activated normally. When lesions of subbranches supplying the anterior wall and the ROVT are present, only a slight degree of delay is observed, with a minor superior shift of the terminal forces.

Despite the detailed observations of the effects of lesions on each RB subdivision, the correlation between ECG findings and level of RBBB is far less precise than the same correlation in LB hemiblocks.

This poor correlation is certainly due to the anatomic difference between the 2 branches. There is no large and recognizable branch system supplying a specific area of the right ventricle as is the case for anterior and posterior LB fascicles.

Although the level of block cannot be reliably predicted by ECG analysis, subtle electrocardiographic changes have been correlated with progressive RB conduction delay, introducing the concept of *incomplete RBBB* (**Fig. 10**). A diminution of S wave in V2, followed by slurring of the upstroke in the same lead, are considered the first subtle signs of RB delay (**Fig. 11**). As delay progresses, an r′ appears in V1 or V2, initially of low voltage, then increasing with time to become larger than the S wave, and finally assuming an rSR′ morphology. The overall QRS duration is not increased above 0.11 seconds with the R′ not wider than 0.04 seconds. Complete RBBB will induce a more marked widening of the QRS and in particular of the R′ and a superior shift of terminal vectors (**Fig. 12**).

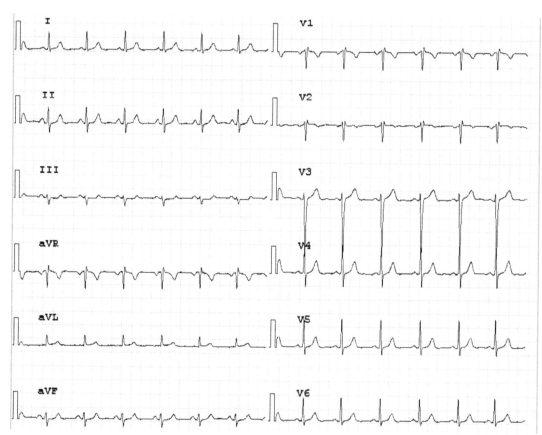

Fig. 10. Incomplete RBBB. Rhythm is sinus with QRS showing a clear r′ in V1/V2. This ECG is consistent with initial stage of RB disease.

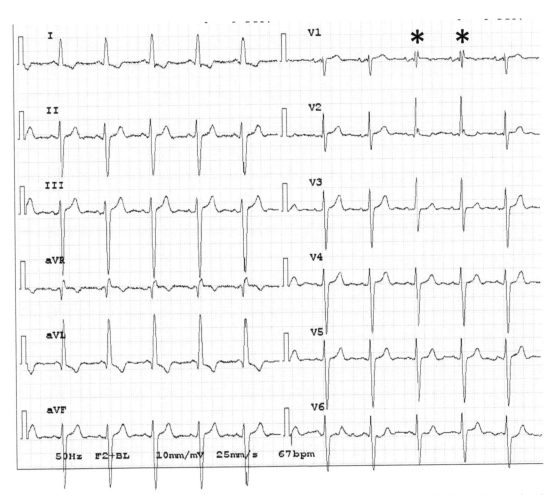

Fig. 11. LAFB and intermittent IRBBB. Dominant rhythm is sinus; note in beat 8 and 9 (*asterisks*) evidence of early RB delay with the appearance of r′ in V1/V2 and a right anterior axis shift evidenced by an increased R voltage in V2/V3. The shift in axis suggests that the delay in the RB is more marked than previous figure, probably because of more extensive HPS disease in keeping also with the presence of LAFB.

The mechanism of these progressive ECG findings is attributed[13] to an initial delay of RV paraseptal activation, normally inscribing the initial r in V1-V2. Being delayed, this vector will now occur synchronously with the much larger LV free wall activation, and given its opposite direction, it will diminish the overall magnitude of the LV vector. The decrease in amplitude is reflected by a small decrease in the voltage of S wave in the same leads. With more severe interruption of conduction, the RV free wall will end its depolarization after the completion of LV free wall activation, therefore inscribing a late positive vector r′ in the first 2 chest leads. As delay increases, this late vector becomes more prominent and acquires larger voltage. When the RB is completely blocked, the R′ in V1 will be notched and wider than 0.04 seconds, reflecting an increase in muscle to muscle conduction. At the same time, the delayed activation of the RVOT will generate a late vector directed upright and responsible for the inscription of the terminal S waves in V5-V6.

Based on these observations, a particular ECG pattern characterized by QRS prolongation to 0.11 seconds with a terminal r′ in V1 and S wave in V5 or V6 has been associated with a delay in the RB conduction and named "incomplete RBBB."

This pattern is not a fully accepted ECG entity. An alternative point of view suggests that any delay in activation of the RV free wall occurring after completion of LV depolarization can cause an incomplete right bundle branch block (IRBBB) pattern. Causes of this pattern could include not only RB electrical delay but also RV hypertrophy with increased duration of RV activation time because of increased wall thickness.

Animal studies, and more cogently, a large electrocardiographic-pathologic correlation[14] study

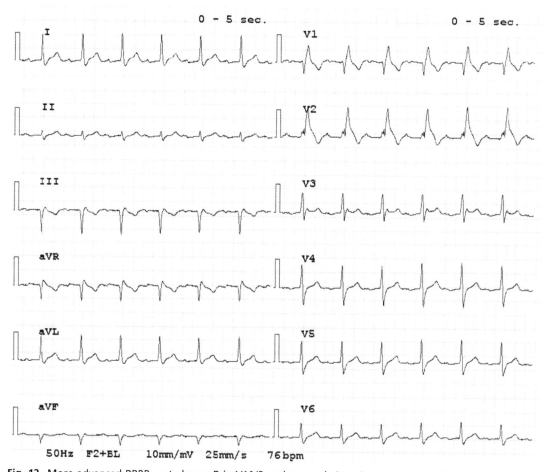

Fig. 12. More advanced RBBB: note larger R in V1/V2 and more obvious S waves in the left precordial leads.

showed, in fact, that electrocardiographic evidence of IRBBB was associated with a histologically normal RB and evidence of RV hypertrophy.

Along the same logic, a short duration of LV depolarization can leave the terminal vectors of RV depolarization unopposed. This reasoning would therefore explain the juvenile, physiologic pattern of IRBBB observed in infancy whereby a changing ratio of right to left ventricular wall thickness causes a shorter duration of LV activation when compared with RV.

Isolated RBBB is considered a benign lesion because it is associated with a modest increased risk of all-cause mortality in the general population. This risk increases in the presence of preexisting MI or congestive heart failure, but the predictive value of RBBB is unclear in the presence of advanced cardiovascular disease.

COMBINED BLOCKS
Bifascicular and Trifascicular Blocks

Almost 100 years ago, a group of researchers working on animals observed, following surgical interruption of RB and anterior LB fibers, changes in the ECG of RBBB and marked S wave in lead III.

The observation of bifascicular block was extended to humans with studies correlating anatomopathologic findings and similar ECG patterns.

RBBB with LAFB is by far the most common combination and is observed in clinical practice with a prevalence of almost 1%, with LAFB usually preceding RBBB. On the contrary, block or delay of the left posterior fascicular block (LPFB) in association with RBBB is rare possibly because of the larger size of this fascicle.

The anatomopathologic lesions observed in RBBB and LAH usually involve the penetrating portion of His at the level of the central fibrous body. The lesions can occur either alone or in combination with more distal disease in the proximal RB, or in the anterior LB branch at the upper end of the interventricular septum. In the small number of pathologic studies reporting on the causes of bi-fascicular block, degenerative disease was slightly more common than septal MIs. Although the first cause tended to be centrally located, MI tended to induce extensive destruction of the RB and LAF peripheral ramifications.

The correlation between vector changes associated with bifascicular block and the resultant ECG features has been studied in detail (see **Fig. 6**; **Fig. 13**).

In "pure" RBBB, the first 60 to 80 milliseconds of the QRS are normal, because during this period the intact LB depolarizes the septum and part of the LV free wall. If a left hemiblock is associated with RBBB, septal activation will be carried out by unopposed depolarization of the unblocked fascicle. The ECG findings will be simply the association of the features described singularly for each component of the bifascicular block (see **Box 1**).

The risk of progression from bifascicular to complete heart block and the identification of high-risk individuals has been the subject of multiple studies with conflicting results. The study with the longest follow-up of patients with "high-risk bundle branch block"[15] observed that patients with bifascicular conduction disease are at increased risk of death and sudden death when compared with patients with normal conduction. Careful evaluation of the mode of death in these subjects suggests that progression to complete heart block occurs at a rate of approximately 1.2% per year. These studies also suggest a limited role of the ECG in the identification of patients with chronic bifascicular or trifascicular block at high risk of death due to heart block.

This is because of the limited correlation of 12-lead ECG abnormalities and severity of conduction system disease as demonstrated, in some cases, by a normal ECG despite extensive disease in 2 or 3 fascicles. Furthermore, the ECG cannot reliably distinguish between bundle or fascicular delay and complete conduction block. A slowing of conduction through a functionally altered bundle branch may not have the same clinical implications of a complete block, but it will produce the same electrocardiographic pattern. Our diagnosis of complete LBBB, for example, is based on specific ECG features and implies a complete anatomic disruption of continuity in the LB. In reality, any slowing of conduction, in bundles or fascicles, which allows unopposed propagation of a wavefront from the other intact branch, will generate the same vectors regardless of the nature of conduction delay. Transseptal activation takes place in 40 to 60 milliseconds; hence, any conduction delay, complete or incomplete, longer than this interval will result in the same ECG morphology of "complete bundle branch block."

The same mechanism is behind the large number of reports of alternating RB and LBBB (**Fig. 14**) or anterior and posterior fascicular block (**Fig. 15**).

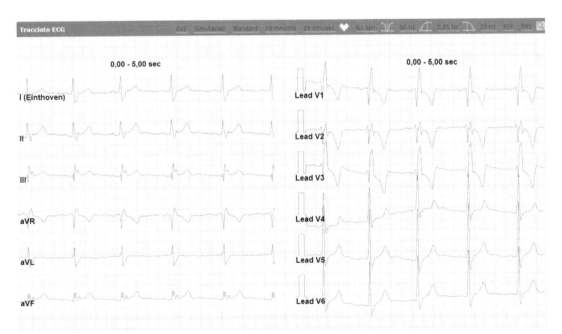

Fig. 13. Complete RBBB: The patient underwent surgery for congenital cardiomyopathy. Note the marked delay of RV activation with late R′ in V1/V2 and S waves in left precordial leads. As expected in RBBB, the initial 80 milliseconds of depolarization are normal. These changes are consistent with severe proximal RB lesion possibly because of surgical moderator band resection.

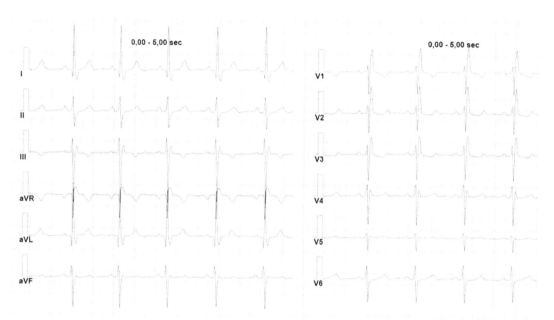

Fig. 14. RBBB and LAFB. Note the rapid deflection of the QRS in the first 60 milliseconds. The features of both blocks are clearly present.

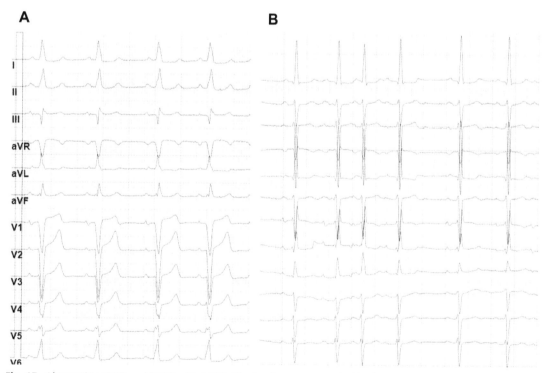

Fig. 15. Alternating LBBB and RBBB with LAFB. The tracings are recorded in the same patient a few hours apart. Tracing A shows LBBB, whereas tracing B illustrates an RBBB with LAFB. These findings demonstrate that the ECG findings of BBB may, at times, represent a delay of HPS conduction of unclear severity. Several factors may affect the degree of delay, including heart rate. In this case, the sinus rate of tracing A is faster than the one in B, but a shift in BBB due to rate is unlikely in view of the APC in B conducted with unchanged ECG morphology. In any case, this tracing is consistent with very advanced HPS disease.

The explanation for these findings is that there is no complete block but instead a conduction delay of variable degree affecting more than a single branch/fascicle. Because slowing of conduction is dynamic and not fixed, several factors can influence the relative branch delay. These changing conditions can shift the majority of conduction from one branch to the other producing the electrocardiographic appearance of alternating blocks.

As conduction delay and complete block carry different prognostic implications, the inability of distinguishing between the 2 limits the ECG value in predicting the progression of conduction disease.

Despite the limited number of studies following a large number of patients with RBBB and LAFB, there is a general agreement on the overall low mortality, morbidity, and progression to CHB associated with this condition.

As previously mentioned, LPH is almost invariably associated with RBBB, and this combination indicates a more extensive conduction system involvement.

In fact, when this combination is present, it is very likely that the anterior division of the LBB is also involved, as shown in a study whereby 30% of the patients with LPH and RBBB had clinical evidence of trifascicular disease. In this group, 60% of them developed CHB; in all cases, this was preceded by PR prolongation and frequently by Adams-Stokes seizures, suggesting further deterioration of conduction in the remaining LAF. RBBB with LPH are more likely to be associated with degenerative myocardial disease than coronary artery disease, the opposite of what is observed in RBBB with LAH.

Deterioration of conduction most often begins with LAFB, progresses to bifascicular block, and in some cases, to complete heart block.

An intermediate stage before this final step is trifascicular block (**Fig. 16**). Trifascicular block is a stage characterized by a variable association of block and delay affecting all 3 components of the conduction system.

The standard 12-lead ECG is unfortunately unable to predict precisely the extent or the progression

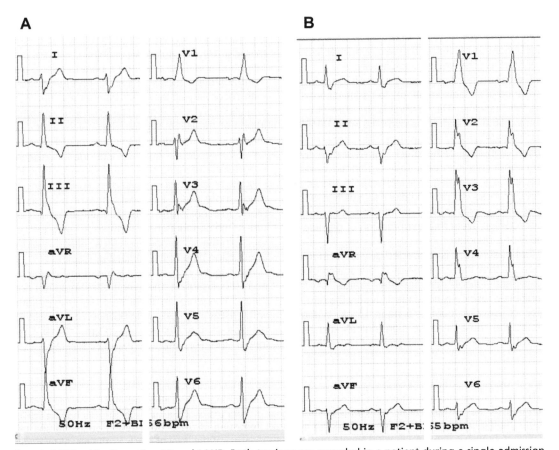

Fig. 16. RBBB with alternating LP and LAHB. Both tracings are recorded in a patient during a single admission. Sinus rhythm with RBBB accompanied by LPFB (tracing A) and LAFB (tracing B). The observations made in **Fig. 15** apply to this case.

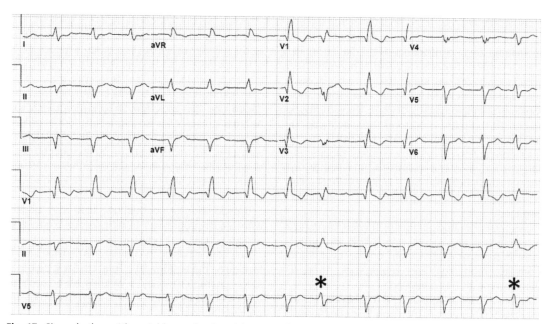

Fig. 17. Sinus rhythm with variable conduction delays in trifascicular block (RBBB and LAFB). Note slight QRS narrowing in beat 1 and shortening of PR decreased R′ voltage and right axis shift in beat 8 and 13 (*asterisks*). These findings suggest an incomplete trifascicular block with occasional improvement of conduction. The axis change does not represent a shift from LAFB to LPFB but most likely is just a variation of the left fascicular recruitment.

from bifascicular to trifascicular block unless transient evidence of alternating main bundle or fascicular block is observed serendipitously.

The PR is the other parameter often used, in the presence of bifascicular block, to define disease in the third fascicle. This interval is the sum of conduction time through the atrium, the Atrio-Ventricular Node (AVN) and HP system. The latter is only a small component of the total PR time, and HP system conduction can be greatly prolonged without substantially affecting this interval. On the other hand, marked PR prolongation is usually associated with a delay in AVN conduction, a markedly more benign event than progression of disease in the R or L bundle.

This observation is supported by several studies showing that the PR interval in bifascular block does not reliably predict the status of the unblocked fascicule, nor does it identify the patient likely to develop complete heart block. Without doubt, the most ominous sign indicating a high likelihood of progression to complete AV block is the presence of spontaneous alternating BBB (see **Fig. 14**), particularly if associated with PR prolongation and if observed on a beat to beat basis.

Intracardiac studies assessing conduction time with recording of the H-V[a] interval are far more specific than ECG in quantifying conduction alterations of the HPS. In general, patients with ECG evidence of isolated fascicular or BBB have normal conduction time. As conduction disease progresses affecting other components of the HP system, evidence of increased HV timing becomes much more likely. ECG evidence of bifascicular block does not inform us of the true extent and nature of the conduction impairment, whereas HV interval, in the same condition, is a reflection of the conduction time of the remaining fascicle.

As long as one of the LB fascicles maintains normal conduction, the overall HV should not prolong.[16] Therefore, an abnormal HV time in patients with RBBB and LAD is indicative of trifascicular disease in the His-Purkinje (**Figs. 17–19**). The longer the HV interval, the more likely is the

---

[a]The HV interval (normal 30–55 milliseconds), recorded positioning a recording catheter across the upper portion of the tricuspid valve, represents the sum total of conduction time through the His bundle (BH), both bundle branches, and peripheral Purkinje network. Recording of the depolarization of the RB and LB common branch is feasible, allowing a more precise quantification of the level of block. With present technologies, it is not possible to record the potential from the anterior and posterior division of the LB. RB and LB recordings are simultaneous, but endocardial activation of the LV side of the septum is approximately 10 milliseconds earlier than the right side.

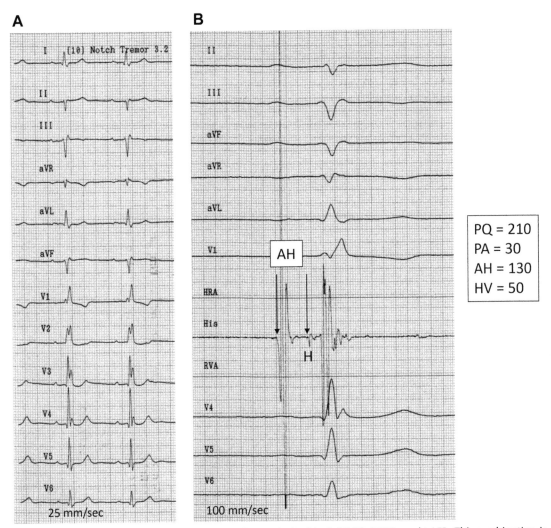

A

I   [10] Notch Tremor 3.2
II
III
aVR
aVL
aVF
V1
V2
V3
V4
V5
V6
25 mm/sec

B

II
III
aVF
aVR
aVL
V1   AH
HRA
His   H
RVA
V4
V5
V6
100 mm/sec

PQ = 210
PA = 30
AH = 130
HV = 50

Fig. 18. Tracing A: Sinus rhythm, first-degree atrioventricular block (AVB), RBBB, and LAFB. This combination is often defined as trifascicular block and considered to represent more advanced HPS disease. The severity of the conduction defect cannot be assessed from this surface ECG. Tracing B: The first 7 and the last 3 represent ECG tracings as marked. The ninth tracing represents intracardiac recordings of obtained in the region of the AV junction. Clearly defined are the atrial (A) electrogram followed by study the recording of the common bundle of His (H) and ventricular activation (V). The tracing shows that the delay causing the PR prolongation is due to a slowing within the AVN (prolonged AH).

progression to CHB, to the point that a value of 100 ms is considered, by some authorities, an indication for Permanent Pace Maker (PPM) placement even in asymptomatic patients.

Just recording an abnormal HV time does not precisely localize the site of delay in the HPS, which includes the main stem LB, the posterior division of the LB, or the peripheral ramification of the Purkinje system. Furthermore, occasionally, a normal HV interval can be observed in patients with clinically and pathologically significant chronic conduction disease, manifest at times with intermittent AV block and syncope.

On the contrary, a prolonged HV interval can be seen in patients with normal ECG if the delay occurs in the common bundle, so-called intra-His block, before the trifurcation.

WHEN ELECTROCARDIOGRAPHY IS NOT ENOUGH
Functional Bundle Branch Block, Normalization of Bundle Branch Block

Block or delay of conduction resulting in ECG manifestations of BB aberrant conduction can be functional or fixed. As the authors have previously described, multiple pathologic conditions can cause persistent propagation delays or blocks in different parts of the conduction system.

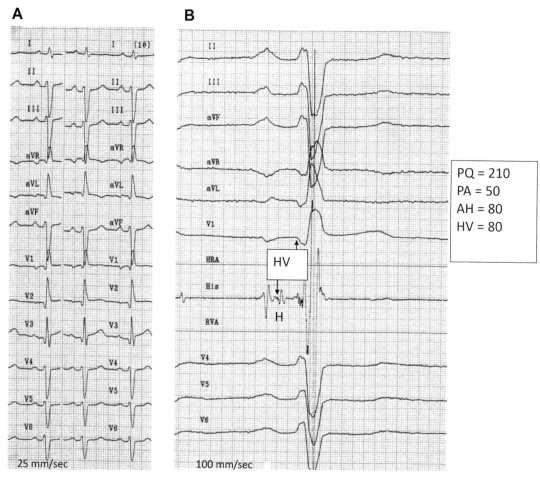

Fig. 19. Tracing A: Sinus rhythm, first-degree AVB, RBBB, and LAFB. Tracing B: The intracardiac study in this case shows that the delay causing the PR prolongation is localized between the recording of H and the V localizing, demonstrating a slowing of HPS conduction (prolonged HV).

In functional block, conduction is temporarily interrupted because of inadequate recovery of one or more subdivision of the HPS. Premature stimulation of fibers not fully recovered (phase 3 block) explains the aberrancy, which accompanies a premature beat. Inadequate recovery of resting potential is also observed during stimulation at a rate that prevents full recovery of excitability (rate-related block).

Less common mechanisms of functional block include bradycardia-dependent block (phase 4 block), usually manifested as LBBB, where loss of resting membrane potential renders the cells less excitable when depolarized by normal sinus beat or by serendipitous retrograde penetration of a premature beat. Although rate-related aberrancy and phase 4 are pathologic phenomena, phase 3 aberrancy is a physiologic behavior.

A complete analysis of a functional conduction abnormality requires invasive evaluation of the conduction system. During an electrophysiology study, it is possible to assess the responses to anterograde and retrograde prematurity, the effect of rate on action potential duration and the differences in functional refractoriness between divisions and subdivisions of the HPS. These studies have allowed the demonstration of the dynamic nature of the block and the shifting of its anatomic site during aberration.

Another phenomenon, which often requires intracardiac evaluation to elucidate its mechanism, is the normalization of a preexisting BBB by a premature ventricular beat. There are several possible explanations for this event[13]:

1. The premature beat originates from the opposite ventricle and, occurring in late diastole, fuses with the antegrade impulse conducted with BBB to generate a normal, more often near normal, beat.

2 A premature supraventricular beat reaches the bifurcation of the common bundle at the time

corresponding with the end of the T wave of the preceding conducted beat, coinciding with the supernormal phase of the blocked bundle. During this small time window during repolarization, an impulse reaching the blocked bundle will conduct better than expected, without delay and therefore normal QRS.

3. A premature beat, supraventricular or fascicular with retrograde conduction, engages the healthy bundle conducting with delay, because of prematurity. If this delay is similar to the pre-existing delay of the affected bundle, the normal sequence of depolarization is restored with normalization of the ECG. This is often, but not always, accompanied by a prolongation of the PR if there is a marked slowing of the HPS conduction time.

Although the first mechanism discussed can be surmised by skillful analysis of the ECG or rhythm strips to identify parasystolic or repetitive premature ventricular contractions, the other 2 require intracardiac recordings and detailed analysis of the functional properties of each bundle.

REFERENCES

1. Durrer D, van Dam RT, Freud GE, et al. Total excitation of the isolated human heart. Circulation 1970;41:899.

2. Strauss DG, Selvester RH. The QRS complex—a biomarker that "images" the heart: QRS scores to quantify myocardial scar in the presence of normal and abnormal ventricular conduction. J Electrocardiol 2009;42:85–96.

3. Padanilam BJ, Morris KE, Olson JA, et al. The surface electrocardiogram predicts risk of heart block during right heart catheterization in patients with preexisting left bundle branch block: implications for the definition of complete left bundle branch block. J Cardiovasc Electrophysiol 2010;21:781–5.

4. Vassallo JA, Cassidy DM, Miller JM, et al. Left ventricular endocardial activation during right ventricular pacing: effect of underlying heart disease. J Am Coll Cardiol 1986;7:1228.

5. Bacharova L, Szathmary V, Mateasik A. Electrocardiographic patterns of left bundle-branch block caused by intraventricular conduction impairment in working myocardium: a model study. J Electrocardiol 2011;44:768.

6. Rowlands DJ. Left and right bundle-branch block, left anterior and left posterior hemiblock. Eur Heart J 1984;5(suppl A):99–105.

7. Willems JL, Robles de Medina EO, Bernard R, et al. Criteria for intraventricular conduction disturbances and pre-excitation. World Health Organizational/International Society and Federation for Cardiology Task Force Ad Hoc. J Am Coll Cardiol 1985;5:1261.

8. Schamroth L, Bradlow BA. Incomplete left bundle branch block. Br Heart J 1964;26:285–8.

9. Rosenbaum M, Elizari MV, Lazzari JO. The hemiblocks. Oldsmar, Florida: Tampa tracings; 1970.

10. Bayes de Luna A, Riera AP, Baranchuk A, et al. Electrocardiographic manifestation of the middle fibers/septal fascicle block: a consensus report. J Electrocardiol 2012;45:454.

11. MacAlpin RN. In search of left septal fascicular block. Am Heart J 2002;144:948.

12. Horowitz LN, Edmunds LH, Alexander IA, et al. Postoperative right bundle branch block: identification of three levels of block. Circulation 1980;62:319.

13. Schamroth L, Meyburgh DP, Shamroth CL. The early signs of right bundle branch block. Chest 1985;86:180.

14. McAnulty JH, Rahimtcola SH, Murphy E, et al. Natural history of "high-risk" bundle branch block. N Engl J Med 1982;307:137.

15. Narula OS, Javier RP, Samet P, et al. Significance of His and left bundle recordings from the left heart in man. Circulation 1970;42:385.

16. Akhtar M, Gilbert C, Al-Nouri M, et al. Site of conduction delay during functional block in the His-Purkinje system in man. Circulation 1980;61:1239–48.

Role of Surface Electrocardiograms in Patients with Cardiac Implantable Electronic Devices

Emanuela T. Locati, MD, PhD[a],*, Giuseppe Bagliani, MD[b],
Alessio Testoni, MS[a], Maurizio Lunati, MD[a],
Luigi Padeletti, MD[c,d]

KEYWORDS

- Electrocardiogram • Cardiac pacing • Pacemaker • Implantable cardioverter-defibrillator
- Cardiac resynchronization • Pacing mode • Cardiac arrhythmias • Syncope

KEY POINTS

- Surface electrocardiograms play an essential role in establishing indications for cardiac implantable electronic devices, and in the evaluation of patients already implanted.
- Surface electrocardiograms remain the critical tool to detect device malfunction, evaluate programming and function, verify the automatic arrhythmia analysis and the delivered electric therapy, and prevent inappropriate intervention.
- For a correct interpretation of the surface electrocardiograms (both baseline 12-lead and ambulatory) it is mandatory to have information on the cardiac implantable electronic device characteristics and programming.
- Ambulatory monitoring can be useful in patients with symptoms suggestive of device malfunction when routine device interrogation does not reveal the reason for the corresponding clinical symptoms.

INTRODUCTION

Surface electrocardiograms (ECGs), both baseline 12-lead ECG and ambulatory ECG monitoring (AECGM), not only play an essential role in establishing indications for pacemaker (PM) implantation, but also for the evaluation of patients with cardiac implantable electronic devices (CIED). Current CIEDs (PMs, implantable cardiac defibrillators [ICDs], and cardiac resynchronization devices [CRTs]) have prolonged memory capabilities (often defined as Holter functions) and remote monitoring capabilities, allowing the evaluation of electrical properties and detection of arrhythmias.[1–5] Nonetheless, the availability of sophisticated self-analysis and prolonged memory capabilities cannot replace the analysis of surface ECG, which remains critical to detect device malfunction, evaluate the device programming and function, verify the arrhythmia analyses, and minimize the risk of inappropriate interventions.[6–10]

Disclosure: The authors have nothing to disclose.
[a] Electrophysiology Unit, Cardiovascular Department, Niguarda Hospital, Piazza Ospedale Maggiore, 3, Milano 20162, Italy; [b] Cardiology Department, Arrhythmia Unit, Foligno General Hospital, Via Massimo Arcamone, 06034 Foligno (PG), Italy; [c] Heart and Vessels Department, University of Florence, Largo Brambilla, 3, Florence 50134, Italy; [d] Cardiovascular Department, IRCCS, Multimedica, Via Milanese 300, 20099 Sesto San Giovanni, Italy
* Corresponding author. Cardiovascular Department, Cardiology 3, Electrophysiology, ASST GOM Niguarda, Piazza Ospedale Maggiore, 3, Milano, Milan 20162, Italy.
E-mail address: emanuelateresa.locati@ospedaleniguarda.it

Card Electrophysiol Clin 10 (2018) 233–255
https://doi.org/10.1016/j.ccep.2018.02.012
1877-9182/18/© 2018 Elsevier Inc. All rights reserved.

cardiacEP.theclinics.com

Over the years, CIEDs evolved considerably from simple life-saving PMs to highly sophisticated multichamber devices performing near-physiologic stimulation and complex arrhythmias analysis and, in the case of ICDs, delivering antitachycardia therapy. Several automatic algorithms have been developed from the "rate-responsive (R-R) function," adapting the heart rate response during physical activity through special sensors; to the "minimizing ventricular pacing" function, favoring the emergence of spontaneous beats, to the "rate-smoothing" functions, reducing the cycle length fluctuations in case of frequent supraventricular or ventricular arrhythmias and of heart rate drops, to prevent symptoms and arrhythmogenesis. The knowledge of those complex functions is crucial to evaluate the correct function of the devices and to avoid erroneous diagnosis of device malfunctions.

Finally, in the last decades, CRT devices aimed to resynchronize the left ventricular mechanical activity in heart failure patients have been developed, and according to the current guidelines, the surface ECG is the essential tool to identify patients eligible for a CRT procedure, and to verify the correct function of CRT systems.[2,8,9]

ROLE OF SURFACE ELECTROCARDIOGRAMS TO ESTABLISH INDICATIONS FOR CARDIAC IMPLANTABLE ELECTRONIC DEVICE IMPLANTATION

Surface ECG plays a crucial role in the identification of patients requiring CIED—PM, ICD, and CRT.[1,2,8] Specifically, AECGM monitoring may provide valuable information regarding the type of device to be implanted in terms of single versus dual chamber. As examples, DDD pacing with preferential algorithms to minimize ventricular pacing (MVP) may be preferred in patients with sick sinus syndrome with preserved A-V conduction. The detection of frequent, even asymptomatic, episodes of atrial arrhythmias and/or bradyarrhythmias in patients referred for an ICD implantation may suggest that a dual chamber device should be preferred, because these patients may require permanent pacing if antiarrhythmic drugs are to be administered during follow-up, or for tracking the tachyarrhythmia burden, for better discrimination of supraventricular versus ventricular tachyarrhythmias. AECGM may also be useful in CRT candidates, particularly in patients with permanent persistent atrial fibrillation, in whom the analysis of the ventricular rate response can contribute to optimize the response to biventricular pacing. In patients with poorly controlled ventricular response, A-V node ablation may be recommended at the time of or after CRT implantation, the so-called ablate-and-pace strategy.[1,2,8]

ELECTROCARDIOGRAPHIC METHODOLOGIES USED IN THE EVALUATION OF PATIENTS WITH CARDIAC STIMULATION

The main ECG modalities to evaluate the correct CIED function are the following.

a. Baseline 12-lead ECG, alone or in conjunction with the use of device programmer, remains the starting point of every electrophysiologic investigation in patients with CIEDs, because it can provide critical and immediate information on the basic functions of pacing and sensing and on the type of pacing mode.[1–4]

b. AECGM, or Holter monitoring, lasting from 24 hours to several days, and recently up to 3 to 4 weeks, can be useful to correlate symptoms suggestive of arrhythmias or device malfunctioning, or to optimize the device programming.[6,7,9] AECGM is no longer used as a routine test after CIED implantation, owing to the availability of sophisticated autoanalysis algorithms. Myopotential inhibition, crosstalk, and PM-mediated tachycardia (PMT), that is, the PM disfunctions more frequently detected by AECGM, are now less frequently encountered, and may be detected and notified by remote monitoring.[5,10] AECGM can also contribute to the evaluation of the correct performance of advanced systems, such as sequential A-V pacing systems with special rate-adaptive pacing algorithms, or ventricular resynchronization systems with biventricular stimulation.[6–10]

c. ECG monitoring during exercise stress testing is rarely used nowadays in the current evaluation of patients with cardiac stimulation, and it is mainly used to verify the correct programming of rate adaptive algorithms.

d. Remote CIED control is now the technique of choice to monitor the patients with CIEDs, allowing the timely detection of changes in the pacing and sensing functions, the identification of electrocatheter malfunctions, the evaluation of the correct diagnosis and therapies of supraventricular and ventricular arrhythmias, and the performance of CRT functions.[5,8,10]

BASIC PRINCIPLES OF INTERPRETATION OF SURFACE ELECTROCARDIOGRAMS IN PATIENTS WITH A CARDIAC IMPLANTABLE ELECTRONIC DEVICE

Most current CIEDs include the ability to sense and/or stimulate both the atrial and ventricular chambers. When the device does not detect a heartbeat within a predefined interval, it

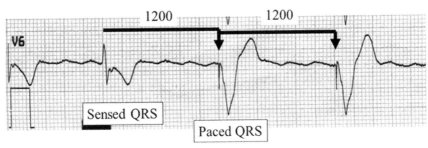

Fig. 1. Sensing and pacing functions in a single chamber pacemaker (VVI). The spontaneous ventricular event is sensed by the pacemaker, and a stimulus is triggered after a programmed time interval (1200 milliseconds in this case), correspondent to a low rate of 50 bpm.

stimulates the atrium or the ventricle by an electric impulse at the programmed duration and voltage. The sensing and pacing activity is continuously carried on a beat-to-beat basis. A simple classification code including 5 positions allows a quick identification of the device type and mode of sensing and pacing operations.[11] The first 3 code positions (I, II, and III) are related to the antibradycardia functions, the fourth position (IV) concerns the rate modulation, and the fifth code position (V) identifies multisite pacing parameters.

Noteworthy, for a correct interpretation of the surface ECG (both baseline 12-lead ECG and AECGM) it is mandatory to have information on the CIED characteristics and programming.

Evaluation of the Sensing Function

The sensing function represents the CIED ability to detect the spontaneous activity of a cardiac chamber, either atrial or ventricular (**Fig. 1**) The sensing threshold is widely programmable to allow the exclusion of noise signals, which can be external signals (eg, external electrical sources or muscular contractions), or intracardiac signals from a different chamber (the so called far-field signals), that may cause malfunctions or may be misinterpreted as arrhythmias. The oversensing of external or intracardiac signals misinterpreted as spontaneous normal cardiac activity may induce pathologic pauses provoked by an abnormal retention of a due pacing stimulus.

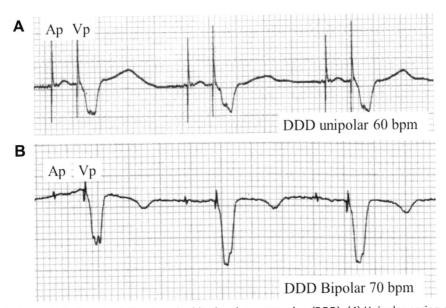

Fig. 2. Unipolar and bipolar stimulation in a double-chamber pacemaker (DDD). (*A*) Unipolar pacing configuration: both atrial and ventricular spikes are evident. (*B*) Bipolar pacing configuration: atrial and ventricular spikes have lower amplitude when compared with the unipolar configuration. Ap, atrial stimulation; Vp, ventricular stimulation.

Evaluation of the Pacing Function

The pacing function represents the CIED ability to deliver electrical pulses activating a given cardiac chamber. On surface ECG, artificial stimulation (often defined as spike) has a needlelike or quadric wave appearance, usually distinguishable from the spontaneous electrical activity.

Pacing artifact in unipolar or bipolar stimulation configuration

The spike amplitude primarily depends on the stimulation configuration (**Fig. 2**). In the presence of a unipolar configuration, the stimulus is provided between the electric pole at the apex of the lead and the metal generator can, which can be visible as a relatively high-voltage deflection on the surface ECG. Conversely, in presence of a bipolar configuration, the stimulus is delivered between the 2 electric poles, both placed at the tip of the lead, resulting in a substantially lower voltage deflection on surface ECG. Sometimes, the bipolar spike amplitude on surface ECG is so low to require a change to unipolar configuration for better visualization.

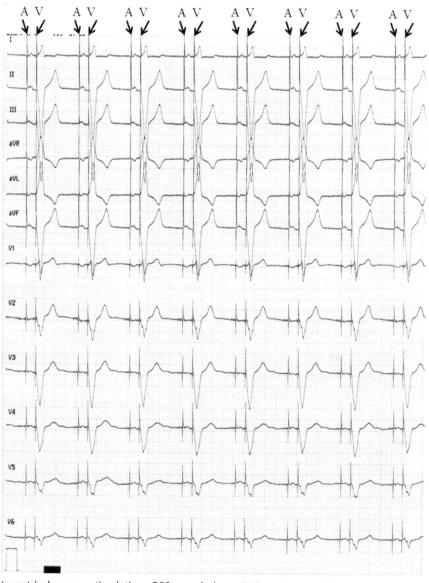

Fig. 3. Right ventricular apex stimulation: QRS morphology. DDD pacing can be recognized after the regular sequence of stimulation in the atrium (A) and in the ventricle (V). The impulse originates from the apex of the right ventricle and spreads to the ventricular myocardium with a left ventricular conduction delay; therefore, the QRS morphology is a left-type bundle branch block. The axis in the frontal plane is markedly deviated to the left.

Atrial and ventricular depolarization waveforms after artificial pacing

The lead for atrial pacing is commonly placed into the right appendage; thus, the atrial depolarization after the atrial pacing is often hardly visible on the surface ECG. Alternative sites for the atrial pacing lead are possible (eg, the interatrial septum), but they are less used. The ventricular depolarization induced by ventricular pacing is usually well-evident on the ECG and its morphology depends on the site of stimulation. Commonly, the right ventricular lead is placed in the apex of the right ventricle. In this case, the ventriculogram is characterized by a left intraventricular conduction delay morphology with an axis directed from the bottom to the top and toward left (ie, marked left axis deviation; **Fig. 3**).

The concepts of fusion and pseudofusion

The fusion phenomenon results from the competition between the spontaneous and artificial induced activation of the ventricles, giving rise an intermediate QRS morphology on ECG surface (**Fig. 4**). In the presence of a very delayed electric impulse, unable to depolarize the perilead portion of the myocardium and consequentially any portions of the cardiac chamber, a pseudofusion phenomenon is observed. In this case, despite the ventricular stimulation, the depolarization morphology is similar to the spontaneous QRS (**Fig. 5**). The fusion and pseudofusion morphologies should be correctly recognized, to avoid misinterpretation as abnormal PM function.

The hysteresis function

To avoid a competition between spontaneous and paced rhythms, the spontaneous rhythm can be favored, activating the so-called hysteresis function, by which a pacing rate inferior to the programmed lower rate is allowed (**Fig. 6**). The hysteresis is the difference between the programmed lower rate and the effective heart rate leading to pacing activation. The hysteresis can be modulated from 10 up to or 30 bpm (generally 10 bpm). This function can be applied both to single and dual chambers devices.

Response to the application of a magnet

The simple analysis of the ECG changes induced by placing a magnet on the device allows the immediate diagnosis of the mode of operation of any CIED. Under the magnet effect, the system loses the sensing function and commutates to the asynchronous pacing mode (A00, V00, D00) at the maximum amplitude of the stimulus. The ECG analysis allows to identify whether is a single or dual chambers stimulation (**Fig. 7**). The pacing heart rate induced by the magnet application is called the magnetic frequency and it is a marker of the battery charge level. A decreased magnetic frequency can be suggestive of the need of device replacement. The asynchronous mode of pacing mediated by an external magnet can be used also to avoid an inappropriate PM inhibition during surgeries requiring the use of electrosurgical devices. The asynchronous stimulation induced by a magnet can generate dangerous ventricular arrhythmias; therefore, its use requires appropriate precautions, and continuous ECG monitoring is recommended during magnet inhibition.

Evaluation of the Programming Mode

The basic ventricular on-demand pacing mode is defined as VVI (or in case of rate responsive adjustment, VVIR), which is used when no synchronization with the atrial beat is required, such as in patients with permanent atrial fibrillation. The equivalent atrial pacing mode is AAI(R), which can be used when the atrioventricular conduction is

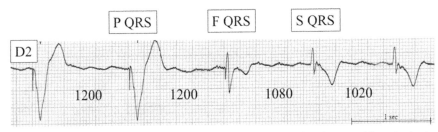

Fig. 4. Paced, fused, and spontaneous QRS. The basic rhythm is atrial fibrillation with a single-chamber pacemaker (VVI) set to an LRI of 50 bpm (ie, cycle length of 1200 milliseconds). The first 2 ventricular complexes are paced (P QRS), as shown by the presence of spikes, followed by depolarization complexes with a 180-ms duration and monophasic and negative morphology in the inferior lead. The last 2 narrow QRS are spontaneous, because no spike can be detected. The third QRS has a fusion morphology between the paced and spontaneous, because its duration is only slightly increased (100 milliseconds). The fusion is also evident at the ventricular repolarization; the T wave is positive in the stimulated beats, whereas it is negative when the QRS is spontaneous, and it is much less negative in case of fusion QRS beats.

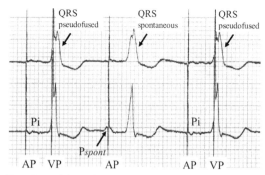

Fig. 5. Atrial and ventricular "pseudofusion." The tracing includes 3 cardiac cycles in the presence of a dual-chamber pacemaker (DDD; leads D1 and D2). *Atrial pacing:* The pacemaker delivers atrial stimulation (AP) in all 3 cardiac cycles, but only in the first and third cycles the atrial depolarizations are induced (P_i); in the second cardiac cycle, the spontaneous atrial activity (P_{spont}) and the atrial spike constitute an atrial pseudofusion. *Ventricular pacing:* The pacemaker delivers a stimulation to the ventricle (VP) only at the first and third cardiac cycles without change of the QRS morphology (ventricular pseudofusion).

preserved but the sinoatrial node is impaired, as in sinus node disease or sick sinus syndrome. When the atrioventricular conduction is also impaired, as in the A-V block (AVB), the PM is required to sense the atrial beat, and to trigger a ventricular beat after a normal delay (100–200 milliseconds), unless a spontaneous beat already occurred. This can be achieved by a single pacing lead with a sensing electrode in the right atrium and a sensing and pacing electrode in the right ventricle, defined as the VDD mode, or by positioning 2 catheters, in the right atrium and ventricle, both with pacing and

sensing capabilities, defined as DDD mode. Nowadays, both AAI(R) and VDD(R) mode are infrequently used, whereas DDD(R) mode is the most commonly used, because it covers all the possible pacing options, although it requires separate atrial and ventricular leads, and careful programming for optimal results.

Single chamber pacing: AAI(R) and VVI(R)

In single-chamber pacing mode, only 1 cardiac chamber is paced, the right atrium in the AAI mode and the right ventricle in the VVI mode, respectively. After the detection of spontaneous activity, the device is inhibited, and the stimulus is delivered after a predetermined interval from a previous either spontaneous or induced event, according to a programmable rate interval (the lower rate interval [LRI]). The AAI mode is now rarely used, and the VVI mode is generally limited to cases with atrial fibrillation associated to low ventricular response. Very recently, new intracardiac wireless VVI pacing systems have been proposed (Micra by Medtronic [Minneapolis, MN], and Nanostim by St. Jude Medical [St. Paul, MN]), which can be used in patients with low response permanent atrial fibrillation, or in patients still in sinus rhythm with advanced AVB, but with contraindications to a traditional lead pacing system, such as very elderly patients.[12] In case of sinus rhythm with AVB, the VVI stimulation is asynchronous with respect to sinus activity, and the ventricular stimulation is triggered when the LRI is attained (**Fig. 8**).

Dual-chamber pacing: DDD(R)

The DDD pacing mode is meant to reproduce the physiologic sequence and timing occurring in a

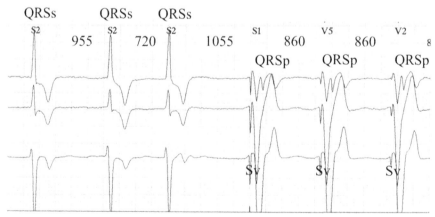

Fig. 6. "Hysteresis function" in a VVI pacemaker. The intrinsic rhythm is atrial fibrillation, the first 3 complexes are spontaneous beats (QRSs), whereas the last 3 complexes are stimulated beats (QRSp). The pacemaker triggers the first beat after an interval of 1055 milliseconds, longer than the basic stimulation rate (860 milliseconds interval), owing to the presence of the "hysteresis function," which is meant to favor the preferential onset of the spontaneous rhythm.

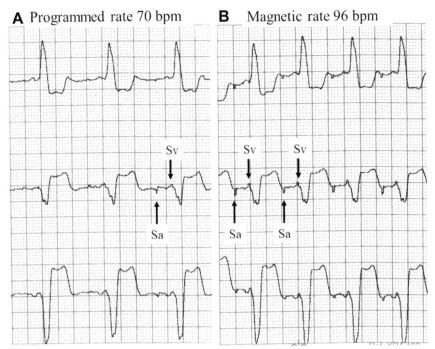

Fig. 7. The magnetic frequency of a pacemaker. (*A*) An artificial atrial and ventricular stimulation at a rate of 70 bpm is present. (*B*) The application of a magnet induces a stimulation at a rate of 96 bpm, which corresponds with the magnetic frequency.

normal heart. A dual-chamber device detects (by the sensing function) the spontaneous activity both in the atrium and in the ventricle. In case of spontaneous activity, the device is inhibited, whereas in the absence of spontaneous activity, when the heart rate falls below a predetermined frequency or LRI, the device sequentially paces the atria and ventricles according to a programmable rate interval. The A-V delay, the interval

between the atrial and ventricular activation, is widely programmable. On the surface ECG, a patient implanted with a dual chamber device with DDD/DDDR pacing mode can show at 4 different pacing patterns (**Fig. 9**):

a. When both atrial activity and conduction to the ventricles are normal, both atrial and ventricular PM channels are inhibited (AS-VS);

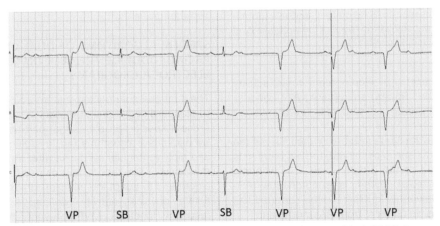

Fig. 8. Asynchronous VVI stimulation in case of sinus rhythm with complete A-V block (AVB). In case of intrinsic sinus rhythm with complete AVB, the VVI stimulation (VP) is asynchronous with respect to sinus beats (SB) with high-grade AVB, and the ventricular stimulation is triggered when the lower rate interval is attained.

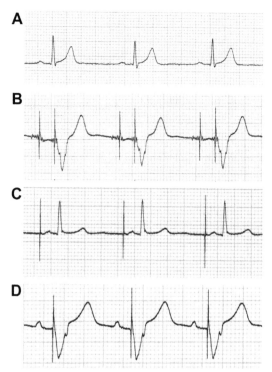

Fig. 9. Different pacing modalities and correspondent electrocardiographic (ECG) findings in dual-chamber pacemaker (DDD). (*A*) In the presence of normal atrial activity and normal atrioventricular conduction, both atrial and ventricular pacing is inhibited; therefore, no spike can be detected (AS-VS). (*B*) In the presence of incompetent sinus activity (below the lower rate interval [LRI]) and delayed atrioventricular conduction, both atria and ventricles will be stimulated, showing the classic ECG pattern consistent with 2 stimuli with the corresponding paced depolarization (atrial and ventricular, respectively), separated by the programmed AV interval (AP-VP). (*C*) The atrial rate is below the LRI and the A-V conduction is preserved and the pacemaker stimulates the atria, but not the ventricles (AP-VS). (*D*) The atrial rate is preserved but the A-V conduction is compromised, and the spontaneous atrial depolarization triggers the ventricle stimulation (VAT mode, or AS-VP).

b. When there is an incompetent sinus activity (below the LRI) and an impaired A-V conduction, both atria and ventricles are stimulated (AP-VP);

c. When the atrial rate falls below the LRI, but the A-V conduction is preserved, the right atrium is stimulated at the programmed LRI, whereas the ventricular rhythm is spontaneous (AP-VS). Noteworthy, in this case the surface ECG pattern is no different from AAI mode; and

d. When sinus atrial activation is preserved, but the A-V conduction is altered, after a spontaneous P wave, a ventricular spike appears,

followed by a stimulated ventricular depolarization (AS-VP).

Autocapture and Autothreshold Algorithms

As the patient's condition changes, the pacing thresholds may change, requiring different parameters to be monitored regularly and modified, if necessary. Therefore, algorithms to maintain adequate safety margins for pacing output and to optimize device longevity have been developed to minimize the risk of pacing failure and to reduce management costs.

The autocapture algorithms automatically manage the pacing thresholds in all the chambers that can be stimulated (right atrium, right ventricle, and left ventricle), by monitoring the pacing pulse capture to the myocardium and adjusting the output, if necessary.

Every day, generally at night (but the testing time can be programmed otherwise), the device performs a capture test in the available chambers. Usually, the pacing threshold test begins at an amplitude lower than the last measured amplitude, or at the same amplitude if it was below a predetermined value. Before starting the autocapture test, the device verifies if the patient is in stable sinus rhythm. During the test, the device checks if the myocardium capture is present and, at the first pulse not followed by an activation, it stimulates the heart with a backup pulse; then, it optimizes the threshold output within a predetermined range.

An autocapture test, when recorded on AECGM, can be easily misinterpreted as a possible severe malfunction of capture, if the analyzer is not aware that the autocapture test is a correct and essential device option. In some cases, the autocapture test can give rise to symptoms (generally palpitations), and the AECGM can contribute to exclude arrhythmias, and to correctly correlate symptoms with autocapture tests.

SPECIFIC ALGORITHMS OF DUAL-CHAMBER PACING (DDD) IDENTIFIABLE ON SURFACE ELECTROCARDIOGRAMS

The dual-chamber pacing systems, albeit superior to standard single-chamber pacing systems, may present specific problems that can be prevented by dedicated algorithms (eg, avoiding cross-talk and high ventricular response after atrial tachyarrhythmias). More recent devices also have specific algorithms to adapt the stimulation rate to the patient's physical activity (defined as the rate response function), MVP, prevent the onset of atrial fibrillation, avoid sudden heart rate drops, and test automatically the atrial and ventricular capture threshold. The specific activity of those

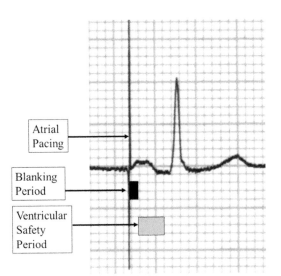

Atrial Pacing

Blanking Period

Ventricular Safety Period

Fig. 10. The blanking period and the "ventricular safety period." After an atrial stimulation, a blanking interval is generated in the ventricular channel, preventing its inhibition by the atrial depolarization. The subsequent interval is defined as "window of cross-talk detection," in which each sensed event is followed by a ventricular safety pacing or "committed pacing."

algorithms can be evaluated and correctly recognized on surface ECG, particularly during AECGM. However, if the analyzer is not aware of such programs, in some cases they may be erroneously interpreted as device malfunction.

The Blanking Period and the Ventricular Safety Pacing (or "Committed Pacing")

One of the main problems with a dual-chamber PM is the possibility that the ventricular channel can be inhibited by atrial depolarization. This is the phenomenon of cross-talk, a potentially dangerous situation that may cause asystole in patients without a spontaneous heart rhythm. The probability of cross-talk also depends on the amplitude of the atrial depolarization and it is, therefore, more likely in case of unipolar atrial stimulation. To avoid cross-talk, a blanking period is present in the ventricular channel, starting with the atrial depolarization and generally lasting 15 to 50 milliseconds. During the blanking period, the sensing of the ventricular channel is abolished (**Fig. 10**). After the blanking period, to avoid that, the ventricular electrical activity may be inappropriately inhibited, a further period was introduced, during which the PM responds to any sensed event by "ventricular safety pacing." This mode of pacing is usually defined as "committed" and is characterized by a particularly short atrioventricular interval (usually 110 milliseconds; **Fig. 11**).

Pacing Algorithms to Control High Ventricular Pacing Rates

The A-V sequential stimulation, typical of DDD pacing, is a mechanism by which the PM stimulates the ventricular chambers after a spontaneous atrial depolarization. In case of rapid atrial tachyarrhythmia, specific functions have been introduced to avoid high ventricular rates triggered by rapid atrial rates. The primary function performing such protection is the maximum tracking rate, which is based on the Wenckebach phenomenon relative to the A-V sequence, that is, the delivery of ventricular stimulus is progressively delayed until when the rate increase, and an atrial activity is no longer followed by a stimulus conducted to the ventricle (**Fig. 12**). This function is made possible by the introduction of the postventricular atrial refractory period (PVARP), that is, a period of refractoriness

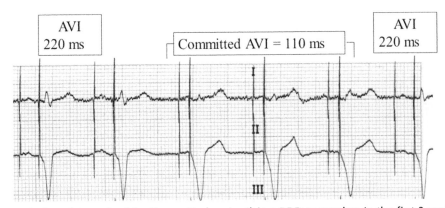

Fig. 11. "Ventricular safety pacing" (or "committed pacing") in a DDD pacemaker. In the first 2 cardiac cycles, both atrial and ventricular stimulations are present (with an A-V interval of 220 milliseconds). In the following 3 cardiac cycles, the ventricular safety pacing (or committed pacing) occurs, characterized by an A-V interval of 110 milliseconds. In the last cardiac cycle, the A-V interval returns to baseline (220 milliseconds).

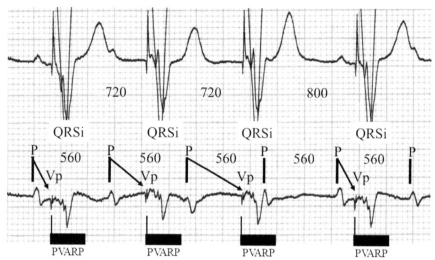

Fig. 12. Mechanism of decremental atrioventricular conduction (Wenckebach-like) in DDD mode. An atrial tachycardia (PP cycle of 560 milliseconds) is conducted to the ventricles at the "maximum tracking rate" (720 milliseconds cycle). The pacing cycles are irregular (720–720–800 milliseconds), and the longest cycle is due to the fourth P-wave not being conducted to the ventricles, as it falls within the "postventricular atrial refractory period" (PVARP). The following P wave is regularly sensed and triggered to the ventricle according to the programmed A-V interval. The A-V interval shows a Wenckebach-like trend, with a progressive prolongation up to a blocked P wave.

of the atrial channel after a ventricular depolarization. During the PVARP, the PM cannot sense any atrial activity. During an atrial tachyarrhythmia, when an atrial depolarization wave falls within the PVARP, it is not perceived and therefore it does not trigger a ventricular stimulation, and this prevents fast atrial tachyarrhythmia to be conducted with a 1:1 ratio to the ventricles (**Fig. 13**).

When an atrial tachycardia stabilizes at high frequencies, the 2:1 AVB can be reached, as such phenomenon is made possible by the occurrence of atrial depolarization alternatively falling into the PVARP. In most current dual-chamber devices, both the maximum tracking rate value and the 2:1 AVB value can be programmed separately.

Rate-Responsive Algorithms and Automatic A-V Intervalrate Responsive Shortening

In patients with chronotropic incompetence, the heart rate that cannot adapt to their needs during physical activity, and typical symptoms may be shortness of breath, fatigue, and lack of tolerance to even modest efforts (such as climbing few

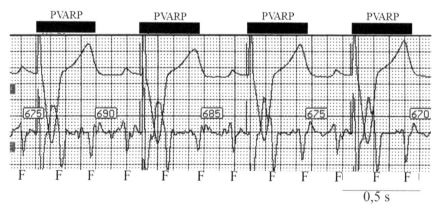

Fig. 13. Atrial flutter with 3:1 atrioventricular conduction in a patient with a DDD pacemaker. Protective mechanism against high ventricular rates. The atrial recording (esophageal lead) shows an atrial flutter (F-F cycle 230 milliseconds) conducted to the ventricles by the pacemaker with atrioventricular ratio of 3: 1. Such degree of block occurs because 2 F waves out of 3 occur within the postventricular atrial refractory period (PVARP).

steps). The R-R function allows the pacing system to increase the frequency of stimulation in response to the level of patient's physical activity.

The R-R devices are equipped with specific sensors to detect physical activity, which can be based on different parameters, including movement, muscle tremors, oxygen saturation, pH, respiratory rate, and QT interval duration. The R-R algorithm can increase the stimulation frequency until a maximum programmed value, according to specific protocols that can be adapted to the patient's needs. Generally, it is possible to program the maximum pacing rate, as well as the slope of the heart rate increase. Most R-R devices also have algorithms that automatically shorten the A-V interval as the frequency of stimulation increases.

The correct ECG interpretation of the R-R phenomenon is not difficult, if the device programming parameters are available. In some cases, the AECGM can be useful to correlate patient's symptoms, for example, palpitations, owing to an inappropriate activation of the R-R function, as an example at rest or during light activity (**Fig. 14**).

Automatic Lower Resting Rate Algorithm, or "Sleep" Function

A special algorithm can automatically reduce the stimulation rate below the basal lower rate when the patient is at rest or during sleep, based on the level of activity automatically sensed by the sensor. This algorithm is useful to avoid unnecessary pacing during rest or sleep. Therefore, if the algorithm is active, on AECGM it can be observed that the heart rate at rest or during sleep is lower than the programmed lower rate.

Algorithms to Prevent Sudden Heart Rate Drops

Because spontaneous sudden heart rate drops may give rise to presyncope or syncope in susceptible patients, special algorithms have been developed to activate the atrial stimulation when a sudden decrease of heart rate is perceived, even if the lower rate is not attained. The aim of such algorithms is to avoid sudden decreases in the heart rate, and to smooth the heart rate fluctuations.

The activity of such algorithms can be recognized on AECGM when an atrial pacing is observed at heart rate above the lower rate, independent of the patient's level of activity. In some cases, the AECGM can be useful to correlate patient's symptoms, for example, syncope or presyncope, or palpitation, owing to an inappropriate activation of the heart rate drop function (**Fig. 15**), as example during sleep or rest. In such cases, AECGM can be useful to attain an optimal programming of the heart rate drop function.

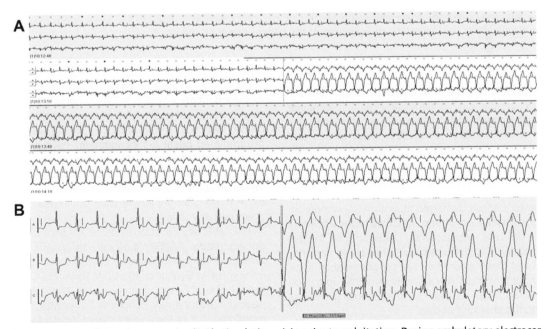

Fig. 14. Inappropriate rate-responsive (R-R) stimulation giving rise to palpitation. During ambulatory electrocardiographic monitoring, the patient with a dual chamber pacemaker with DDDR programming became symptomatic for palpitations (*A*); owing to an inappropriate R-R ventricular stimulation (*B*) in the absence of significant patient activity. Palpitations disappeared when the programming was changed to DDD mode.

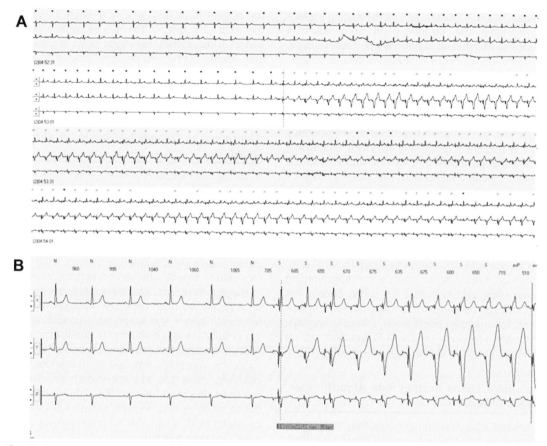

Fig. 15. Inappropriate activation of the rate drop function during sleep giving rise to palpitations. Inappropriate activation of the heart rate drop function during sleep, symptomatic for palpitation (*A*). The activity of such algorithms can be recognized on ambulatory electrocardiographic monitoring, because A-V pacing is observed at a heart rate above the lower rate, independent of the patient's level of activity (*B*).

Algorithms to Minimize Ventricular Pacing

In patients with intact or intermittent spontaneous A-V conduction, unnecessary right ventricular pacing may be associated with an increased risk of atrial fibrillation, congestive heart failure, and left ventricular dysfunction.[1] Therefore, various algorithms have been developed with the specific goal of optimizing ventricular pacing—as examples, the MVP algorithm (by Medtronic) or the ventricular intrinsic preferred algorithm (by Abbott-St. Jude Medical), or others, specifically developed by the different manufactures. Depending on the device model and the manufacturer, some parameters of these algorithms are programmable, such as the maximum A-V delay (extendible up to 600 milliseconds), as well as the checking interval and the checking cycles.

The main feature of the ventricular intrinsic preferred algorithm is to promote the patient's intrinsic A-V conduction. To do so, the ventricular intrinsic preferred algorithm, periodically adds a programmable delta to the basic A-V interval (A-V interval hysteresis). In the presence of intrinsic A-V conduction, a prolonged A-V interval is maintained; in the absence of intrinsic conduction, the device switches to dual chamber pacing with the programmed basal A-V conduction. The function of this algorithm can be detected on the surface ECG of AECGM in the presence of atrial pacing followed by spontaneous ventricular conduction with an A-V conduction longer than the basal programmed A-V delay.

The MVP algorithm consists of an atrial-based pacing mode [AAI(R)], designed to switch to a dual-chamber pacing mode [DDD(R)] only in presence of an AVB [annotated as AAI(R)<==>DDD(R) mode]. The MVP algorithm provides AAI(R) mode pacing, while the A-V conduction is continuously monitored. If 2 of the 4 most recent atrial intervals are not followed by a ventricular event, the MVP identifies a missed A-V conduction and automatically switches to DDD(R) pacing mode (see

Fig. 15). Thereafter, the device periodically checks if there is spontaneous A-V conduction, to return to the AAI(R) mode. Usually, the first check occurs 1 minute after the switch. If the next A-A interval is followed by a sensed ventricular beat, the check is successful, and the device remains in AAI(R) mode. Instead, if the A-A interval is not followed by a sensed ventricular beat, the check is unsuccessful and device switches back to dual-chamber pacing mode. The time between subsequent checks doubles, if each one check fails (from 2 minutes up to 16 hours). In patients with complete AVB, the device operates in dual-chamber mode pacing persistently, and every 16 hours the device checks A-V conduction with a single dropped ventricular beat (**Fig. 16**).

It is important to be aware of the presence of such algorithms to minimize ventricular pacing (MVP) when evaluating AECGM, because the correct operation of those algorithms can be erroneously interpreted as PM malfunction, for example, when the maximum A-V delay is so long to imitate an AVB, or when the atrial pacing is followed by a pause owing to missed ventricular pacing during checks (see **Fig. 16**).

Algorithms to Prevent Atrial Fibrillation

Potential causes of atrial tachyarrhythmias include mostly premature atrial contractions, resulting in long sinus pauses and ectopic premature beats originating from multiple atrial sites. To counteract

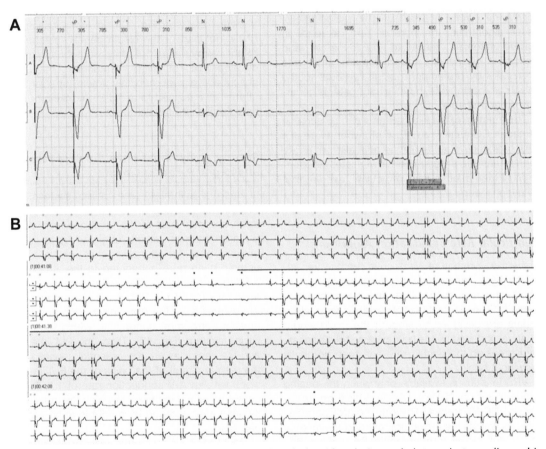

Fig. 16. Function of the "minimize ventricular pacing" (MVP) algorithm during ambulatory electrocardiographic monitoring (AECGM). Operation of the MVP algorithm during AECGM. The A-V conduction is continuously monitored, and the algorithm periodically checks if there is spontaneous A-V conduction, to return to the AAI(R) mode (A). Because 2 of the 4 most recent A-A intervals were not followed by a ventricular event, the MVP identified a missed A-V conduction and automatically switched to DDDR pacing mode. Thereafter, the device periodically checked if there was spontaneous A-V conduction (usually the first check occurs 1 minute after the switch). In this case, because the A-A intervals were not followed by a sensed ventricular beat, the check was unsuccessful, and the device switched back to dual-chamber pacing mode (B). The time between subsequent checks generally doubles, if each subsequent check fails (from 2 minutes up to 16 hours). Noteworthy, periodic MVP checks could be easily misdiagnosed as pacing failures.

this potential mechanism favoring the onset of atrial fibrillation, algorithms have been developed to maintain continuous atrial pacing (>90%), at a rate slightly higher than the sinus rhythm. As examples, some of those algorithms are the atrial preference pacing (by Medtronic) or atrial fibrillation suppression (by Abbott-St. Jude).

By such algorithms, the device responds to changes in sinus atrial cycles by accelerating the pacing rate until reaching a constantly paced rhythm. After each nonrefractory atrial sensed event, the device decreases the atrial pacing rate by a programmed value, and this progression continues until the pacing rate is slightly higher than the spontaneous sinus rate, resulting in a stable atrial paced rhythm. Such an atrial rate is maintained for the number of the programmed beats, then the pacing rate decreases slightly, to search for the next atrial intrinsic activation. Because of those algorithms, the increase and decrease in pacing intervals result to be dynamic and controlled. Generally, the maximum atrial rate attainable by preference pacing is equal to the maximum pacing rate, but this parameter is generally programmable.

The function of these algorithms can be seen on surface ECG (mainly on AECGM), when there is a high incidence of atrial pacing activation at a rate higher than the programmed lower rate, independent of the patient's level of activity (even at rest or during sleep).

Ventricular Rate Stabilization Algorithms

Generally, premature ventricular beats are followed by a compensatory pause, giving rise to short–long sequences, that may be arrhythmogenic.[13] The ventricular rate stabilization algorithms are designed to smooth the cycle length changes induced by the postextrasystolic pauses, by increasing the pacing rate and then gradually slowing it back.

VRS function is available only when the pacing mode is set on DDD(R), DDI(R), VVI(R) on AAI(R) <==>DDD(R) modes. The rate control parameters, as well as the maximum rate and the interval increment, are all programmable. So, when a PVC occurs, the device paces the ventricle at the previous pacing interval plus the programmed interval increment. In dual chamber devices, the VRS triggers an atrial pacing to maintain the A-V synchronicity. Then the VRS increases the pacing rate until the upper programmed pacing rate is reached or when a new ventricular activity is sensed. An upper limit is set for VRS function, to avoid a sustained high heart rate for extended time.

PACEMAKER-MEDIATED ARRHYTHMIAS

The PM-mediated arrhythmias are conditions in which the pacing system participates in the trigger and/or in maintenance of the arrhythmias. The PMT can be divided in 2 subgroups, depending on the role played by the stimulation system: atrial tachyarrhythmias passively conducted to the ventricles and reentry arrhythmias have the pacemaker as an integral part of a circuit.

Atrial Tachyarrhythmias Passively Conducted to the Ventricles

Fast atrial arrhythmias (atrial flutter, atrial tachycardia, or atrial fibrillation) can be sensed by the atrial lead of the PM and consequently transferred to the ventricle up to the programmed maximum tracking rate (see **Fig. 13**). In those cases, the PM is not part of the electrogenetic mechanism of the arrhythmia, but only contributes to the development of high ventricular rates. As described elsewhere in this article, special algorithms are designed to avoid the tracking of atrial arrhythmias into the ventricles.

Reentry Arrhythmias Have the Pacemaker as an Integral Part of a Circuit

In such arrhythmias, also called endless loop tachycardia (ELT), or PMT, the stimulation system is an essential part of the electrogenetic circuit. Such arrhythmias usually originate by an atrial r ectopic beat (or in some case or ventricular ectopic beat) retro-conducted to the atria. When a premature atrial depolarization is sensed by the atrial channel of the PM, it will be conducted to the ventricles by the PM, and it will return to the atria by retrograde conduction within the nodo–Hisian system (**Fig. 17**). Thus, the PM, the atria and the ventricles are the essential constituent of the reentry circuit at the basis of the ELT mechanism, with an A-V conduction rate of 1:1. **Fig. 18** shows an example of ELT in which the atrial activity has been recorded by a double atrial esophageal lead.

Most PMs have automatic systems for the interruption of such arrhythmias after a fixed number of beats. Also, many PMs can extend the PVARP after an atrial premature beat, with the aim to prevent ELT.

PMT and ELT can be perceived by patients as palpitations, and AECGM can be useful in correlating PMT with patient's symptoms (**Fig. 19**), and to optimize the programming to avoid PMT onset.

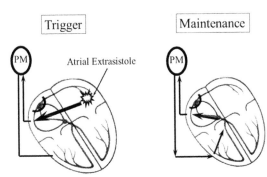

Fig. 17. Pacemaker (PM)-mediated tachycardia (PMT) or endless loop tachycardia (ELT): trigger and maintenance. The diagram shows the trigger mechanism and the subsequent maintenance of a reentry PMT. The trigger is usually an atrial ectopic beat, which is sensed and triggered to the ventricles by the pacemaker. The impulse comes back to the atria through a retrograde conduction within the nodo–Hisian conducting system, and it is sensed as normal by the atrial lead and then triggered to the ventricle, creating the self-maintained PMT (or ELT). The pacemaker forms the anterograde (atrium to ventricle [A → V]) limb of the circuit, and the nodo-Hisian system forms the retrograde limb (ventricle to atrium [V → A]) of the circuit.

ELECTROCARDIOGRAPHIC SIGNS OF BIVENTRICULAR PACING

The main purpose of the biventricular pacing is to resynchronize the areas of myocardium that

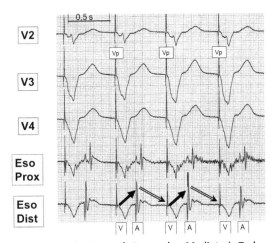

Fig. 18. Mechanism of Pacemaker-Mediated Tachycardia (PMT) or endless loop tachycardia (ELT). Surface and esophageal ECG leads contribute to identification of the electrogenetic mechanism of PMT. The ventricular depolarization induced by the pacemaker (Vp) is retro-conducted to the atria through the A-V conduction system (*dark arrow*). The atrial depolarization (A) is sensed by the atrial lead of the pacemaker with consequent depolarization of the ventricles (*double arrow*).

spontaneously depolarize late, with the aim to restore their contractile function. To better understand the ECG pattern of biventricular pacing, it should be reminded that the pattern of right ventricular pacing is characterized by a left intraventricular conduction delay morphology with marked left axis deviation (see **Fig. 3**). As to the left ventricular pacing ECG pattern, the stimulation of left ventricle generates an activation front directed from the left to the right leading to an essentially negative QRS in D1. This right axis deviation in the frontal plane is associated with a typical morphology in V1 with a positive QRS initial component (**Fig. 20**). During biventricular pacing, owing to the fusion of 2 activation fronts (left and right), the QRS duration is shorter than after a single left or right stimulation (**Fig. 21**). Biventricular ECG pattern is characterized by an initial QRS negativity (or Q-wave) in D1 and an initial QRS positivity (R waves) in V1, both generated by the left ventricular pacing contribution. The QRS axis in the frontal plane is intermediate between the left pacing axis directed from the bottom to the right, and the right pacing axis directed upward to the left. The timing programmability of both right and left ventricular channels are completely independent and a wide range of fusion morphologies between left and right ventricular activity can occur (**Fig. 22**). An early activation of the left ventricular chamber (LV -30 milliseconds vs RV; see **Fig. 22B**) provoke more evident Q wave in D1 and R wave in V1, peculiar signs of the left ventricular activation. Conversely, when the left ventricular activation is progressively delayed (see **Fig. 22D**, LV+30 milliseconds vs RV) both Q wave in D1 and R wave in V1 gradually reduce, until when they disappear (see **Fig. 22E**, LV+60 milliseconds vs RV), and QRS morphology becomes similar to that observed after isolated right ventricular pacing. The QRS axis in the frontal plane is directed: (a) to the top and right side when the ventricular stimulation is simultaneous (LV 0 milliseconds vs RV); (b) down and to the right side when the left ventricular stimulation is anticipated (LV -30 milliseconds vs RV); and (3) up and toward left side when the right ventricular stimulation occurs earlier (LV +30 milliseconds vs RV).

The surface ECG, and particularly AECGMG, can be useful in patients with CRT, because it can verify the changes in QRS morphology, indicating effective resynchronization. Also, in case of frequent VPBs, AECGM can contribute to verify the impact of the VPBs burden on the resynchronization. Benefits from CRT depend mostly on the effectiveness of biventricular pacing and programming should ensure the maximum (>95%) of biventricular pacing.[1–4,8,14]

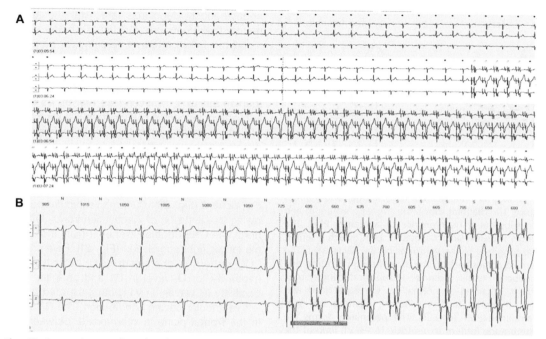

Fig. 19. Pacemaker-mediated tachycardia (PMT) recorded by Holter monitoring. Recording of PMT episode lasting for several second by Holter monitoring, while the patient was symptomatic for palpitations (*A*). Sudden DDD pacing activation, presumably after an atrial depolarization sensed by the pacemaker (*B*). PMT was abolished by reprogramming the postventricular atrial refractory period, and the patient became asymptomatic thereafter.

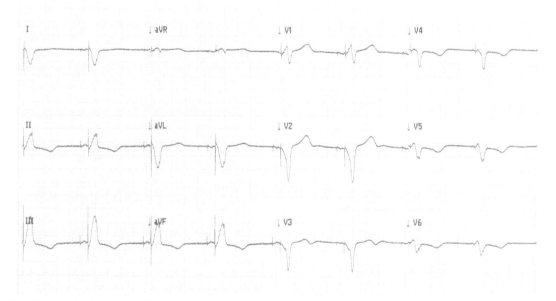

Fig. 20. A 12-lead electrocardiograph in left ventricular stimulation. The figure refers to an electrocardiogram in which ventricular pacing is performed from the lateral wall of the left ventricle. This mode of stimulation generates an activation front directed from left to the right with a QRS essentially negative in the derivations exploring the left ventricle (D1, A-VL, V5, V6) and positive in lead V1. The Q wave in D1 and the R wave in V1 are characteristics of the stimulation from the lateral wall of the left ventricle.

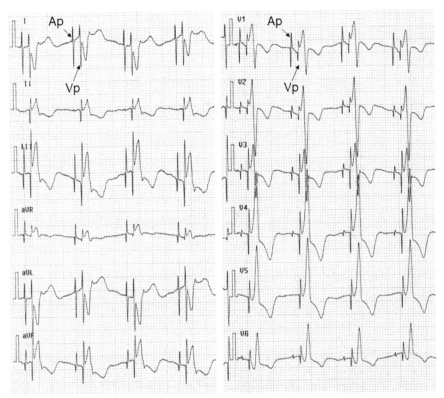

Fig. 21. A 12-lead electrocardiograph showing atrial and biventricular pacing (unipolar). The electrocardiogram shows a unipolar pacing in which an atrial stimulus (Ap) is followed by a ventricular stimulus (Vp) provided by a system of simultaneous biventricular pacing (first generation). The induced QRS is the result of a fusion between the left and right ventricular depolarization. The Q wave extension D1 and an R wave in lead V1 are typically generated by left ventricular depolarization. The QRS axis in the frontal plane is intermediate between the left ventricular pacing axis directed from the bottom to the right and the right ventricular pacing directed upward to the left.

According to the European Heart Rhythm Association/Heart Rhythm Society expert consensus on CRT, AECGM monitoring is recommended to document ventricular or atrial arrhythmia that might not have been detected by the device, or to verify the proper arrhythmia classification performed by the device.[4] AECGM can also be useful to evaluate the presence of pacing fusion and pseudofusion beats, which may lead to overestimation of the effective biventricular pacing delivered by a CRT device.[4,8,14] In CRT patients with atrial fibrillation and more than 90% biventricular pacing, analysis of Holter monitoring may reveal a high prevalence of fusion and pseudofusion beats that lessen CRT response. Therefore, AECGM evaluation is recommended, especially in nonresponders or in patients who initially responded to CRT and then deteriorated during follow-up. Even in cases of a high percentage of biventricular pacing capture, intermittent loss of LV capture, or frequent fusion and/or pseudofusion beats competing with paced beats detected by AECGM, may forecast inadequate response to CRT.[4,8]

IDENTIFICATION OF PACEMAKER MALFUNCTIONS BY ELECTROCARDIOGRAPHIC MONITORING

A PM malfunction can occur for an alteration of both sensing and pacing function, either alone or in combination, and surface ECG, mainly AECGM, can be the tool of choice to identify suspected PM dysfunctions.[4,6]

Impairment of the Pacing Function

A defect in the pacing function is usually characterized by the inability of the pacing electrical pulse to depolarize the cardiac chamber in which the lead is positioned. The surface ECG shows the presence of spikes not followed by depolarization waves. Pacing malfunctions can occur both at the

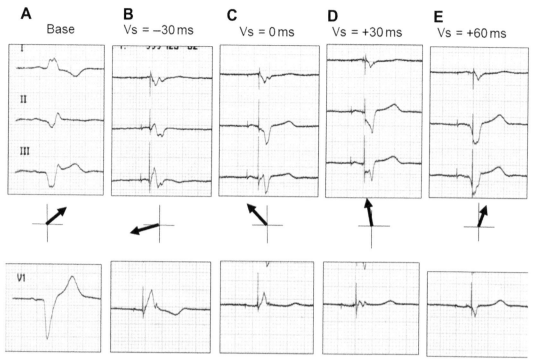

Fig. 22. Electrocardiographic changes of the QRS by biventricular pacing by different LV-RV timing. The morphology of the QRS varies with the time sequence of the stimulation of the 2 ventricles. This figure shows the morphologic variations of the QRS in leads D1, D2, D3, and V1 and the *Arrows* show the direction of the vector in the frontal plane with a second-generation biventricular pacing. (*A*) At baseline, in spontaneous sinus rhythm a typical left bundle branch block is present (QRS duration of 180 milliseconds). (*B*) The stimulator is programmed so that the left ventricular pacing anticipates the right ventricular pacing of 30 milliseconds; therefore, the typical signs of left ventricular stimulation appear (Q wave in lead D1 and R wave in lead V1). D3 shows a positive QRS typically associated with right axis deviation. (*C*) Left and right ventricular pacing are delivered simultaneously. The QRS morphology is identical to a first-generation biventricular pacing. Compared with *B*, the R wave amplitude in V1 and Q wave in D1 are reduced, because the left ventricular component is reduced. For the same reason, the QRS axis in the frontal plane moves upward, as shown by the QRS morphology in D3. (*D*) The left ventricular pacing is delayed of 30 milliseconds with respect to the right ventricular pacing; there is a further reduction of the R wave amplitude in V1 and of the Q wave in D1. The QRS axis in the frontal plane shifts to the left, becoming negative in D3. (*E*) The left ventricular pacing is markedly delayed (60 milliseconds), and the global ventricular depolarization is almost completely determined by right ventricular pacing. The QRS morphology becomes similar to the one observed in isolated right ventricular pacing.

atrial (**Fig. 23**) and ventricular levels (**Fig. 24**). Lead dislodgment or rupture, fibrosis at the site of insertion, and battery discharge are the main causes of loss of pacing.

Impairment of the Sensing Function

Alterations in the sensing function may occur either for the PM inability to detect the intrinsic depolarization of the chamber in which the lead is placed (undersensing), or for an excess of sensing (oversensing) resulting in an erroneous inhibition of the pacing. The undersensing defect is characterized on the surface ECG by an emission of spikes despite the presence of spontaneous rhythm. This alteration can appear both at the atrial (**Fig. 25**) and at ventricular levels (**Fig. 26**).

The oversensing defect occurs when electrical signals extraneous to the cardiac chamber lead (muscle tremors, or external electric interferences, or lead rupture, or other pathologic conditions) are sensed by the device (**Fig. 27**). Oversensing is a potentially dangerous phenomenon because the consequent cessation of pacing can provoke a prolonged asystole in PM-dependent patients (**Fig. 28**). In patients with ICD and CRT defibrillator, oversensing can induce an incorrect detection of fast ventricular arrhythmias, potentially leading to inappropriate shocks (**Fig. 29**).

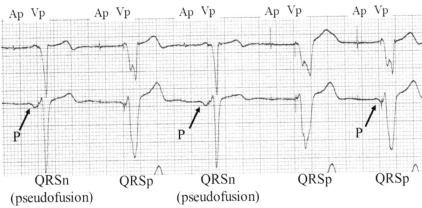

Fig. 23. Impaired atrial pacing in DDD pacing. A dual-chamber pacemaker with DDD mode programming delivers both atrial (Ap) and ventricular (Vp) spikes. An impaired pacing function at the atrial level is observed, because the atrial stimuli (Ap) are not followed by a corresponding atrial depolarization; occasionally, spontaneous P wave appears. The pacemaker constantly paces the ventricles, but only in the first and in the third complexes does the spontaneous atrial activity (P) seem to reach the ventricles, generating a QRS of normal morphology (pseudofusion).

ROLE OF SURFACE ELECTROCARDIOGRAPHS IN THE EVALUATION OF PATIENTS WITH CARDIAC IMPLANTABLE ELECTRONIC DEVICES WITH SYMPTOMS AND ARRHYTHMIAS

Notably, PM dysfunctions are a rare cause of syncope or presyncope (<5% in most studies), whereas other causes for syncope, including arterial hypotension or supraventricular or ventricular arrhythmias, are more frequently observed in PM patients with a history of syncope or presyncope.[9,15,16] Nonetheless, intermittent loss of capture or oversensing of external noise may lead to clinically significant pauses, which can be revealed by AECGM. Thus, AECGM monitoring can be useful in patients with symptoms suggestive of device malfunction, particularly syncope and presyncope, when routine interrogation does not reveal the reason for the corresponding clinical symptoms.

An evaluation of atrial and ventricular arrhythmia by device software and retrieved diagnostics may not always be complete.[16] As an example, atrial arrhythmias may be underestimated by monochamber devices (such as an ICD with a single right ventricular catheter), although they can be better characterized and quantified by AECGM to guide for proper treatment. Also, patients in whom arrhythmia counters show frequent PVCs may be treated with ablation procedure, which may be guided by 12-lead AECGM to evaluate the exact morphology of PVCs and/or episodes of ventricular tachycardia.

Even though the results of new clinical studies have provided new evidence for the optimal programming of ICD and CRT devices to reduce inappropriate intervention,[17,18] AECGM monitoring and exercise testing, together with data stored by remote monitoring, may still be useful in individual optimization of ICD settings in some difficult cases.[9]

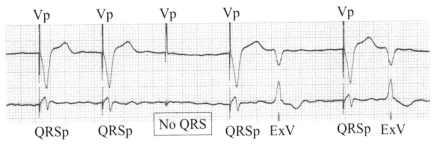

Fig. 24. Impairment of ventricular pacing in a VVI pacemaker. The basic rhythm in atrial fibrillation with VVI pacing (Vp). The first 2 beats are regularly paced in VVI mode, whereas the third ventricular stimulus (Vp) is not followed by an appropriate ventricular depolarization. The fourth ventricular stimulus regularly paces the ventricles, and the next ventricular ectopic ventricular beat is normally sensed by the pacemaker, which waits until the predefined interval (the lower rate interval) before releasing a new ventricular stimulus.

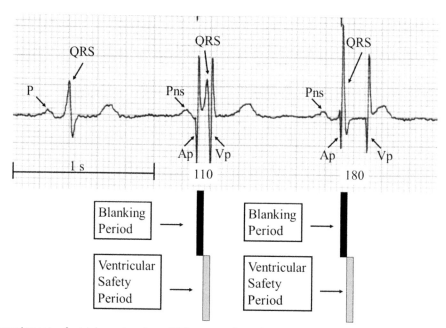

Fig. 25. Impairment of atrial sensing in a DDD pacemaker, the blanking and ventricular safety periods. A sequence of 3 cardiac cycles in a patient with a dual chamber pacemaker (DDD) is shown. In the first cardiac cycle, a normal activation (P-QRS) is sensed by the pacemaker, which is correctly inhibited. In the second cardiac cycle, owing to a transient loss of atrial sensing, the P wave is not sensed (Pns) and an atrial pacing (Ap) is delivered; the next spontaneous QRS, originating from the nonsensed P wave, falls within the window of detection of cross-talk, giving rise to a ventricular safety pacing (Vp); in this committed pacing, typically the A-V interval lasts 110 milliseconds. Also, in the third cardiac cycle the P wave is not sensed; therefore, an atrial stimulus is delivered (Ap). The subsequent spontaneous QRS falls in the blanking period and, therefore, is not perceived by the pacemaker; a ventricular stimulus (Vp) at the A-V interval (180 milliseconds) is delivered.

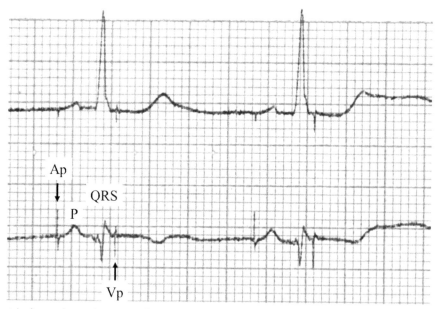

Fig. 26. Ventricular undersensing. Loss of ventricular sensing in a DDD pacemaker. The ventricular channel lost the ability to sense the spontaneous activity of the ventricles. A ventricular stimulus (Vp) is delivered after the spontaneous QRS.

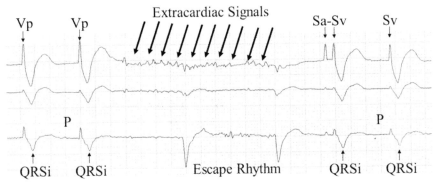

Fig. 27. Pauses owing to ventricular oversensing in a DDD pacemaker during Holter recording. Holter recording of a patient with DDD pacemaker. Electrical signals of extracardiac origin (*arrows*) inhibit the emission of the stimuli, generating pause, with the emergence of a ventricular escape rhythm.

ROLE OF SURFACE ELECTROCARDIOGRAPHS IN THE EVALUATION OF PATIENTS AFTER EXPLANT OF THE CARDIAC IMPLANTABLE ELECTRONIC DEVICE

As the number of implantable devices increase, the number of patients undergoing explants for device problems and/or infections is increasing. The need for reimplantation can be established even before explantation, by the monitoring of symptoms and ECG changes with the device programmed at a pacing rate below the patient's intrinsic rate. Both European and American

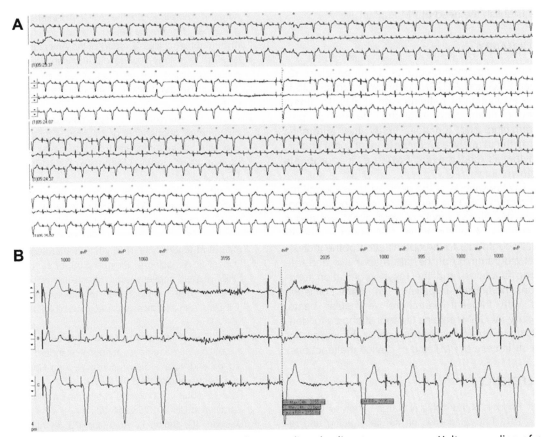

Fig. 28. Pauses owing to oversensing during Holter recording, leading to presyncope. Holter recording of a pacemaker-dependent patient with a dual chamber pacemaker, showing 2 consecutive pauses (3.5 and 2.0 s) provoking presyncope (*A*). The pauses were due to oversensing of muscular contraction, with inhibition of atrial and ventricular pacing (*B*).

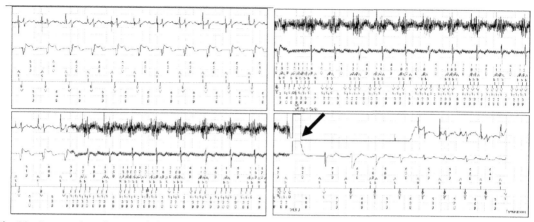

Fig. 29. Oversensing of external electrical noise, leading to a misdiagnosis of ventricular fibrillation and inappropriate shock in a patient with a cardiac resynchronization device. Remote monitoring (Holter function) showing the recording of oversensing of external electrical noise (on both channels), misdiagnosed as ventricular fibrillation, leading to 35J inappropriate shock (*arrow*). RA, right atrium; RV, right ventricle.

guidelines emphasize that, after device removal, careful reassessment of the indications for reimplantation should be performed on an individual basis to determine the risk–benefit ratio and to reestablish the need of PM implant.[1,4,9,18]

SUMMARY

Surface electrocardiograms, both baseline 12-lead ECG and AECGM, play an essential role in the evaluation of patients with CIEDs, to detect device malfunction, evaluate the device programming and function, verify the automatic arrhythmia analyses, correlate symptoms and arrhythmias, and prevent PMT and inappropriate interventions.

The knowledge of the new complex algorithms of current CIEDs is necessary to properly recognize the device functions and avoid erroneous diagnosis of malfunctions. AECGM may specifically contribute to the optimization of the individual programming of the rate responsive and rate drop functions, and the resynchronization functions, particularly in patients with atrial fibrillation or with frequent premature ventricular beats. Finally, AECGM remains the tool of choice to identify and correlate symptoms to arrhythmias, particularly in case of PMT and of device malfunctions.

REFERENCES

1. Brignole M, Auricchio A, Baron-Esquivias G, et al. 2013 ESC guidelines on cardiac pacing and resynchronization therapy. The Task Force on Cardiac Pacing and Resynchronization Therapy of the European Society of Cardiology (ESC). Developed in collaboration with the European Heart Rhythm Association (EHRA). Europace 2013;15: 1070–118.

2. Epstein A, DiMarco JP, Ellenbogen KA, et al, Heart Rhythm Society. 2012 ACCF/AHA/HRS focused update incorporated into the ACCF/AHA/HRS 2008 guidelines for device-based therapy of cardiac rhythm abnormalities: a report of the American College of Cardiology Foundation/American Heart Association Task Force on Practice Guidelines and the Heart Rhythm Society. J Am Coll Cardiol 2013; 61:e6–75.

3. Varma N, Auricchio A. Recommendations for post-implant monitoring of patients with cardiovascular implantable electronic devices: where do we stand today? Europace 2013;15(Suppl 1):i11–3.

4. Wilkoff BL, Love CJ, Byrd CL, et al, American Heart Association. 2015 HRS/EHRA/APHRS/SOLAECE expert consensus statement on optimal implantable cardioverter-defibrillator programming and testing. Heart Rhythm 2016;13:e50–86.

5. Dubner S, Auricchio A, Steinberg JS, et al. ISHNE/EHRA expert consensus on remote monitoring of cardiovascular implantable electronic devices (CIEDs). Ann Noninvasive Electrocardiol 2012;17: 36–56.

6. Barold SS. Usefulness of Holter recordings in the evaluation of pacemaker function: standard techniques and intracardiac recordings. Ann Noninvasive Electrocardiol 1998;3:345–79.

7. Ritter P. Holter in monitoring of cardiac pacing. Prog Cardiovasc Dis 2013;56:211–23.

8. Daubert JC, Saxon L, Adamson PB, et al. 2012 EHRA/HRS expert consensus statement on cardiac resynchronization therapy in heart failure: implant and follow-up recommendations and management. Heart Rhythm 2012;9:1524–76.

9. Steinberg JS, Varma N, Cygankiewicz I, et al. 2017 ISHNE-HRS expert consensus statement on ambulatory ECG and external cardiac monitoring/telemetry. Ann Noninvasive Electrocardiol 2017;22(3). https://doi.org/10.1111/anec.12447.

10. Andrikopoulos G, Tzeis S, Theodorakis G, et al. Monitoring capabilities of cardiac rhythm management devices. Europace 2010;1:17–23.

11. Bernstein AD, Daubert JC, Fletcher RD, et al. The revised NASPE/BPEG generic code for antibradycardia, adaptive-rate, and multisite pacing. PACE 2002;25:260–4.

12. Tjong FVY, Reddy VY. Permanent leadless cardiac pacemaker therapy: a comprehensive review. Circulation 2017;135:1458–70.

13. Locati ET, Bagliani G, Padeletti L. Normal ventricular repolarization and QT interval: ionic background, modifiers, and measurements. Card Electrophysiol Clin 2017;9(3):487–513.

14. Kamath GS, Cotiga D, Koneru JN, et al. The utility of 12-lead Holter monitoring in patients with permanent atrial fibrillation for the identification of non-responders after cardiac resynchronization therapy. J Am Coll Cardiol 2009;53:1050–5.

15. Ofman P, Rahilly-Tierney C, Djousse L, et al. Pacing system malfunction is a rare cause of hospital admission for syncope in patients with a permanent pacemaker. Pacing Clin Electrophysiol 2013;36: 109–12.

16. Kumor M, Baranowski R, Kozluk E, et al. Is the diagnostic function of pacemakers a reliable source of information about ventricular arrhythmias? Cardiol J 2010;17:495–502.

17. Lunati M, Proclemer A, Boriani G, et al, Clinical Service Cardiological Centres. Reduction of inappropriate anti-tachycardia pacing therapies and shocks by a novel suite of detection algorithms in heart failure patients with cardiac resynchronization therapy defibrillators: a historical comparison of a prospective database. Europace 2016; 18(9):1391–8.

18. Locati ET. New direction for ambulatory ECG recording following 2017 HRS-ISHNE expert consensus. J Electrocardiol 2017;50:828–32.

Ectopic Beats
Insights from Timing and Morphology

Giuseppe Bagliani, MD[a,b,]*, Domenico Giovanni Della Rocca, MD[c],
Roberto De Ponti, MD, FHRS[d], Alessandro Capucci, MD[e],
Margherita Padeletti, MD[f], Andrea Natale, MD, FACC, FHRS[c,g,h,i,j,k]

KEYWORDS

- Ectopic beats • Premature atrial beats • Premature junctional beats • Premature ventricular beats
- Atrial fibrillation • Electrocardiography • Arrhythmias

KEY POINTS

- Premature complexes are electrical impulses arising from sites other than the sinus node, which can cause contractions of the heart.
- Premature electrical impulses can arise from atrial, junctional, or ventricular tissue.
- Premature atrial beats are much more frequent than those arising in the atrioventricular junction, but less frequent than premature beats from the ventricles.
- Surface electrocardiogram (ECG) analysis of premature beats is of pivotal importance to predict the site of origin of the ectopic focus.

INTRODUCTION

Premature complexes are electrical impulses arising from sites other than the sinus node, which can cause contractions of the heart. The sinus node normally initiates cardiac activation, as a result of a faster intrinsic rate of automaticity; however, premature electrical impulses can arise from atrial, junctional, or ventricular tissue, leading to premature heart beats. The most common mechanism promoting the development of a premature beat is increased automaticity. Premature atrial beats (PABs) are much more frequent than those arising in the

Premature junctional beats (PJBs) but less frequent than Premature ventricular beats (PVBs). The aim of this article was to review the main electrocardiogram (ECG) features of premature complexes and discuss their implications in clinical practice.

PREVIOUS CONSIDERATIONS AND DEFINITIONS

Significant insights for diagnosis and localization of ectopic beats can be obtained via the analysis of the coupling interval and the post-extrasystolic pause (**Fig. 1**); they both result from the

Disclosures: A. Natale has received speaker honoraria from Boston Scientific, Biosense Webster, St. Jude Medical, Biotronik, and Medtronic, and is a consultant for Biosense Webster, St. Jude Medical, and Janssen. G. Bagliani, D.G. Della Rocca, R. De Ponti, A. Capucci, and M. Padeletti have nothing to disclose.
[a] Arrhythmology Unit, Cardiology Department, Foligno General Hospital, Via Massimo Arcamone, Foligno, Perguia, Italy; [b] Cardiovascular Diseases Department, University of Perugia, Perugia, Italy; [c] Texas Cardiac Arrhythmia Institute, St. David's Medical Center, 3000 N Interstate Hwy 35 #700, Austin, TX 78705, USA; [d] Cardiology Department, University of Insubria, Via Ravasi, 2, 21100 Varese, Italy; [e] Cardiology and Arrhythmology Clinic, Marche Polytechnic University, University Hospital "Ospedali Riuniti", Via Conca, 71, Torrette, Ancona 60030, Italy; [f] Cardiology Department, Mugello Hospital, Viale Resistenza, 60 - 50032 Borgo San Lorenzo (FI), Italy; [g] Department of Biomedical Engineering, University of Texas, Austin, TX, USA; [h] Interventional Electrophysiology, Scripps Clinic, La Jolla, CA, USA; [i] MetroHealth Medical Center, Case Western Reserve University School of Medicine, Cleveland, OH, USA; [j] Division of Cardiology, Stanford University, Stanford, CA, USA; [k] Electrophysiology and Arrhythmia Services, California Pacific Medical Center, San Francisco, CA, USA
* Corresponding author. Via Centrale Umbra, 17, Spello, Perugia 06038, Italy.
E-mail address: giuseppe.bagliani@tim.it

Card Electrophysiol Clin 10 (2018) 257–275
https://doi.org/10.1016/j.ccep.2018.02.013
1877-9182/18/© 2018 Elsevier Inc. All rights reserved.

Abbreviations	
AD	Afterdepolarization
AV	Atrioventricular
LBBB	Left bundle branch block
LV	Left ventricle
PAB	Premature atrial beat
PJB	Premature junctional beat
PSVB	Premature supraventricular beat
PVB	Premature ventricular beat
RBBB	Right bundle branch block
RV	Right ventricle
SA	Sinoatrial
SHD	Structural heart disease
SoO	Site of origin
VT	Ventricular tachycardia

interactions between the ectopic focus and the conduction system of the heart.

Coupling Interval

The coupling interval is the interval between the dominant heart beat and a following ectopic beat. In an ECG recording several premature beats, the coupling interval may be fixed or variable. Coupling intervals are classified as fixed (**Fig. 2**) if their difference is <120 ms in the same patient, or variable (**Fig. 3**) if it is >120 ms. Ectopic beats with a fixed coupling interval are likely due to foci depending on the normal sinus rhythm, such as the normal beat influences the development of an ectopic beat. Ectopic beats displaying variable coupling intervals result from a protected ectopic focus, which is not related to the baseline rhythm. The ectopic focus is not depolarized by the sinus impulses, usually because of a unidirectional entrance block. Premature complexes with variable coupling intervals originate in a so-called parasystolic focus (**Fig. 4**).

Post-extrasystolic Pause

The post-extrasystolic pause is the interval between the ectopic complex and the following sinus complex. Post-extrasystolic pause can be classified as follows:

- Fully compensatory (**Fig. 5**): the ectopic impulse frequently does not reach and reset the sinus node and the distance between the QRS complex preceding the premature beat and the following complex is twice the sinus cadence
- Not fully compensatory (**Fig. 6**): the ectopic impulse reaches and depolarizes the sinoatrial (SA) node, therefore resetting the sinus cycle. In this scenario, a pause following the ectopic beat does not compensate its prematurity
- Absent because of interpolation of the premature beat into 2 perfectly normal cardiac cycles (**Fig. 7**)

Distribution

On the basis of timing distribution, premature beats can display a repetitive sequence and be classified as follows (**Fig. 8**):

- Bigeminal: a repetitive sequence of a sinus and a premature beat
- Trigeminal: a repetitive sequence of 2 sinus and a premature beat
- Quadrigeminal: a repetitive sequence of 3 sinus and a premature beat Complexity (**Fig. 9**):
- Couplet: in the occurrence of 2 consecutive ectopic beats
- Tachycardia: if there are 3 or more consecutive ectopic beats

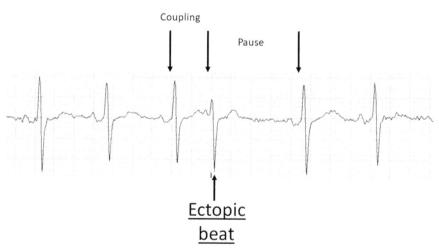

Fig. 1. How to measure the coupling interval and the post-extrasystolic pause of an ectopic beat.

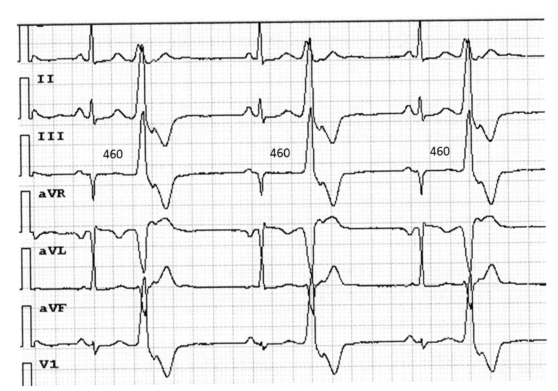

Fig. 2. Fixed coupling intervals of bigeminal PVBs.

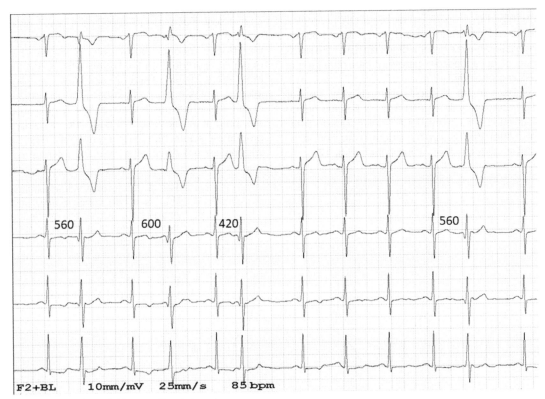

Fig. 3. PVBs with variable coupling intervals.

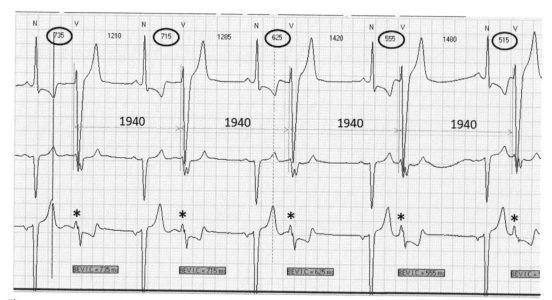

Fig. 4. Parasystolic distribution of PVBs. Asterisks indicate a sequence of PVBs with variable coupling intervals; the intervals between the ectopic beats is regular (1940 ms).

PREMATURE SUPRAVENTRICULAR COMPLEXES

Premature supraventricular beats (PSVBs) are premature complexes of supraventricular origin that arise above His bundle division and particularly from the atria (**Fig. 10**) or the atrioventricular junction (**Fig. 11**). A PSVB generates a QRS complex similar to that during sinus rhythm, even if both a preexisting bundle branch block (BBB) or the presence of an accessory pathway can change the QRS morphology.

PABs can be unifocal or multifocal, appear at random intervals or after 1, 2, or 3 sinus beats, resulting in a bigeminal, trigeminal, or quadrigeminal rhythm. PSVBs also can occur in pairs or be repetitive, as a result of reciprocation (**Fig. 12**).

Mechanisms

PABs are more frequently caused by a microreentry in the atrial fibers, but sometimes the circuit is macro-reentrant. In other cases, PABs can be caused by an increase in the automaticity or triggered by electric activity (post-potentials). Conversely, PJBs are frequently the result of an ectopic focus or an aborted reentrant atrioventricular (AV) junctional tachycardia. Because their origin is dependent on the baseline heart rhythm, most PSVBs have a fixed or nearly fixed coupling interval, which is the distance from the beginning of the previous sinus P wave to the beginning of the premature ectopic P' (**Fig. 13**). However, premature supraventricular complexes (PSVCs) with an extremely variable coupling interval may

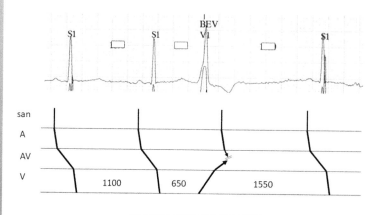

Fig. 5. Electrophysiologic explanation of a fully compensatory post-extrasystolic pause: the premature beat does not reach the sinus node, whose electrical activity remains unchanged. On the ECG, the sum of the coupling interval and the pause (650 + 1550 ms) is equivalent to 2 basic cycles (1100 + 1100 ms).

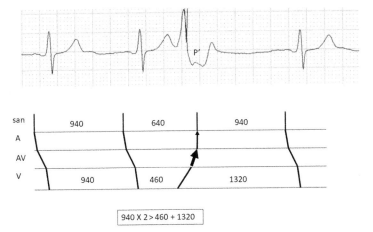

Fig. 6. Electrophysiologic explanation of a not fully compensatory post-extrasystolic pause: the ectopic impulse reaches and depolarizes the sinus node, therefore resetting the sinus cycle. The sum of the coupling interval and the pause (460 + 1320 = 1780 ms) does not compensate the prematurity and is less than 2 basic cycles (940 + 940 = 1880 ms).

originate from an automatic focus. Those are called parasystoles and result from an independent automatic focus, which is protected to be depolarized from the basic rhythm. PSVBs rarely fulfill the ECG criteria for atrial parasystole, such as variable coupling interval, interectopic intervals of P′ being multiples and observation of possible atrial fusion complexes (**Fig. 14**).

Electrocardiogram Findings

A premature "normal" QRS complex generally characterizes a PSVB. The ECG is able to differentiate between an atrial or junctional origin of a supraventricular beat: in case of a PAB, a clear P wave (P′ wave) always precedes ventricular activation. Differently from PABs in the PJBs, the atria are not involved in the focal mechanism; a retrograde P wave can be recorded just before (**Fig. 15**) or after the QRS (**Fig. 16**). A PAB is characterized by a premature ectopic P, which is generally followed by a QRS complex with a normal or slightly prolonged PR interval due to conduction on the slow pathway of the AV node (**Fig. 17**). If the coupling interval of the PAB is very short, the atrial activation

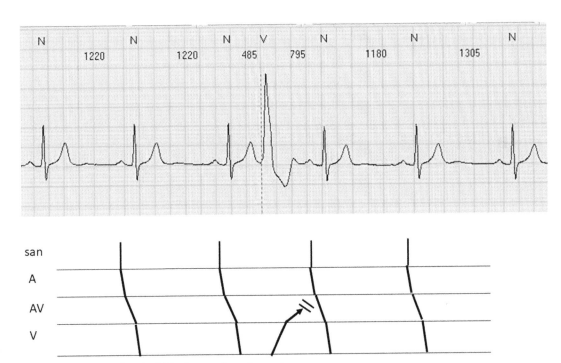

Fig. 7. A PVB interpolated within 2 normal cardiac cycles.

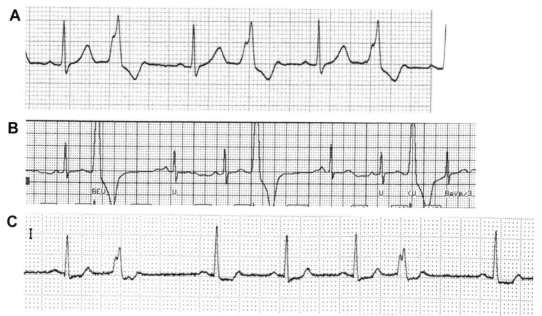

Fig. 8. Example of repetitive sequences of premature beats: on the basis of sequence distribution, premature beats can be classified as bigeminal (*A*), trigeminal (*B*), and quadrigeminal (*C*).

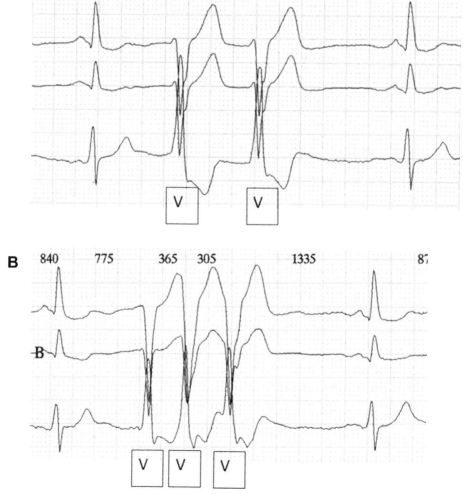

Fig. 9. Complex PVBs organized in a couplet (*A*) and a run of "nonsustained" VT (*B*).

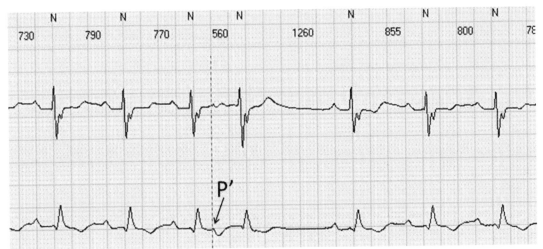

Fig. 10. The ectopic P wave (P′) of a PAB is followed by a long PR interval and a normal QRS complex. The pause is fully compensatory.

can block in the AV junction (see **Fig. 17**). The prematurity of the PAB may widely vary: early complexes may be superimposed on the previous T wave (see **Fig. 17**), whereas late complexes may occur just before the next sinus beat (**Fig. 18**).

P wave morphology
Although the difference might be slight, the P′ wave morphology generally shows a different pattern from the sinus P wave. When the prematurity is very late, an atrial fusion complex can be observed, which is the result of the combined atrial activation from the ectopic focus and the sinus node. A fusion P wave has an intermediate morphology, which reflects both that of the sinus and of the ectopic complex.

The surface ECG can help localize the site of origin (SoO) of the ectopic focus, but is significantly less accurate than the use of a large array of intracardiac and surface electrodes. Several reasons may hinder the correct localization of the source of ectopic activity. First, ectopic foci located at divergent sites can

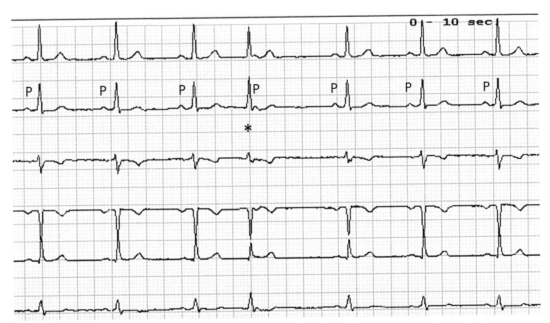

Fig. 11. A PJB: asterisk indicates a premature normal QRS. The sinus P-P sequence remains constant.

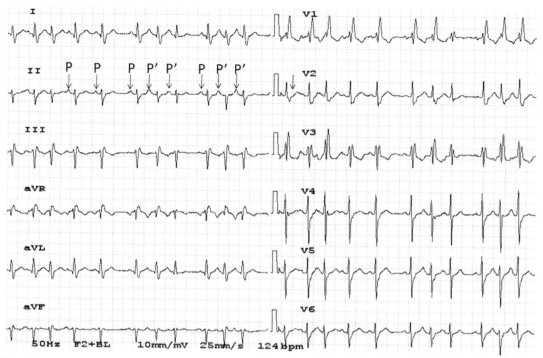

Fig. 12. Recurrent couplets of PABs (P'-P') and short sequences of sinus beat (P).

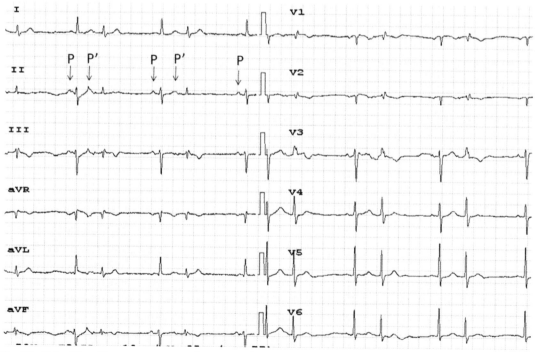

Fig. 13. PABs (P') with a constant coupling interval, bigeminal distribution and aberrant conduction (RBBB pattern).

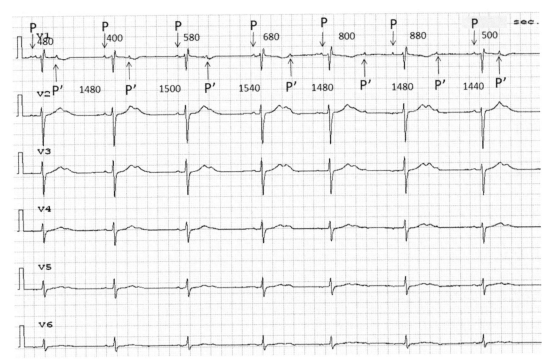

Fig. 14. An example of atrial parasystole. Normal sinus rhythm is present (P-P = 1400 ms). The activity of an automatic focus (P′) is clearly evident and its electrical activity is independent from sinus depolarizations (P-P′ interval varies from 400 to 880 ms); the interectopic intervals (P′-P′) show only little variation (1440–1560 ms).

produce similar P wave patterns.[1] Second, impulses arising from the same site can result in different P wave patterns, as a result of differences in intra-atrial and interatrial conduction.

A sinus P wave has a duration less than 120 ms and an amplitude less than 0.25 mV. Its axis in the frontal plane varies from 0 to +75°, with most falling between +45° and +60°. A normal atrial

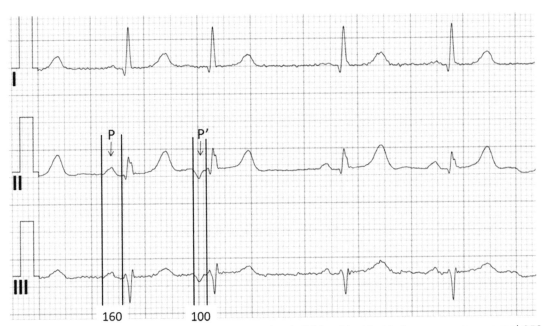

Fig. 15. PJB: a retrograde atrial activation (P′, negative in D2–D3) is evident just before a premature normal QRS (P′-R = 100 ms). The very short P′R interval excludes an atrial origin of the premature beat.

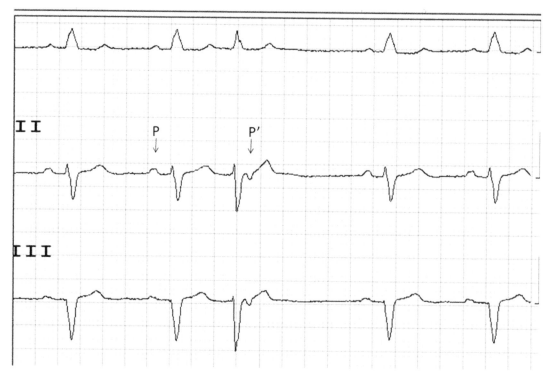

Fig. 16. PJB with retrograde atrial activation (P'), which follows a normal premature QRS complex.

activation has a rounded shape, and is positive in inferior and left precordial leads, which can also display a minimal notched pattern of the apex, as a result of the activation timing of the 2 atria. In lead V1, the P wave is positive or biphasic (positive-negative).

PACs may originate in different sites.[2] P wave configuration in leads I and V1 can be used to differentiate right from left atrial foci, whereas inferior lead (II, III, aVF) patterns can help discriminate

superior or inferior foci. If the focus is near the sinus node, the ectopic P wave simulates the sinus P wave pattern. A sinus P wave, as well as an ectopic one arising near the sinus node, is usually positive-negative in the right precordial leads. However, they may be positive if the late negative component is isoelectric or negative if the early positive component is isoelectric. A negative or biphasic P wave in lead I and a positive P wave in lead V1 predicts a left atrial origin (pulmonary

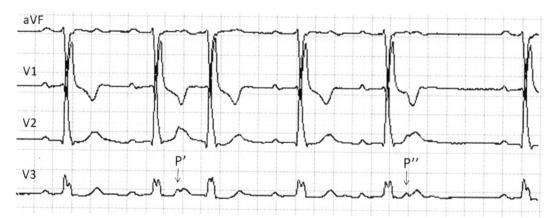

Fig. 17. PABs conducted to the ventricles and blocked in the AV junction. Two ectopic atrial beats (P' and P'') are superimposed on the previous T wave. P' is conducted to the ventricles and displays a long P'R interval. P'' is earlier than P' and is blocked at the level of AV node. The following pause mimics sinus node disease.

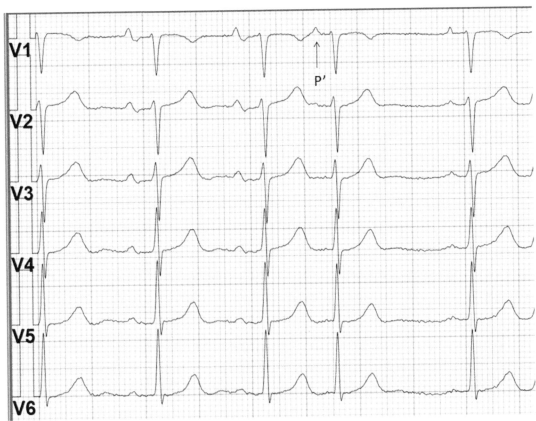

Fig. 18. PAB: the P′ wave follows the end of the previous T wave.

veins), whereas a positive P wave in lead I and a negative one in V1 predicts a right atrial site.[3] A negate or biphasic P wave in lead aVL indicates a left superior pulmonary vein focus. In case of a right atrial site, a negative P wave in lead aVR indicates an ectopic beat arising from crista terminalis; if the P wave in aVR is positive, P wave configuration in leads V5 and V6 can help differentiate between a tricuspid (positive P waves) or a septal (negative P waves) SoO.

If the focus is near the AV junction, the ectopic P wave is inverted in the inferior leads. These findings are similar to those described in case of an ectopic P wave originating in the AV junction (always negative in II, II, and aVF leads). However, an atrial ectopic P wave resulting from a focus in close proximity to the AV junction can be differentiated from a premature AV junctional complex in that the PR interval is usually ≥120 ms.

PR interval
The PR interval of PABs is usually ≥120 ms and may be normal or longer (usually no shorter) than in normal sinus complexes. The PR interval tends to lengthen when the coupling interval is short (see **Fig. 17**); at some point, a very early premature

complex may not be conducted to the ventricles. If the ectopic beat occurs relatively late and the focus is near the SA node, the PR interval is usually similar to the PR interval of the sinus complex. However, it may become shorter if the focus is near the AV node. As previously mentioned, both PABs arising in close proximity to the AV junction and PJBs have negative P waves in the inferior leads, but the PR interval is usually ≥120 ms in case of atrial foci and less than 120 ms if the origin of the ectopic beat is in the AV junction. Additionally, if the conduction of PJBs to the atria is slow, the P′ may be hidden within the QRS, or occur just after the ventricular complex (see **Fig. 16**). Foci arising from atrial epicardial sites usually display a longer PR interval, compared with those from endocardial sites.[4]

Conduction to the ventricles
Conduction of PABs to the ventricles usually does not differ from that of a normal sinus beat. However, 2 other different ways of AV conduction may occur: aberrant intraventricular conduction (**Fig. 19**) and blocking (see **Fig. 17**) in the AV junction, leading to a pause. Aberrant intraventricular conduction is more likely to occur when the RR

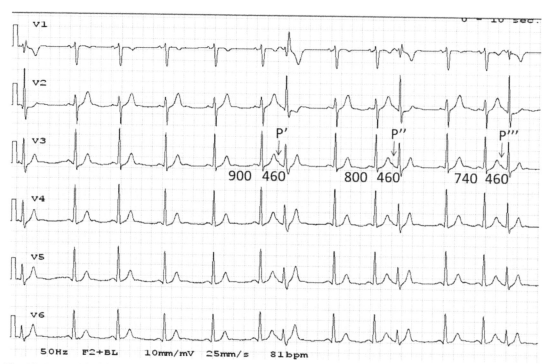

Fig. 19. PABs with different degrees of intraventricular conduction delay. P′, P″, and P‴ have similar coupling intervals (460 ms) but a long RR interval (900 ms) preceding the first ectopic beat (P′) promotes the occurrence of a complete RBBB. P″ and P‴ are conducted with an incomplete RBBB.

interval preceding the ectopic beat is long and the premature impulse appears early (a short RP′ interval). Different degrees of intraventricular conduction delay are possible depending on the prematurity of the ectopic atrial beat (see **Fig. 19**). In the occurrence of aberrant conduction, the QRS pattern has frequently a right BBB (RBBB) morphology, as a result of the relatively longer refractory period of the right branch. Conversely, a left BBB (LBBB) morphology is more common in patients with heart disease and with various QRS morphologies. As previously mentioned, PSVBs may be isolated or occur in runs. When a run of supraventricular tachyarrhythmia occurs, the first premature beats of the run might show a sustained aberrant morphology due to the refractory periods of some sections of the specific conduction system. This aberrant intraventricular conduction represents a slow adaptation of the conduction system to the sudden change in the heart rate, as a result of the Gouaux-Ashman phenomenon. The phenomenon was first described by Gouaux and Ashman in 1947[5] as an aberrant conduction due to a rapid change in QRS cycle length. If a sudden lengthening of the QRS cycle occurs, the subsequent impulse with a normal or shorter cycle length may be conducted with aberrancy, causing diagnostic confusion with PVBs. The Gouaux-

Ashman phenomenon is dependent on the effects of heart rate on the electrophysiological properties of the conduction system, and specifically on the relative refractory period of the components of the conduction system distal to the AV node. Because the refractory period depends on the heart rate and the changes with the R-R interval of the preceding cycle, if a shorter cycle follows a long cycle, the supraventricular impulse may reach the His-Purkinje system while one of its branches is still in the refractory period (relative or absolute). As a result, the impulse is likely to be blocked or conducted with aberrancy. In case of aberrant conduction, the RBBB pattern is more common than the LBBB one, owing to the longer refractory period of the right bundle branch.

In the latter scenario, such as in case of a blocked PSVB leading to a pause, the blocked ectopic complex should not be confused with a second-degree AV block. As a rule, the concealed atrial ectopic complex slightly modifies the preceding T wave and the pause between 2 QRS complexes is similar to that observed when in-between there is an atrial premature complex.

Post-extrasystolic pause

Ectopic impulses arising from supraventricular sites can easily reach and depolarize the SA node, therefore resetting the sinus cycle. As a result, the cycle length after the PSVB is longer than that of the basic sinus rhythm but, unlike that usually observed after PVBs, the pause is not fully compensatory (see **Fig. 19**). In some cases, an ectopic impulse reaching and resetting the SA node can depress the rhythmicity of the sinus node. In the absence of a retrograde depolarization of the SA node, its rhythmicity is undisturbed and the pause is fully compensatory. The PSVB also can be interpolated between 2 normal sinus P waves, as a result of a slow sinus rate and a retrograde SA block.

Premature atrial beats and risk of atrial fibrillation

PABs are a benign phenomenon; however, in some circumstances, they may have a pivotal role in the development of sustained supraventricular arrhythmias. Atrial ectopic foci may trigger atrial fibrillation (AF) and play an important role in disease pathogenesis. Considerable data have suggested that catheter ablation targeting ectopic atrial activity in patients with AF reduces arrhythmia recurrences.[6] Additionally, a correlation between PABs and incident AF in patients without a history of this arrhythmia has been demonstrated in both patients with recent cryptogenic stroke and in the general population.[7,8] From an electrophysiologic standpoint, the main mechanisms in AF are ectopic/triggered activity and reentry. AF can be initiated by 1 or multiple atrial ectopic complexes frequently falling into the atrial vulnerable period. This is the initial mechanism responsible for most cases of paroxysmal AF, especially in patients without structural heart disease (SHD). Those frequent PABs generally have very short coupling intervals, and trigger AF when one of them falls in the atrial vulnerable period. Ectopic activity depends by early afterdepolarizations (ADs) and delayed ADs. Delayed ADs depend on Ca2+-handling abnormalities and favor early ADs.

Reentry circuits can occur around anatomic obstacles when each point of the pathway has sufficient time to regain excitability before the arrival of the next impulse. The wavelength, which results from conduction velocity × effective refractory period, controls the likelihood of anatomic reentry. As a result, the relationship between atrial size and size of reentry circuits is pivotal for the perpetuation of the arrhythmia. Of note, focal ectopic firing also can arise from micro-reentry circuits, rather than from triggered activity. Experimental models have demonstrated that AF can be initiated by a single, automatic focus, as demonstrated by topical application of aconitine to the atrial appendage. In the laboratory, AF also can be induced by rapid pacing, stimulation during the vulnerable period, and isoproterenol and acetylcholine infusion. Compared with that induced by a single focus, which can disappear when the atrium is isolated by the focus, AF initiated by rapid pacing is attributed to a multitude of independent wavelets coursing around islands at different stages of excitability. Yang and colleagues[9] analyzed the PABs during the 5 minutes preceding the onset of paroxysmal AF: patients with high PAB activity had fewer and shorter episodes of AF compared with those with high activity. The first were classified as "trigger fibrillators," whereas the latter, which display a higher AF burden, as a consequence of a high atrial substrate factor, were classified as "substrate fibrillators."

Clinical Implications

PSVBs are a common finding in clinical practice. Among 100 healthy young male and female patients, 24-hour Holter ECG showed PSVBs in 60% of the population, specifically 56% of men[10] and 60% of women.[11] The vast majority of patients experiencing PSVCs do not have any organic heart disease. However, PABs may trigger or terminate any type of atrial and junctional reentrant tachycardia (**Fig. 20**); those kinds of sustained arrhythmias are less frequently triggered by PJBs, which more commonly may be the origin of a junctional tachycardia due to ectopic focus. Although PSVBs are generally benign, it is pivotal to determine their frequency and association with any etiologic factor, their behavior during exercise, and if they are associated with paroxysms of other supraventricular arrhythmias. In patients without manifest heart disease, PSVBs may be triggered by emotional stress, fatigue, digestive problems, smoking, and alcohol and coffee intake, and their prevalence and number increase with increasing age, as well as in the presence of SHD (eg, ischemic heart disease, cor pulmonale) or other comorbidities (eg, thyroid dysfunction, drugs, digitalis intoxication). PSVBs are commonly documented in patients with atrial disease or enlargement; if they are very frequent and premature, and if runs are documented, PSVBs are known to precede the establishment of AF (specifically those arising in the pulmonary veins) or atrial flutter.

PREMATURE VENTRICULAR COMPLEXES

PVBs are premature complexes of ventricular origin, therefore displaying a different, prolonged QRS pattern compared with that of the baseline rhythm. Conventionally, the ectopic activity originates distal to the bifurcation of the His bundle.

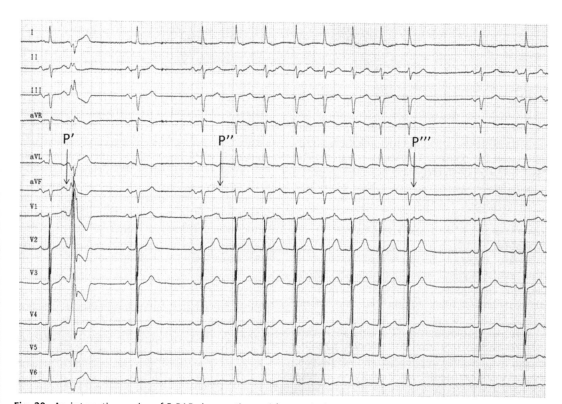

Fig. 20. An interesting series of 3 PABs in a patient with ventricular preexcitation. P′ reveals a ventricular preexcitation (short P′R interval and wide QRS complex). P″ induces a reciprocating tachycardia retrogradely involving the bundle of Kent and P‴ interrupts the same tachycardia.

Foci lying within the His bundle are excluded from the definition, even if this structure is located in the interventricular septum, as well as arrhythmias using an accessory pathway. PVBs can be unifocal or multifocal or appear at random intervals or after 1, 2, or 3 sinus beats, resulting in a bigeminal, trigeminal, or quadrigeminal rhythm. PVBs also can occur in pairs or be repetitive. If PVBs are repetitive, they can form pairs or runs of ventricular tachycardia (VT). As a rule, a VT lasting for more than 30 seconds is classified as sustained.

Mechanisms

PVBs can be caused by extrasystolic or parasystolic mechanisms. Extrasystoles are much more common, and generally show a fixed (**Fig. 21**) or nearly fixed coupling interval (**Fig. 22**); **Fig. 22** shows as a minimal variation of the coupling interval is also able to change the ventriculo/atrial relationship. The mechanism of ectopic ventricular beats may be due to a reentrant mechanism (usually micro-reentry, but sometimes branch-to-branch, or scar-related), and less frequently to triggered activity (post-potentials); in this case the appearance of the VPB depends on a critical range of heart rate (**Fig. 23**). Parasystoles are due to an

ectopic focus, which is protected from the baseline rhythm, as a result of a unidirectional entrance block of the site. In case of parasystole, the coupling intervals are highly variable and the interectopic intervals are multiples of each other (**Fig. 24**). Parasystolic foci can only activate the ventricular myocardium, if the muscle is not in the absolute refractory period, and sometimes exhibit a certain degree of exit block (2:1, 3:1, or Wenckebach-type). As a result, not all parasystolic complexes can be detected in the ECG recording.

Electrocardiogram Findings

PVBs display a premature onset compared with the expected baseline rhythm. The QRS complex has an abnormal duration and pattern, and shows secondary changes of the ST segment and the T wave. Retrograde conduction to the atria may or may not occur (see **Fig. 22**). Because the ectopic impulse frequently does not reach and reset the sinus node, the post-extrasystolic pause is usually fully compensatory (the distance between the QRS complex preceding the PVB and the following complex is twice the sinus cadence). Of note, if the sinus rate is slow, sometimes the

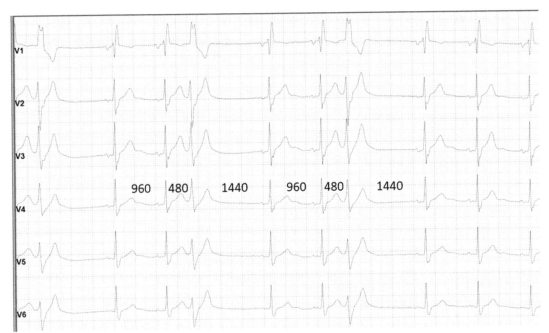

Fig. 21. PVBs displaying a fixed coupling interval and a fully compensatory pause.

following sinus stimulus can be conducted toward the ventricles, even if the PVB enters the AV junction by retrograde concealed conduction in the fast pathway of the AV node; as a result, the sinus front will across the AV node using the slow pathway and the PR interval is consistent. In this type of "interpolated beat" the RR interval containing the VPB is longer than a basal RR interval (**Fig. 25**).

Duration of the QRS complex

The QRS duration of PVBs is the result of the ectopic focus SoO and the characteristics of myocardial tissue. The QRS duration is usually ≥120 ms. This occurs when ectopic foci originate in the Purkinje network or in the ventricular muscle. A wider QRS complex also occurs when the coupling interval is short, as a result of the partial refractoriness of the encountered tissue during impulse conduction. In some cases, foci arise from 1 of the 2 main branches of the bundle of His or in 1 of the 2 divisions of the left bundle branch. In these cases, the QRS duration is <120 ms (narrow fascicular PVB) and the observed pattern may be similar to that of an intra-ventricular conduction block. Of note, patients

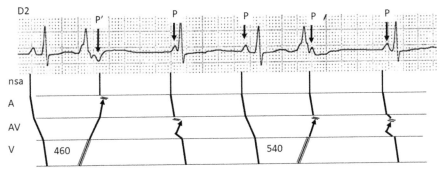

Fig. 22. PVBs with variable coupling intervals; this figure shows how a minimal variation of the coupling interval (460–540 ms) may change the ventriculo/atrial relationship. The first PVB (coupling interval. 460 ms) is retroconducted to the atria and resets sinus node activity; conversely, the second PVB (coupling interval. 540 ms) cannot influence the sinus atrial activation. Both PVBs have a fully compensatory pause and a junctional escape beat can arise.

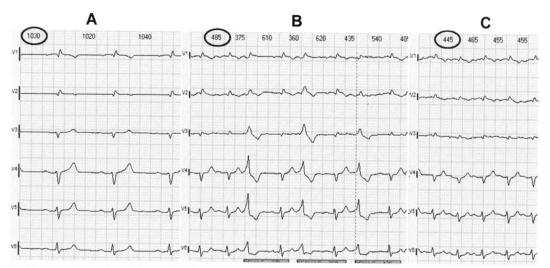

Fig. 23. Cycle-dependent PVBs: a critical range of heart rate may lead to a bigeminal distribution of VPBs (*B*). At lower (*A*) or higher (*C*) heart rates, no VPBs are evident.

with SHD tend to display PVBs with notches and shelves of greater than 40-ms duration and QRS duration greater than 160 ms, which frequently reflect the coexistence of a dilated, globally hypokinetic left ventricle (LV).[12]

Morphology of the QRS complex

PVBs may display different configurations, which usually represent the result of multiple foci causing ectopic beats. However, multiple QRS patters also may be the product of the same

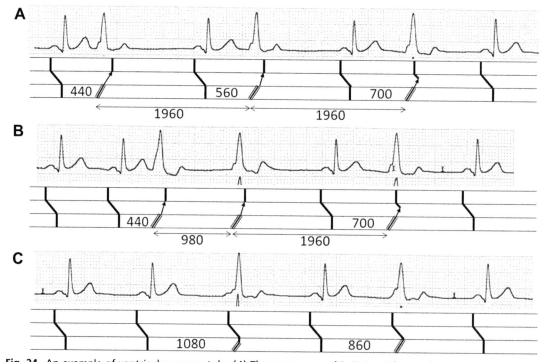

Fig. 24. An example of ventricular parasystole: (*A*) Three monomorphic PVBs with completely variable coupling intervals (440, 560, 700 ms); however, the interectopic intervals are constant (1960 ms). (*B*) The interectopic parasystolic cycle (980 ms). The interectopic intervals are multiple of each other (parasystolic cycle: 980 ms). (*C*) A fusion beat.

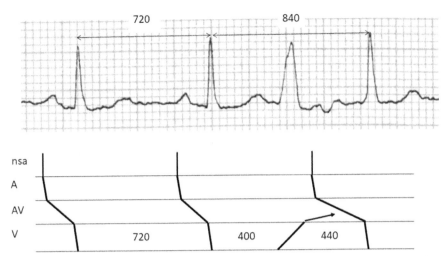

Fig. 25. A pseudo-interpolated PVB: a PVB prolongs the AV conduction time and the PR interval of the following beat results longer. As a consequence, the RR interval containing the PVB is longer than the basal RR interval.

ectopic site, as a result of varying spread of excitation into the ventricles. In this case, which can be commonly described in patients with coronary artery disease, the correct location of the focus SoO can be particularly problematic. Different QRS configurations not caused by multiple ectopic foci can also be observed when (1) the ectopic beat has a long coupling interval, which may lead to several degrees of fusion with the following sinus complex, as well as (2) in couplets, when the second complex can have an additional aberrant conduction secondary to the short RR interval. However, when the coupling intervals are different, different QRS configurations are likely due to multiple foci.

As a general rule, PVBs arising in the right ventricle (RV) generate an LBBB pattern, whereas those arising in the LV generate an RBBB pattern. An accurate analysis of the QRS pattern may provide additional information on the SoO of the ectopic focus. A focus in or near the anterior division of the left bundle branch has a right-ward QRS axis, whereas one in or near the posterior division may display a superior frontal axis. Foci originating from the lateral or inferobasal walls of the LV appear positive in all precordial leads; those originating next to the inferoposterior or superoanterior division of the LBB may have a prominent R wave, frequently with notches in the descending limb of the R wave, without the rsR pattern that is typical of the RBBB.

As previously mentioned, the underlying structural substrate can influence duration and morphology of PVBs. In patients without SHD, ectopic beats of ventricular origin usually have high voltage and a smooth (unnotched) profile of the QRS complex; the ST segment is depressed if the QRS complex is positive, and vice versa, and T waves show asymmetrical branches. In patients with SHD, the ectopic QRS complex is frequently notched and slurred, with a low voltage, and followed by symmetric T waves.

Differential diagnosis between premature supraventricular beats and premature ventricular beats

Premature complexes with wide QRS can result from both supraventricular and ventricular ectopic foci. The first step to differentiate PVBs from PSVBs with aberrant ventricular conduction is finding a P wave preceding the premature QRS complex. The presence of a P wave indicates the supraventricular origin of the ectopic beat. If no P waves can be detected, the focus can be of junctional or ventricular origin. Although the presence of a fully compensatory pause is more likely the result of a PVB, its absence does not allow one to exclude a ventricular ectopy, as a result of retrograde conduction to the SA node. A P wave can be found after the QRS complex in both junctional and ventricular ectopic complexes. This can be either a normal sinus P wave, if no retrograde atrial capture occurs, or a retrograde P wave. In the latter case, an RP interval less than 110 ms is likely due to a PJB, whereas if the interval is ≥200 ms, this is suggestive of a PVB, unless an accessory pathway is present. Another help comes from QRS morphology analysis. The initial forces of an aberrant QRS complex are generally similar to those of the sinus impulse and the pattern has frequently an RBBB morphology. On their side, PVBs tend to display concordant positive or negative precordial leads.

Differential diagnosis of premature ventricular beats in the presence of atrial fibrillation

Differentiation of PVBs during AF with aberrant conduction can be challenging. First of all, the coupling interval may be helpful, as PVBs frequently show a constant coupling interval. Additionally, a longer pause following a wide QRS is generally due to a ventricular ectopy, and results from retrograde penetration of the ventricular impulse into the AV node, which prolongs its refractoriness, hindering anterograde transmission of atrial impulses to the ventricles. Polymorphic wide QRS complexes, especially those displaying various forms of RBBB, generally suggest aberrancy, but also may result from several degrees of fusion among impulses of atrial and ventricular origin.

Clinical Implications

PVBs can be observed in both healthy individuals and patients with heart disease. PVBs can be completely asymptomatic or cause palpitations, chest discomfort, or a transient feeling of absence of pulse. This feeling is more commonly referred by healthy individuals, as a result of a stronger post-extrasystolic potentiation. The frequency of PVBs increases with age, being very common in asymptomatic men after the age of 50. Emotional and physical stress, as well as coffee, alcohol, ginseng, and energy drinks, may promote the development of PVBs. SHD increases frequency and complexity of PVBs, regardless of the degree of LV functional impairment. In healthy individuals, various frequencies of PVBs can be found in approximately 40% to 55% of patients.[10,13] They may increase, decrease, or be totally suppressed by exercise; conversely, they may be triggered by exercise, even if they are absent at rest. In the absence of SHD, the prognosis is excellent; however, it is very uncommon to observe ventricular functional impairment with heart failure. This condition, known as arrhythmia-induced cardiomyopathy, may totally or partially subside after catheter ablation of the ventricular ectopic foci, causing frequent PVBs.[14] Additionally, frequent PVBs, and/or rapid/long runs of PVBs can cause hemodynamic impairment or promote the development of a sustained VT. Patients with SHD show a very high prevalence of PVBs: in patients with chronic ischemic heart disease, their prevalence is approximately 90%, with an estimated risk of developing sustained ventricular arrhythmias 4 times higher than that of healthy individuals.[15] The prevalence of PVBs among patients with an acute coronary syndrome is even higher, reaching 100% of patients, and carrying a very high risk of life-threatening ventricular arrhythmias even several months after the acute ischemic episode. PVBs also are common in patients with cardiomyopathies, and other types of organic heart disease, as well as in patients with digitalis excess.

SUMMARY

Premature beats are commonly found in the general population as well as in patients with SHD. Although frequently benign, they can be responsible for the induction of sustained supraventricular and ventricular arrhythmia. The surface ECG is a valuable tool, which can help identify the SoO of the ectopic focus and suggest eventual clinical strategies to manage these arrhythmias.

REFERENCES

1. Chen SA, Tai CT, Chiang CE, et al. Role of the surface electrocardiogram in the diagnosis of patients with supraventricular tachycardia. Cardiol Clin 1997;15:539–65.
2. Bagliani G, Leonelli F, Padeletti L. P wave and the substrates of arrhythmias originating in the atria. Card Electrophysiol Clin 2017;9:365–82.
3. Michelucci A, Bagliani G, Colella A, et al. P wave assessment: state of the art update. Card Electrophysiol Rev 2002;6:215–20.
4. Waldo AL, Vitikainen KJ, Harris PD, et al. The P wave and the P-R interval: effects of the site of origin of atrial depolarization. Circulation 1970;42: 426–34.
5. Gouaux JL, Ashman R. Auricular fibrillation with aberration stimulating ventricular paroxysmal tachycardia. Am Heart J 1947;34:366.
6. Haïssaguerre M, Jaïs P, Shah DC, et al. Spontaneous initiation of atrial fibrillation by ectopic beats originating in the pulmonary veins. N Engl J Med 1998;339:659–66.
7. Wallmann D, Tüller D, Wustmann K, et al. Frequent atrial premature beats predict paroxysmal atrial fibrillation in stroke patients: an opportunity for a new diagnostic strategy. Stroke 2007;38:2292–4.
8. Dewland TA, Vittinghoff E, Mandyam MC, et al. Atrial ectopy as a predictor of incident atrial fibrillation: a cohort study. Ann Intern Med 2013;159:721–8.
9. Yang A, Ruiter J, Pfeiffer D, et al. Identification of "substrate fibrillators" and "trigger fibrillators" by pacemaker diagnostics. Heart Rhythm 2006;3: 682–8.
10. Brodsky M, Wu D, Denes P, et al. Arrhythmias documented by 24 hour continuous electrocardiographic monitoring in 50 male medical students without apparent heart disease. Am J Cardiol 1977;39: 390–5.

11. Sobotka PA, Mayer JH, Bauernfeind RA, et al. Arrhythmias documented by 24-hour continuous ambulatory electrocardiographic monitoring in young women without apparent heart disease. Am Heart J 1981;101:753–9.

12. Moulton KP, Medcalf T, Lazzara R. Premature ventricular complex morphology. A marker for left ventricular structure and function. Circulation 1990;81:1245–51.

13. Kostis JB, Moreyra AE, Amendo MT, et al. The effect of age on heart rate in subjects free of heart disease. Studies by ambulatory electrocardiography and maximal exercise stress test. Circulation 1982;65:141–5.

14. Della Rocca DG, Santini L, Forleo GB, et al. Novel perspectives on arrhythmia-induced cardiomyopathy: pathophysiology, clinical manifestations and an update on invasive management strategies. Cardiol Rev 2015;23:135–41.

15. Ruberman W, Weinblatt E, Goldberg JD, et al. Ventricular premature beats and mortality after myocardial infarction. N Engl J Med 1977;297:750–7.

Advanced Concepts of Atrioventricular Nodal Electrophysiology
Observations on the Mechanisms of Atrioventricular Nodal Reciprocating Tachycardias

Giuseppe Bagliani, MD[a,b,*], Fabio M. Leonelli, MD[c], Roberto De Ponti, MD, FHRS[d], Luigi Padeletti, MD[e,f]

KEYWORDS

- Atrioventricular node • Electrophysiology • Arrhythmias • Reentrant tachycardia
- Supraventricular tachycardias

KEY POINTS

- Atrioventricular node reentrant tachycardia is a supraventricular arrhythmia easily diagnosed by 12-lead electrocardiogram (ECG).
- The pathways used in the reentry circuits can have multiform presentations (typical or atypical).
- The intracardiac and esophageal recordings supplement the standard ECG to attempt the reconstruction of the reentrant circuits.
- We observe the multiform electrocardiographic aspects to better understand the anatomy and electrophysiology of the atrioventricular node (AVN).

INTRODUCTION

The definition of typical atrioventricular node reentrant tachycardia (AVNRT)[1] postulates the presence of a dual atrioventricular node (AVN) transmission system with a slowly conducting pathway with shorter refractory period (α pathway) and a fast conduction pathway with a longer refractory period (β pathway).[2]

During sinus rhythm the activation wavefront conducts to the ventricles entering both pathways. The faster conducting pathway delivers the impulse to the His-Purkinje system.[3] The wavefront traveling through the slow pathway (**Fig. 1**) blocks finding the lower end of the AVN/His junction rendered refractory by the impulse conducted through the fast pathway: this concealed conduction of the slow pathway into the atrioventricular junction prevents during sinus rhythm the retrograde conduction through the slow pathway.

A premature atrial depolarization can block in the fast pathway and conduct slowly down the slow pathway (**Fig. 2**); in this situation the

Disclosure: The authors have nothing to disclose.
[a] Cardiology Department, Arrhythmology Unit, Foligno General Hospital, Via Massimo Arcamone, Foligno 06034, Italy; [b] Cardiovascular Diseases Department, University of Perugia, Piazza Menghini 1, 06129 Perugia, Italy; [c] Cardiology Department, James A. Haley Veterans' Hospital, University South Florida, 13000 Bruce B Down Boulevard, Tampa, FL 33612, USA; [d] Cardiology Department, University of Insubria, Via Ravasi, 2, 21100 Varese, Italy; [e] Heart and Vessels Department, University of Florence, Largo Brambilla, 3, Florence 50134, Italy; [f] IRCCS Multimedica, Cardiology Department, Via Milanese, 300, 20099 Sesto San Giovanni, Italy
* Corresponding author. Via Centrale Umbra 17, Spello, Perugia 06038, Italy.
E-mail address: giuseppe.bagliani@tim.it

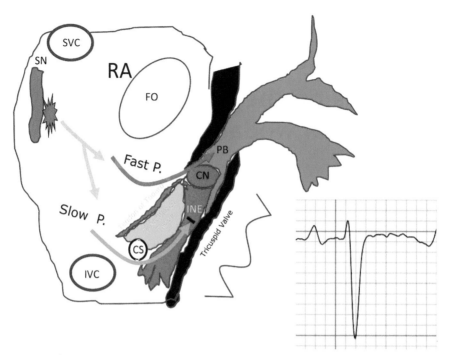

Fig. 1. Propagation of normal sinus rhythm in the junctional region (fast pathway). The red arrows show the fast pathway conduction of the sinus atrial depolarization to the His-Purkinje system. The blue arrow shows the concealed conduction of the slow pathway into the atrioventricular junction. CN, compact node; CS, coronary sinus; FO, fossa ovalis; INE, inferior nodal extension; IVC, inferior vena cava; PB, penetrating bundle; RA, right atrium; SN, sinus node; SVC, superior vena cava. On the electrocardiogram is evident a normal PR interval duration.

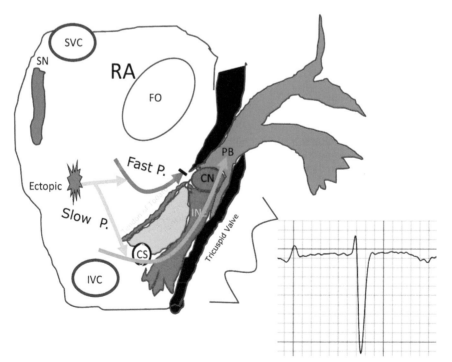

Fig. 2. Propagation of premature ectopic beat in the junctional region (slow pathway) The blue arrow shows the slow pathway conduction of the ectopic atrial depolarization to the His-Purkinje system. The red arrow shows the concealed conduction of the fast pathway. A prolonged PR interval duration is evident.

concealed conduction is in the fast pathway. The conduction change from fast to slow pathway, in some case defined as "jump," is well evident on the surface electrocardiogram (ECG) as a prolonged PR interval (**Fig. 3**). If antegrade conduction is longer than the refractory period of the fast pathway the depolarization wavefront propagates retrogradely and rapidly along the fast pathway. This generates an echo beat with electrocardiographic evidence of a retrograde P at the end of QRS. Repetition of activation along this circuit is the base for typical or slow/fast AVNRT (**Fig. 4**).

Together with this typical form of AVNRT, other, more uncommon, reentrant circuits have been observed,[4] where the fast pathway is used for antegrade conduction and the slow pathway for retrograde conduction (fast/slow) (**Fig. 5**). Furthermore, multiple pathways are observed in a minority of patients generating reentrant circuits with more variable antegrade and retrograde conduction.[5] This complex conduction pattern explains an even rarer form of AVNRT,[6] where both antegrade and retrograde propagation occurs on slow conducting pathways (slow/slow AVNRT) (**Fig. 6**).

The reasons why typical AVNRT represents the arrhythmia circuit in more than 90% of cases are the "preferential conduction" over the slow pathway by premature atrial ectopy (**Fig. 7**) and the favored engagement of the fast pathway by premature ventricular beats. Two reasons account for this strict relationship between pathways and origin of premature beats. First, the longer refractoriness of the fast pathway, which is related to an increased expression of sodium channels in these cells leading to a larger cellular inflow of this ion during depolarization. This requires a longer time to extrude intracellular sodium ions prolonging repolarization and membrane refractory period. Second, the preferential conduction using the fast pathway during premature ventricular beats, retro-conducting to the atria using the His-AVN system. This conduction is determined by the anatomic connections between the proximal His bundle and the fast pathway.

A large number of reported cases of AVNRT do not fit the schematic explanation of a dual pathway AVN conduction system previously presented. It is therefore necessary, at times, to speculate the existence of multiple conducting pathways with different electrophysiologic properties extending within the junctional region.

Furthermore, the atrial and ventricular connections via the His-Purkinje system do not behave as simple electrical conduit. Conduction blocks varying from high degree to 2:1 have

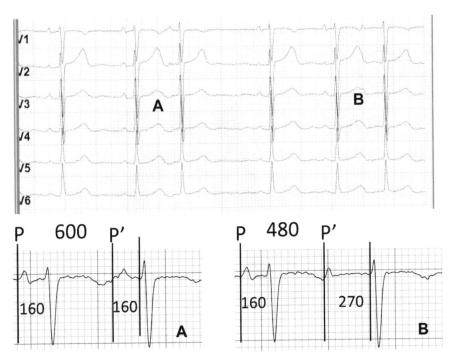

Fig. 3. Ectopic atrial beats with different coupling interval and PR duration. (*A*) P-P' coupling interval of 600 ms corresponds to a normal PR interval (160 ms). The ectopic beat transits through the fast pathway. (*B*) Shorter P-P' coupling interval (480 ms) corresponds to a prolonged PR interval (270 ms). The fast pathway is now refractory and the atrial depolarization conducts through the fast pathway.

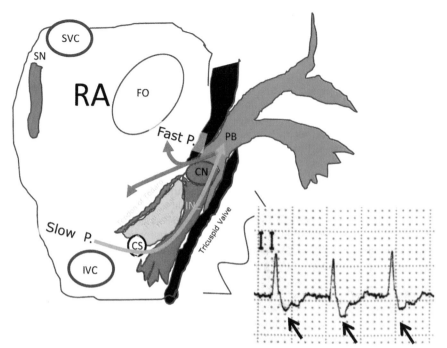

Fig. 4. The circuit of typical or slow/fast AVNRT. Antegrade conduction through the slow pathway and retrograde conduction through the fast pathway. Note the terminal part of retrograde atrial activation at the end of the QRS (*black arrows*).

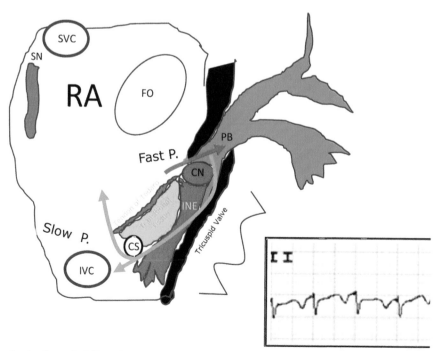

Fig. 5. The circuit of atypical (fast/slow) AVNRT. The antegrade conduction is along the fast pathway (short PR) and retrograde activation via the slow pathway (long R-P).

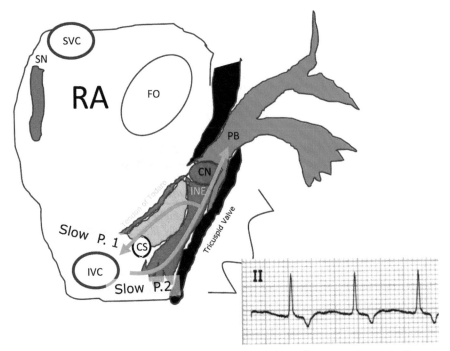

Fig. 6. The circuit of atypical (slow/slow) AVNRT. Both antegrade and retrograde conduction are using two different slow conducting intranodal pathways.

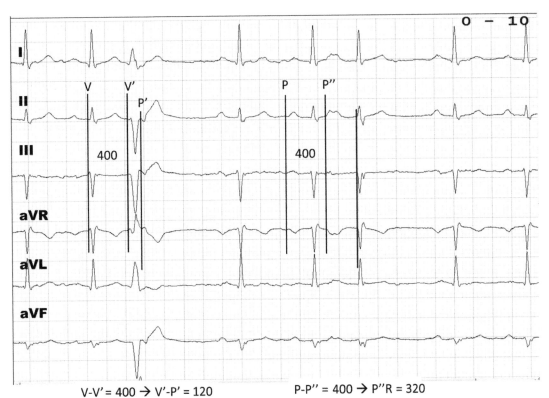

Fig. 7. Preferential conduction of ectopic beats into the AV junction. Different conduction behavior of atrial (PAB) and ventricular (PVB) premature beats through the AVN. Both beats occur with the same degree of prematurity (V-V' = 400; P-P'' = 400 ms); the PVB retro-conducts to the atria with a short V-P interval (V'-P' = 120 ms) suggestive of fast pathway conduction. On the contrary, the PAB conducts to the ventricle through the slow pathway (P''R = 320 ms).

been reported rendering the ECG presentation and the understanding of the arrhythmia circuit more puzzling. Despite its obvious complexities, a close observation of all available ECG tracings is usually sufficient to clarify the mechanism of reentry.

CASE 1
Common Atrioventricular Node Reentrant Tachycardia: Double Physiology of the Atrioventricular Node and Two-Way Sustaining the Circus Movement Tachycardia

The patient is a 40-year-old woman with recurrent episodes of paroxysmal tachycardias (**Fig. 8**). There was initiation of typical AVNRT during an electrophysiologic study (**Fig. 9**). A premature atrial beat introduced at the end of a train of atrial stimuli at CL 600 millisecond blocks in the fast pathway and suddenly conducts to the ventricle using the slow pathway. In the intracardiac recording this is documented by a sudden prolongation in conduction time through the AVN with an increase (jump) of the interval between the atria (A)

and the common His (H). This is followed by a retro conduct beat (A') reaching the atria via the fast pathway and initiates the supraventricular tachycardia (SVT). The retrograde conduction time (H-A' interval) is measured from the H to the retrograde A and is clearly longer than the antegrade (A'-H interval).

CASE 2
Uncommon, Fast-Slow, Atrioventricular Node Reentrant Tachycardia: Three Atrioventricular Node Conducting Pathway?

The patient is a 60-year-old man, healthy and physically fit, complaining of fast regular palpitations at rest and during effort with presyncope. The initial ECG (**Fig. 10**) shows a sinus rhythm with ventricular parasystolic focus (VPC) with variable couple interval to the preceding QRS (500-580-630). A sinus P wave is seen buried in the ST of the VPC. The sinus rate remains unchanged. Absence of sinus node resetting strongly suggests that no retrograde conduction along a fast pathway is present. The patient experiences

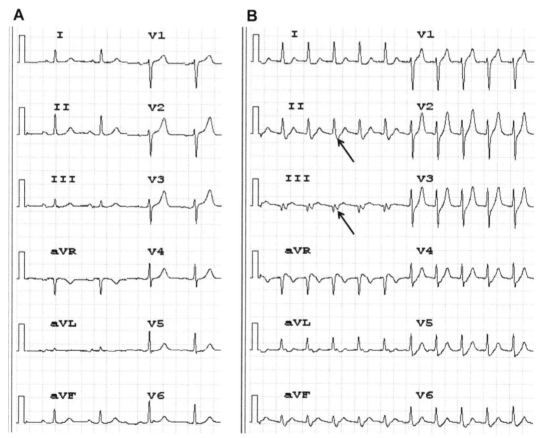

Fig. 8. Case 1, Typical slow/fast AVN reciprocating tachycardia. (*A*) Normal sinus rhythm. (*B*) Tachycardia is shown. Note, in inferior leads, the negative P wave (*arrows*) immediately after the QRS.

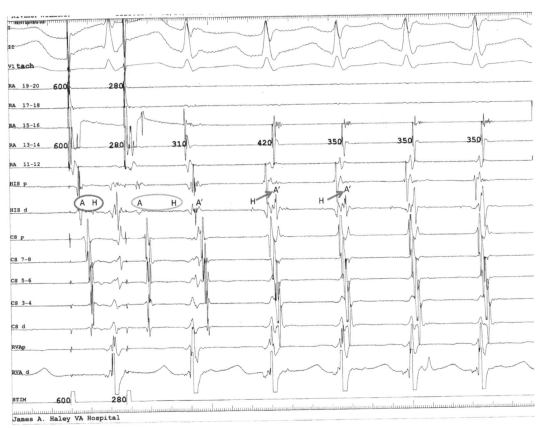

Fig. 9. Case 1, electrophysiologic study in patient with episodes of common AVN supraventricular tachycardia. After a train of atrial stimulation at CL 600 ms a premature atrial depolarization is delivered (coupling 280 ms). The AVN conduction, represented by the AH Interval, during pacing train is 80 ms (*red circle*) in keeping with fast AVN pathway conduction. The premature atrial stimulation finds the fast pathway refractory and it conducts along the slow pathway with an AH of 200 ms (*blue circle*). Antegrade conduction is followed by a retrograde atrial depolarization (A′) via the fast pathway, which is now no longer refractory. Note the short H-A′ of 105 ms (*red arrows*) representing the turnaround time from the lower common pathway to the atria.

an episode of clinical SVT at CL of 580 milliseconds (**Fig. 11**). The arrhythmia is a regular narrow complex tachycardia with a clear retrograde P wave with 1:1 atrioventricular ratio and an R-P interval of 440 milliseconds longer than a P-R of 140 milliseconds. Differential diagnosis includes an atypical slow/fast AVNRT, an atrial tachycardia (AT), and an orthodromic tachycardia using a decremental conducting concealed accessory pathway as in Paroxysmal Junctional Reciprocating Tachycardia (PJRT). The ECG suggests an unusual mechanism of induction (**Fig. 12**; following the last VPC, the T wave shows a "hump" in time with a P-P interval). This sinus beat conducts to the ventricles with a slightly longer P-R (240 milliseconds compared with the usual value of 180 milliseconds) suggesting that the Premature Ventricular Contraction (PVC) has penetrated into the AVN slowing the following antegrade conduction along the fast pathway. These observations suggest a macro reentry that includes the AVN

and practically excludes an AT, which is unlikely to be induced by a normal sinus beat. This mechanism is confirmed by an esophageal recording that documents the beginning of a nonsustained run of SVT. The possibility of a slow conducting retrograde AP is ruled out by observing the response of the SVT to a VPC (**Fig. 13**). The premature beat does not alter the tachycardia cycle length (CL) leaving P-P and subsequent R-R interval unchanged. This could only happen if the ventricle is not a necessary link of the arrhythmia. In orthodromic tachycardia premature capture of the ventricle would have affected the reentrant circuit. An early VPC would have probably terminated the arrhythmia by blocking in a refractory AP; a later timed VPC could have retro-conducted via the AP to the atria advancing (or delaying in the case of a decremental AP) the next P. Having already excluded an AT as a mechanism of this arrhythmia, AVNRT remains the only possible candidate.

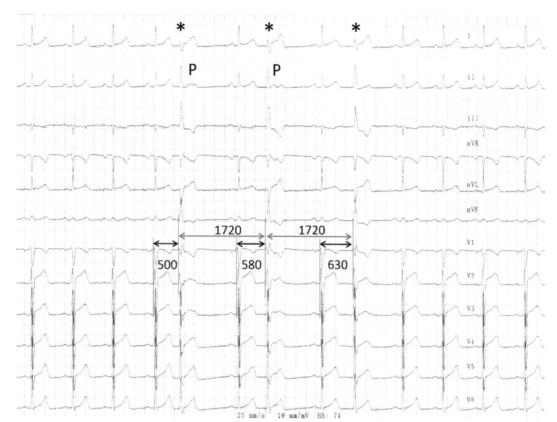

Fig. 10. Case 2, sinus rhythm and parasystolic ventricular focus in patient with recurrent palpitation. The figure shows a sequence of five beats of normal sinus origin. Then three ectopic beats (*asterisk*) with completely variable coupling (500-580-630). Note the presence of undisturbed sinus P waves (P) occurring after the parasystolic QRS. The absence of resetting of the sinus node strongly suggests the absence of a retro-conducting fast pathway.

A treadmill stress test was also performed to assess the mechanism of the elevate heart rates reported by the patient. The patient was in SVT CL 520 milliseconds at the beginning of the test. As the effort increased, the CL of the tachycardia shortened to reach 310 milliseconds. The retrograde conduction is the part of the reentrant circuit most sensitive to the effect of catecholamines as demonstrated by progressive shortening of the R-P in the face of an unchanged P-R (**Fig. 14**).

CASE 3
A Sinus Rhythm with 1:2 Atrioventricular Ratio and Uncommon, Slow-Slow, Atrioventricular Node Reentrant Tachycardia: Three Atrioventricular Node Pathway

The patient is a 40-year-old man without previous cardiac history evaluated because of symptoms of irregular palpitations. The initial ECG (**Fig. 15**) demonstrates an irregular rhythm with clear P waves and variable R-R interval occurring in couplets. Measuring the P-P interval, it shows sinus

rhythm at CL 640 milliseconds with a premature narrow complex QRS occurring 400 milliseconds from previous QRS. Every ventricular depolarization is preceded by a sinus P wave with the exception of the premature beat.

Although the mechanism of the premature QRS could be explained by junctional ectopy, the fixed relationship with the previous P and QRS suggests a dependence of the ectopic beat from the previous normal sinus beat. During the same evaluation the patient was observed to have periods of nonsustained SVT with a cycle length of 560 milliseconds (**Fig. 16**). The arrhythmia is characterized by an R-P interval shorter than the P-R interval (respectively, 140 milliseconds and 420 milliseconds). AVNRT or orthodromic tachycardia is suggested by the termination of the arrhythmia with a P wave. Interestingly, the previously discussed ectopy reoccurs as soon as the tachycardia is terminated suggesting a possible link between the two observations.

During electrophysiological study (EPS), the phenomenon is explained **Fig. 17**. The recording

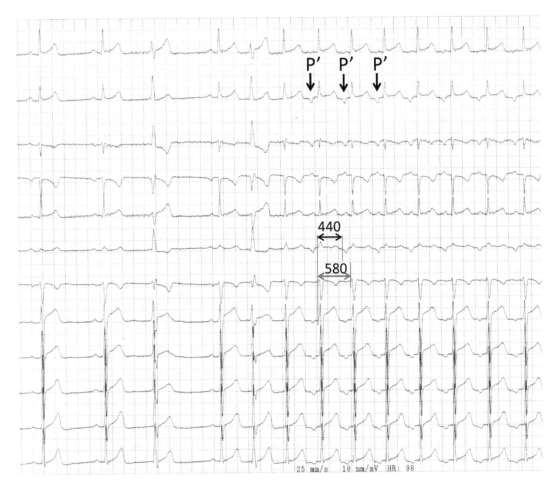

Fig. 11. Case 2, initiation of SVT following a parasystolic ventricular beat. Episode of clinical SVT at CL of 580 ms. The arrhythmia is a regular narrow complex tachycardia with a clear retrograde P wave with 1:1 atrioventricular ratio and an R-P′ interval of 440 ms, longer than a P′-R of 140 ms. Usually, a VPC to induce SVT needs to penetrate one arm of a possible reentry circuit (AVN or AP) or retro-conduct prematurely to the atria to induce atrial tachycardia. In this case no clear retro-conducted atrial depolarization is evident (see **Fig. 12** and text for further explanation).

shows how a sinus beat is conducted to the ventricle with a short A-H of 80 milliseconds using the fast pathway. This is followed by another ventricular beat preceded by a His deflection. A coincidental sinus beat occurs at the time of the ventricular depolarization and conducts to the ventricle using a slow pathway with an A-H of 260 milliseconds. The ventricular depolarization is followed by an echo beat with a long H-A of 150 milliseconds. The most likely explanation for these findings is that the first sinus beat conducted to the ventricle twice using a fast pathway for the first V (A-H = 80 milliseconds) and a slow pathway for the second ventricular depolarization (A-H = 410 milliseconds). The subsequent sinus beat, occurring at the time of the V, conducts to the ventricle using the same slow pathway (similar

A-H of 260 milliseconds). This suggests that the previous antegrade beat penetrated the fast pathway retrogradely but could not depolarize the atria already activated by the slightly earlier sinus beat.

Finally, the echo beat occurs because the retrograde activation is earlier than the subsequent sinus depolarization. With sufficient time, the retrograde activation returns to the atria using a slow pathway with a long turnaround time (H-A interval of 150 milliseconds). **Fig. 18** depicts the end of an episode of tachycardia and the first following sinus beat. The tachycardia is regular with mean RR interval of 400 milliseconds; the retro-conducted P wave (negative in inferior leads) is clearly evident after the QRS. The antegrade and retrograde pathway of the reentry circuit

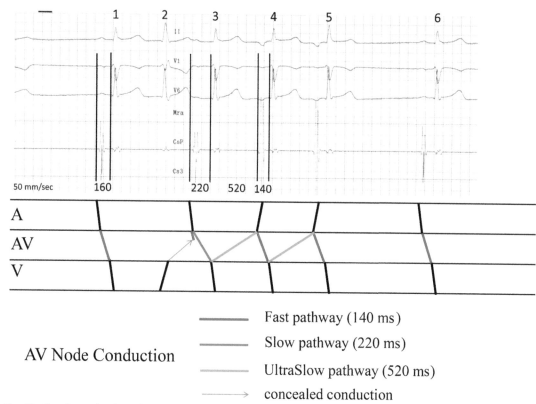

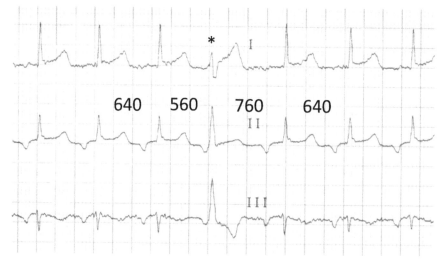

Fast pathway (140 ms)

Slow pathway (220 ms)

UltraSlow pathway (520 ms)

→ concealed conduction

AV Node Conduction

Fig. 12. Case 2, mechanism of induction of a nonsustained episode of supraventricular tachycardia and the role of ectopic ventricular beat. Same case of **Fig. 11**. Beat 1 is a normal sinus conducted QRS. The esophageal recording confirms the induction mechanism suspected on the ECG analysis. VPC (beat 2) is followed by a sinus beat, which conducts to the ventricles (beat 3) with a prolonged A-V interval in keeping with retrograde AVN penetration by the preceding ventricular beat. The sinus origin of the P is confirmed by its morphology on ECG and esophageal recording and the P to esophageal recording time. The possibility of fast pathway antegrade conduction being modulated by the VPC cannot be excluded, but in view of the marked prolongation of the PR (220 ms at similar CL) the hypothesis of a slow antegrade conducting pathway (*blue line*) is favored. Two beats[4,5] of the clinical tachycardia follow. Beat 6 is a normal conducted sinus beat.

Fig. 13. Case 2, AVNRT as the mechanism of the arrhythmia. This tracing excludes the possibility of an accessory pathway dependent SVT and confirms AVNRT as the mechanism of the arrhythmia. During the clinical SVT at CL 640 ms a premature VPB (*asterisk*) occurs with a coupling interval of 560 ms. Despite the VPC the tachycardia continues unchanged demonstrating that the ventricle is not a necessary part of the tachycardia. This is inconsistent with an orthodromic tachycardia where a VPC would have either reset or terminate the arrhythmia.

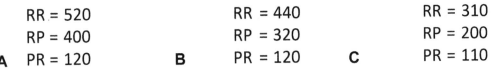

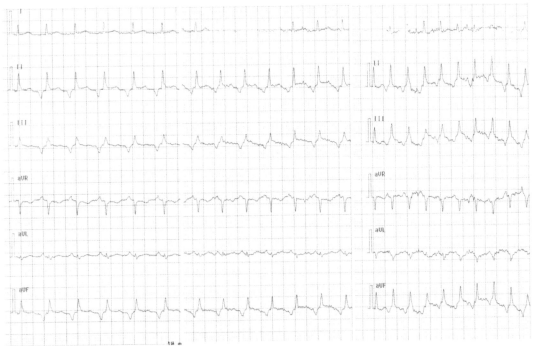

Fig. 14. Case 2, stress test and SVT. The patient developed SVT during stress test. A, B, C are three stages of the ergometric test, respectively basal, intermediate and maximum. As the effort increases there is a progressive shortening of the CL of the arrhythmia (RR) from 520 ms to 310 ms. The decrease in CL is completely accounted for by a shortening of retro-conduction time (R-P) from 400 to 200 ms. Antegrade conduction is mostly unchanged varying from 120 to 110 ms during the increase in SVT rate.

are well characterized, respectively, by the A-H (240 milliseconds) and H-A intervals (160 milliseconds); this sequence suggests a slow-slow AVNRT circuit with the antegrade path particularly slow. A third nodal pathway is evident during sinus rhythm with the shortest interval of the series (A-H interval = 50 milliseconds).

This recording does not exclude an orthodromic tachycardia as the mechanism of the SVT, but previous observations and maneuvers during the study confirmed AVNRT. The tachycardia has been successfully treated with slow pathway ablation.

CASE 4
Transient Atrioventricular 2:1 Block During Atrioventricular Node Supraventricular Tachycardia: The His Alternans Phenomenon

A young soccer player of 14 years of age undergoes a 24-hour Holter monitor to evaluate a complaint of recurrent palpitations. The tracing of **Fig. 19** shows an initial atrial rhythm at cycle length

of 840 milliseconds with PR interval of 110 milliseconds changing into a faster sinus rhythm with a cycle length of 690 milliseconds and PR of 130 milliseconds; a transitional P wave (P1→P2→P3) between the two rhythms let us hypothesize a wandering pacemaker. Three premature atrial beats (P′) induce a regular narrow complex tachycardia (R-R interval 600 milliseconds). The arrhythmia is characterized by an R-P of 320 milliseconds and a P-R of 280 milliseconds. At this point, considering the initiation and the R-P/P-R relation, the most likely diagnosis is AT. **Fig. 20** shows a sudden acceleration of the tachycardia preceded by three aberrant complexes with QRS of similar morphologies but varying QRS width. The SVT continues at a cycle length of 310 milliseconds, doubling the initial heart rate. No clear atrial depolarization is visible. A PVC terminates the arrhythmia **Fig. 21**. The diagnosis rests between an AT with a normalization of a 2:1 exit block or AVNRT with a change in antegrade conduction from 2:1 to 1:1.

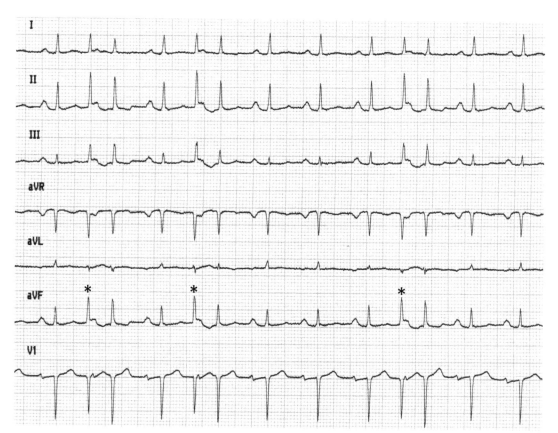

Fig. 15. Case 3, a premature beat of unclear origin. This ECG shows sinus rhythm with CL 640 ms, with a premature R (*asterisk*) of unclear origin. Measuring relevant intervals shows a P to ectopic R (*asterisk*) of 600 ms and an R to ectopic R of 400 ms. These intervals remain the same for the three observed events. The R (*asterisk*) is not preceded by a P wave and initially seems to be an ectopic junctional beat. Timing does not support the hypothesis of a parasystolic focus; furthermore, the fixed relationship with the preceding sinus beat suggests a close mechanistic relationship between these two beats.

The diagnosis was definitively obtained by a transesophageal pacing. Premature atrial stimulation by double stimuli (**Fig. 22**) was followed by an abrupt prolongation of the PQ and induction of the tachycardia with a 2:1 A:V ratio. The tachycardia spontaneously ended by a ventricular premature beat that confirmed definitively the diagnosis of intranodal reentry: the ectopic beat is able to stop the tachycardia without any depolarization of the atria and so excluding the hypothesis of an intra-atrial reentry (**Fig. 23**).

What Is the True Meaning of the 2:1 Atrioventricular Block? His Alternans Phenomenon

Differently from the classical Hisian block, the impaired atrioventricular conduction that commonly realizes during intranodal reentry is not in the bundle of His but in the point of connection between the AVN and the His bundle proper. This explains why the patient was able, during effort, to reach heart rates in sinus tachycardia similar to the AVNRT rates without evidence of conduction block. The explanation, commonly called His alternans, is likely caused by the different inputs into the bundle of His in AVNRT and sinus rhythm.[7] During sinus tachycardia the activation wavefront is transmitted to the anterior portion of the His bundle via the fast pathway (**Fig. 24**A). During AVNRT the antegrade activation proceeds, via the slow pathway, to the posterior portion of the His bundle **Fig. 24**B. This posterior zone of the proximal His bundle has a higher expression of fast conducting/long refractory sodium channels with respect to the corresponding anterior zone: the block in the posterior His bundle, similarly to the one observed in our patient, has a relevant functional component and disappears with the rate-related shortening of the refractory period (see **Fig. 20**).

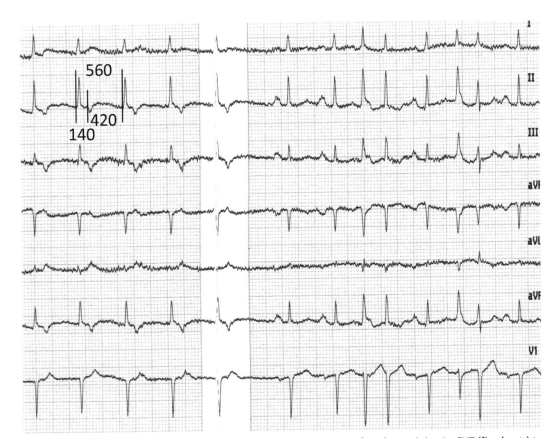

Fig. 16. Case 3, termination of SVT, sinus rhythm, and premature beat of unclear origin. An SVT (five beats) terminates with a retrograde P wave. This strongly suggests an AVNRT or orthodromic tachycardia as the mechanism of the arrhythmia. The SVT has a long PR of 420 ms and an R-P of 140 ms suggesting a retrograde conduction using a slow AVN pathway or a lateral concealed AP. Also note the reoccurrence of the phenomenon described in **Fig. 15**.

CASE 5
Atrioventricular Node Playing Hooky: Is Atrial Tissue Involved in the Reentry Circuit?

The patient is a 64-year-old man with recurrent palpitations, presyncope, and documented regular tachycardia. Baseline ECG shows sinus rhythm with right bundle branch block; during the tachycardia (**Fig. 25**) the morphology of the QRS is identical to sinus rhythm. There is an obvious retrograde P wave at the end of the QRS with retrograde 2:1 ventriculoatrial block. This ECG strongly suggests the presence of AVNRT with fixed right bundle branch block and a 2:1 retrograde block. AT or orthodromic tachycardia could not explain these findings. In AVNRT most of the atrium is not a necessary part of the tachycardia circuit. This can easily be demonstrated by introducing premature atrial stimuli during AVNRT and observing capture of atrial tissue around the AVN without interfering with AVNRT circuit. This observation leads to the controversial issue of whether the

AVNRT reentrant circuit is entirely intranodal or whether some components of the atria or His bundle are required.[8] Although there is no conclusive answer to this question, evidence gathered during surgical or radiofrequency modification of the AVN suggests that some of the reentrant circuit involves tissue above and below the AVN. The extension of the atrial component of the circuit in typical AVNRT is only speculative and some authors have suggested a participation of a portion of up to 3 cm of atrial tissue inferior to the AVN. There is no distinct anatomic structure isolating the AVN and/or immediate subnodal extensions and creating an entrance/exit block to the premature atrial stimuli. An alternative explanation supported by clinical and experimental studies suggests that AVNRT circuit occurs in an area histologically and electrophysiologically defined, which includes compact AVN and bordering transitional cells. This highly anisotropic region would explain the multiple heterogeneous sites of early atrial activation during AVNRT and the different

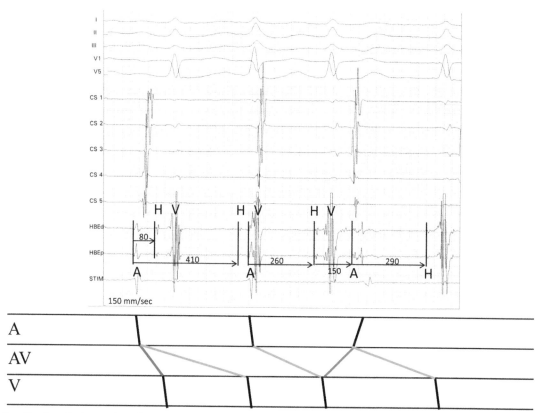

Fig. 17. Case 3, electrophysiologic study: two ventricular beats for one atrial beat. CS decapolar catheter inserted in the coronary sinus; recordings are ordered from distal[1] to proximal.[5] A catheter is positioned across the tricuspid valve to record the His potential distally and more proximally. The rowing ablation/recording catheter (Stim) is positioned close to the sinus node region. An initial sinus beat is followed by normal conduction to the ventricles via a fast pathway (A-H 80 ms, *red line*). The following ventricular beat is preceded by a His and occurs at the same time of another sinus beat. In keeping with previous observations, the most likely explanation is simultaneous antegrade conduction from the sinus beat to the ventricle using both fast (AH = 80) and a slow pathway with an A-H of 410 ms (*green line*): two ventricular beats for one atrial beat. The following sinus beat conducts with a similarly long A-H interval (260 ms) having engaged the slow pathway antegrade and generates an echo beat using a different slow conducting retrograde pathway with an H-A of 150 ms (*blue line*).

regional propagation during fast and slow pathway conduction. It is also conceivable that a change in propagation wavefront would also affect the input into the AVN-His junction determining the selective engagement into slow or fast conduction component of this subnodal junction.

The site of the block here presented is not clearly defined. From animal studies it seems that the most likely site of block is at the superior junction between atrial and transitional tissue. A full EPS confirmed the diagnosis of AVNRT, although it could not document the block. Slow pathway ablation prevented reinduction of the arrhythmia.

SUMMARY

The atrioventricular junction has phylogenetically developed to optimize atrioventricular conduction

to enhance ventricular filling adjusting to different heart rates in circumstances varying from rest to maximal effort. To perform this task the structure of the AVN has developed a complex structure with varying degrees of conduction velocity as is easily surmised by observing the PR variations during different cardiac rates.

Together with this function, the AVN also absolves the task of protecting the ventricles from excessively high heart rate progressively decrementing AV conduction. This property is behind the observed PR prolongation following an atrial premature beat.[9]

To perform the tasks of modulation and filtration of AV conduction according to heart rates requires a high degree of anatomic/functional complexity (expressed in an AV nodal structure).[10] First is a central (AVN body) structure where conduction depends on slow rising AP mediated by calcium

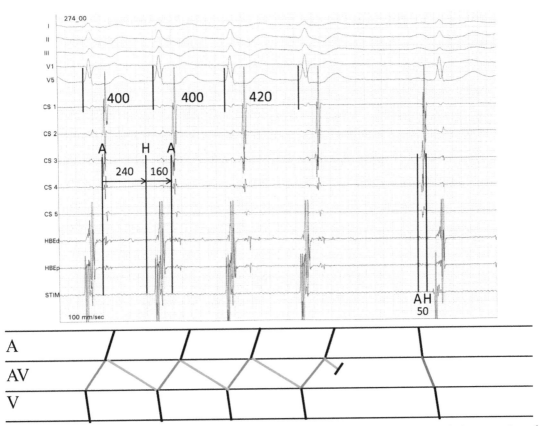

Fig. 18. Case 3, triple nodal conduction. Catheters are situated as in the previous figure with the exception of the Stim catheter now positioned in the right ventricle. The recorded His is of small voltage. The tracing shows termination of AVNRT. The tachycardia is regular with an A-H interval (antegrade) of 240 ms (*green line*) and an H-A (retrograde) of 160 ms (*blue line*) suggesting a slow-slow AVNRT circuit where the antegrade appears very slow. The patient seems to have a third atrioventricular pathway as suggested by an A-H interval of 50 ms (*red line*).

channels. This is the principal slow conducting region. Second is an atrionodal region, where the atrium connects to the AVN via a series of fanlike inputs spreading anteroposteriorly. These cells conduct rapidly using sodium channels especially the anterior input, which partially bypasses the AVN and is responsible for the shortening of the PR interval (fast AVN pathway).

Moving from the anterior toward the posterior conduction velocity decreases in part because of diminished expression of sodium channels and in part because the posterior input traverses the body of the AVN. This region is responsible for the prolongation of the PR (slow AVN pathway).

This hypothesis would account for the different electrophysiologic characteristics of the two AVN pathways. The fast pathway exhibits an "all or none" type of conduction, whereas the slow pathway demonstrates the decremental propagation more specifically associated with AVN conduction.

A pathway is intended as a group of interconnected myocytes with similar anatomic orientation and electrophysiologic properties functioning as an electrical conduit more than a recognizable anatomic structure. This would explain why with a minimal change in direction or velocity of the incoming wavefront, conduction may shift to a "pathway" with dissimilar properties and different exit point. The shift from anterior to posterior input is therefore mostly determined by the delicate balance between different conduction velocities and refractory periods of these two inputs modulated by the parasympathetic system. Given an increased expression of sodium channels, the anterior cells conduct faster but have a longer refractory period compared with the cells of the posterior input. This arrangement explains why in sinus rhythm or sinus tachycardia, under the influence of the sympathetic drive, the impulse is conducted along the fast pathway with shortening of PR.

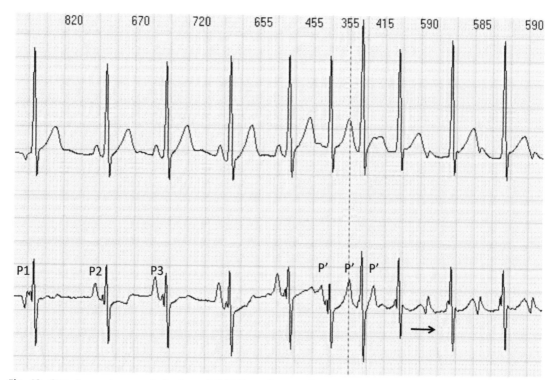

Fig. 19. Case 4, spontaneous induction of SVT. Note the wandering pacemaker (P1-P2-P3) with different rates suggestive a variable autonomic tone. Three atrial premature beats (P') induce the arrhythmia (*arrow*) at CL 600 ms with equal RP and PR intervals.

Furthermore, to explain conduction during normal sinus rhythm and during AVNRT, it is necessary to postulate a common point of contact between the pathway above (upper common pathway) and below (lower common pathway) the AVN. The exact nature and anatomic localization of these two "junction points" is still unclear and remains a highly debated point of contention (see Case 5).

The connections between the fast pathway and the right atrium remain undefined. The exit point of the fast pathway during AVNRT and during ventricular stimulation at the same cycle length is not the same. This is demonstrated in **Fig. 26**, where a close mapping the Koch triangle is performed, in the same patient, in these two situations. During tachycardia (**Fig. 26**A), there are multiple breakthroughs in the upper and mid portion of the AVN region all occurring within a 5-millisecond window. During ventricular pacing (**Fig. 26**B) at the same cycle length, the breakthrough is limited to one well-circumscribed area in the superior aspect of the AVN. This suggests that the exit point of a retrograde conduction in the AVN is determined by its direction and possibly velocity of propagation. A wavefront proceeding from the ventricles into the His engages a closely connected fast

pathway and emerges at the well-defined exit point of this pathway. The retrograde limb of the AVNRT will probably be directed to a less uniform "pathway system," which may represent all or part of the upper common pathway. Given the high anisotropy of this region, once the reentry wavefront emerges into the atrium it disperses into multiple wavelets with different directions. The more inferior wavefront could constitute the input to the "slow pathway' and therefore become part of the circuit. This explains why an ablation in that region renders AVNRT not reinducible.

The third component is the His bundle. The compact AVN continues in the fast conducting His bundle and its bifurcation into right and left branch. Although apparently a uniform structure, His anterior portion seems to be preferentially connected to the fast pathway, whereas the posterior His bundle receives a preferential input from the slow pathway. The clinical cases previously presented (Case 4) require a complex reentrant mechanism and understanding of how an arrhythmia begins and is maintained within the AVN structure.

The existence of two conducting pathways with different electrophysiologic properties is the premise for a reentrant circuit. In normal circumstances a reentry does not occur because conduction

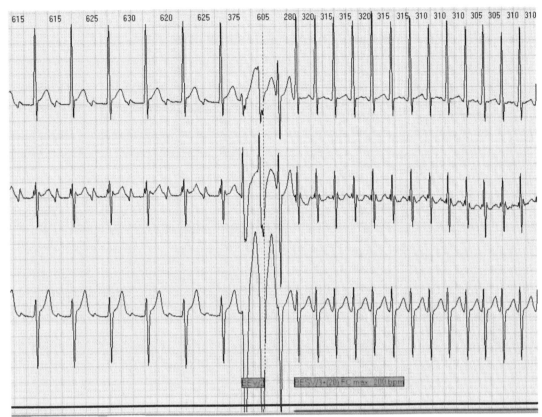

Fig. 20. Case 4, doubling of SVT rate. Sudden doubling of SVT rate. The first three beats at the beginning of the acceleration show aberrancy with progressive accommodation. The arrhythmia continues at CL 300 ms with R-P longer than P-R.

along one input blocks, when they meet at the lower common pathway, the propagation of the impulse in the other. For AVNRT to begin requires a unidirectional block of propagation in one pathway and slow conduction of the same impulse in the other pathway. A critical delay of conduction is required to allow the impulse to find the previously blocked path nonrefractory and propagate retrogradely to the atria and antegradely along the slow pathway (see **Fig. 4**). This type of reentrant circuit is the commonest and for this reason the arrhythmia derived by it is called typical AVNRT (see Case 1). Antegrade conduction along the slow pathway and retrograde using the fast pathway is the most common because of a preferential conduction within the AVN of atria and ventricular ectopic beats. Propagation of ectopic atrial beats, in fact, blocked in the fast pathway because of its shorter refractory period, conduct antegradely using the slow pathway and reenter retrogradely a recovered fast pathway. Ventricular ectopic beats traverse retrogradely the His bundle finding a preferential connection with the fast pathway, and establish the same type of reentry

by finding the slow pathway ready to conduct antegradely. The typical AVNRT can be considered an accentuation of an existing natural set up with two pathways with different connections to the AVN.

A reentrant circuit using the two pathways with opposite direction of propagation (antegrade fast and retrograde slow) is also clinically possible (fast-slow AVNRT). Furthermore, is also possible to observe, albeit uncommonly, two or three more distinct slow pathways with different electrophysiologic properties. This could complicate the mechanism of reentry even further because the options for antegrade and retrograde conduction are increased. Although in this situation, retrograde conduction more often tends to occur in the "slower" pathway located more posteriorly in the region of the proximal coronary sinus, variations have been observed with reentrant circuits using slow pathways to conduct antegradely and retrogradely (slow-slow AVNRT). Cases 2 and 3 show atypical AVNRTs induced by, respectively, and atrial and a ventricular ectopic beat. The circuit in Case 2 is the opposite of the typical reentry

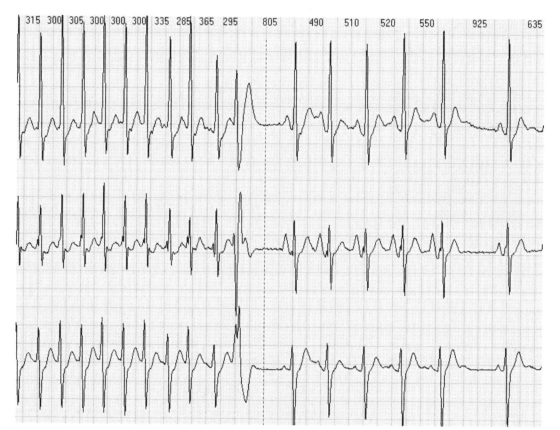

Fig. 21. Case 4, cessation of the arrhythmia. Cessation of the arrhythmia with single VPC. As shown in **Fig. 23**, the VPC terminates the SVT without penetration in the AVN ruling definitely out an AT.

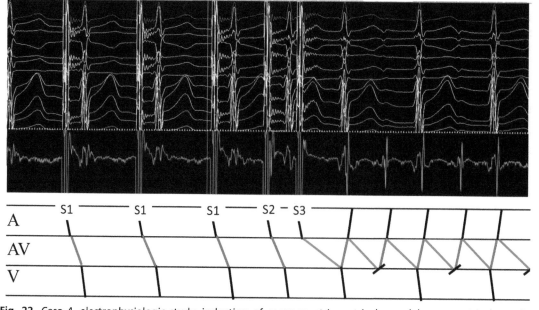

Fig. 22. Case 4, electrophysiologic study, induction of common atrioventricular nodal supraventricular tachycardia with a 2:1 atrioventricular conduction. Electrophysiologic study by transesophageal approach: induction of a supraventricular tachycardia by double premature atrial beat (S2-S3) after a drive (S1). A common atrioventricular nodal tachycardia with a 2:1 atrioventricular conduction was induced.

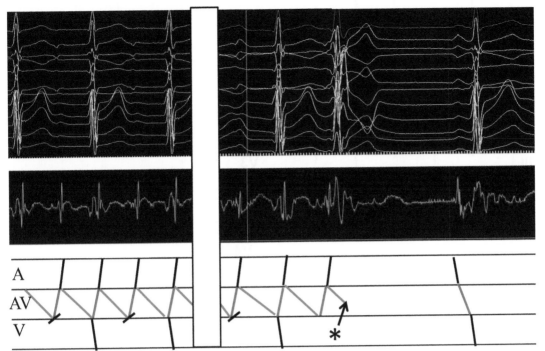

Fig. 23. Case 4: end of tachycardia by a ventricular premature beat: the definitive diagnosis of intranodal reentry. Clinical tachycardia. Spontaneous restoring of the sinus rhythm by a ventricular beat (*asterisk*). Esophageal recording shows that the ventricular premature beat is not conducted to the atria definitively excluding an atrial tachycardia and so confirming the diagnosis of intranodal reentry. The arrows show the fusion into the AV junction between the slow pathway anterograde conduction and the retrograde activation coming from the ectopic beat.

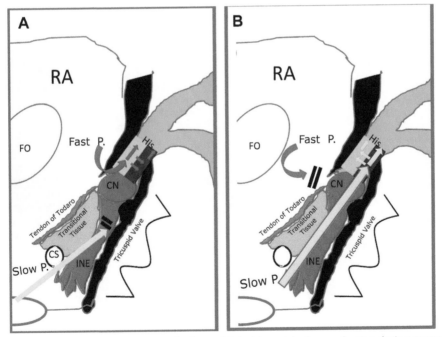

Fig. 24. Case 4, His alternans phenomenon at the base of 2:1 atrioventricular conduction during common AVNRT. The explanation of the 2:1 atrioventricular conduction is caused by the different inputs into the bundle of His in sinus rhythm and AVNRT. (*A*) During sinus rhythm the activation wavefront is transmitted to the anterior portion of the His bundle via the fast pathway. (*B*) During AVNRT the antegrade activation proceeds through the slow pathway, to the posterior portion of the His bundle, which has longer refractory period; this phenomenon is functionally determined and disappears with rate related shortening of the refractory period.

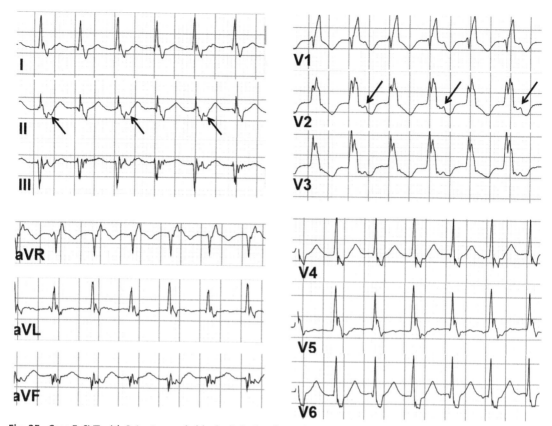

Fig. 25. Case 5, SVT with 2:1 retrograde block clinical tachycardia: the QRS is identical to the one in SR making this an SVT. There is an obvious retrograde P wave (*arrows*) every second beat with a short RP/long PR ratio. Differential rests between AVNRT and junctional tachycardia with retrograde 2:1 block. Clinically AVNRT would be more likely given patient's age and overall normal cardiovascular system and complete regularity of the arrhythmia. The electrophysiological study confirmed dual AV nodal physiology and induction of AVNRT.

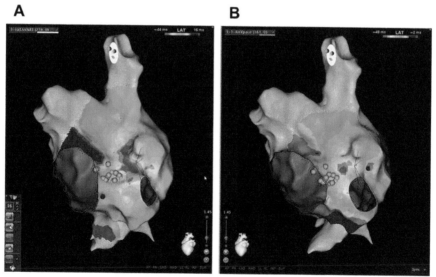

Fig. 26. Electroanatomic atrial mapping comparing common AVNRT and retrograde atrial activation during ventricular pacing. (*A*) Close multipoint mapping of the AVN region during AVNRT. The mapping window is set to show in red the first 3 ms of activation. Yellow points represent the points where a His potential was recorded. This area includes the proximal common bundle of His and the distal compact AVN. There are multiple atrial breakthroughs superior and inferior to the AVN region. The blue dot represents the successful ablation point. (*B*) Atrial exit point during V pacing at same cycle length of the AVNRT. The earliest atrial breakthrough is much more contained and localized in the superior aspect of the AVN in the location of "fast" pathway input. Mapping parameters and definition of the His region as in A.

previously described in that antegrade conduction occurs along the fast pathway, whereas retrograde conduction uses a slow pathway. The data presented in the discussion of this case favor the possibility of a slow pathway conducting antegradely and a very slow pathway conducting retrogradely in the reentrant circuit.

Similar evidence of the existence of multiple AVN pathways is presented in Case 3 where during sinus rhythm with regular rate, the impulse is conducted to the ventricles using a slow and a super-slow pathway. The atypical AVNRT in this case uses two slow pathways. The reasons behind these different reentrant circuits might be caused by the interplay of variable electrophysiologic properties and anatomic structures.

Finally, some observations on the atrioventricular relationship during AVNRT.[8] During AVNRT atrioventricular conduction occurs in most cases on a 1:1 ratio. In rare cases an antegrade block, usually 2:1, is observed or even more uncommonly a similar retrograde block is detected as shown, respectively, in Cases 4 and 5. At times, the antegrade block occurs within the His-Purkinje system often accompanied by evidence of advanced block in this system.[11] Give the normal function of the His-Purkinje system in Case 4, the most likely explanation is the existence of two inputs into the bundle of His and has no relationship with the more common His-Purkinje system blocks. The nature of the block observed in Case 4 is totally benign. Case 5 shows the more uncommon situation of a retrograde block. This event, probably exclusively observed in typical AVNRT, opens the unresolved question of the definition of the extent of atrial tissue participating in the reentrant circuit and consequently of the location of the upper common pathway. It is clear that most right and left atrial tissues are activated as by standards chambers during any type of AVNRT. Both chambers are easily dissociated from the arrhythmia without altering its cycle length. As offered during the discussion of Case 5, the most likely explanation for this rare retrograde block is the possibility of a limited amount of supranodal tissue, still undefined anatomically and electrophysiologically. This region, given the high anisotropy of area, could be sensitive to the propagation velocity and direction of the retrograde wave-front and block the impulse before it reaches atrial tissue proper. This usually happens in a 2:1 fashion but prolonged periods of retrograde block have been previously described.

REFERENCES

1. Kwaku KF, Josephson ME. Typical AVNRT: an update on mechanisms and therapy. Card Electrophysiol Rev 2002;6:414–21.
2. Medkour D, Becker AE, Khalife K. Anatomic and functional characteristics of a slow posterior AV nodal pathway: role in dual-pathway physiology and reentry. Circulation 1998;98:164–74.
3. Bagliani G, Della Rocca DG, Di Biase L. PR interval and junctional zone. Card Electrophysiol Clin 2017; 9(3):411–33.
4. Di Biase L, Gianni C, Bagliani G. Arrhythmias involving the atrioventricular junction. Card Electrophysiol Clin 2017;9(3):435–52.
5. Liu Y, Zhou A, Zhao S. Quadruple atrioventricular nodal pathways involved in orthodromic atrioventricular reentrant tachycardia. Tex Heart Inst J 2010; 37(6):706–9.
6. Katritsis DG, Sepahpour A, Marine JE. Atypical atrioventricular nodal reentrant tachycardia: prevalence, electrophysiologic characteristics, and tachycardia circuit. Europace 2015;17:1099.
7. Zhang Y, Bharati S, Mowrey KA, et al. His electrogram alternans reveal dual-wavefront inputs into and longitudinal dissociation within the bundle of His. Circulation 2001;104(7):832–8.
8. Wellens HJ, Wesdorp JC, Düren DR, et al. Second degree block during reciprocal atrioventricular nodal tachycardia. Circulation 1976;53:595.
9. Pandozi C, Ficili S, Galeazzi M, et al. Propagation of the sinus impulse into the Koch triangle and localization, timing, and origin of the multicomponent potentials recorded in this area. Circ Arrhythm Electrophysiol 2011;4(2):225–34.
10. Kurian T, Ambrosi C, Hucker W, et al. Anatomy and electrophysiology of the human AV node. Pacing Clin Electrophysiol 2010;33(6):754–62.
11. Temple IP, Inada S, Dobrzynski H, et al. Connexins and the atrioventricular node. Heart Rhythm 2013; 10(2):297–304.

P Wave Analysis in the Era of Atrial Fibrillation Ablation

Fabio M. Leonelli, MD[a], Emanuela T. Locati, MD, PhD[b],
Giuseppe Bagliani, MD[c,d,*], Roberto De Ponti, MD, FHRS[e],
Luigi Padeletti, MD[f], Laura Cipolletta, MD[g],
Alessandro Capucci, MD[g]

KEYWORDS

- Atrial fibrillation • Atrial remodeling • Holter recording • P wave

KEY POINTS

- Atrial fibrillation (AF) is a complex arrhythmia not yet completely understood.
- The role of surface electrocardiogram (ECG) is only apparently limited by the disorganized nature of AF.
- Attentive analysis of the ECG can greatly help in the diagnosis and management of AF.
- Electrocardiographic techniques useful in characterizing and managing AF include Holter monitoring and frequency domain analysis of atrial electrograms.

INTRODUCTION

Atrial fibrillation (AF), affecting 1% to 2% of general population, is the most common sustained arrhythmia. It is also related to increased hospitalizations and mortality, causing a significant increase in health care financial resources spent for AF treatment. Its prevalence and incidence of associated morbidity dramatically increases with age.[1] The usual role of the electrocardiogram (ECG) in the management of AF is to diagnose this arrhythmia, to monitor the effects of antiarrhythmic drugs (AADs), and to assess the ventricular response during episodes of AF. In a patient complaining of palpitations, AF episodes can be suspected by simple pulse palpation by the patient or relatives, or by documenting heart rate by using modern sphygmomanometers that are able to identify irregular cardiac rhythms. The suspicion of AF can then be confirmed by a 12-lead ECG, which can differentiate between AF and other irregular rhythms.

More recently, single-lead tracings can be obtained using small tools attached to a smartphone, allowing low-cost continuous monitoring of patients with arrhythmias.

Despite its obvious limitations, surface ECG and its applications remains a very valuable tool, not only in the diagnosis of AF but also in the definition of its proarrhythmic substrate and response to therapy.

[a] Cardiology Department, James A. Haley Veterans' Hospital, Cardiology Department University South Florida, Tampa, FL, USA; [b] Electrophysiology Unit, Cardiovascular Department, Niguarda Hospital, Milan, Italy; [c] Cardiology Department, Arrhythmology Unit, Foligno General Hospital, Foligno, Italy; [d] Cardiovascular Diseases Department, University of Perugia, Perugia, Italy; [e] Cardiology Department, University of Insubria, Varese, Italy; [f] Heart and Vessels Department, University of Florence, IRCCS Multimedica, Sesto San Giovanni, Florence, Italy; [g] Cardiology and Arrhythmology Clinic, Marche Polytechnic University, University Hospital "Ospedali Riuniti", Ancona, Italy
* Corresponding author. Cardiology Department, Arrhythmology Unit, Foligno General Hospital, Foligno, Italy.
E-mail address: Giuseppe.bagliani@tim.it

Card Electrophysiol Clin 10 (2018) 299–316
https://doi.org/10.1016/j.ccep.2018.02.015
1877-9182/18/© 2018 Elsevier Inc. All rights reserved.

THEORY OF ATRIAL FIBRILLATION, TRIGGERS, AND SUBSTRATE (FOCAL ATRIAL TACHYCARDIA, DISPERSION OF REPOLARIZATION, FIBRILLATORY CONDUCTION, ROTORS)

Despite many years of intense research, the mechanism of AF remains imperfectly understood. This is in part because most of the relevant observations have been made in experimentally induced AF in animal models and extrapolated to clinical human AF. There is general agreement that the term AF includes different types of arrhythmia that are clinically defined as paroxysmal, persistent, and permanent. Behind this subdivision, which is based on the duration of AF and its spontaneous ability to return to sinus rhythm (SR), is the fundamental concept of electrical remodeling induced by repetitive of bouts of AF on cardiac tissue.

The term remodeling refers to several changes induced by periods of fast electrical stimulation, such as that observed during paroxysms of AF, on ionic channels expressions, cellular metabolism, and interstitial cardiac tissue. These alterations include downregulation of sodium and calcium channels, and the potassium channel (Transient Outward Potassium Current).

These changes lead to a shortening of the atrial refractory period, loss of physiologic adaptation to increased rates, and a decrease of conduction velocity. The consequences of these changes are an increased inducibility and duration of periods of induced AF, leading to the concept of AF begetting AF.[2]

Finally, the profound electrophysiological abnormalities induced by rapid atrial stimulation in animal models lead to a higher incidence of spontaneous tachycardia often initiated by unstable Ca currents leading to early after depolarizations. This appears to be particularly frequent in myocytes within the pulmonary veins (PVs), Marshall veins, and (possibly) thoracic veins.

Longer periods of AF induce changes in atrial cellular substructure, including accumulation of glycogen, loss of myofibrils, fragmentation of sarcoplasmic reticulum, dispersion of nuclear chromatin, and (more generally) loss of muscle mass. The effects of these functional and structural abnormalities have a wide impact on the propagation of the electrical impulse and atrial mechanics. In humans, a clear relationship between atrial dilatation and AF is commonly observed. Although atrial dilation often precedes AF, atrial diameter has been observed to increase as consequence of this arrhythmia. The enlargement is accompanied by impaired contractility, observed after a few minutes of experimental AF and persisting, in humans, for weeks or even months in atria exposed to prolonged periods of AF.[3]

The physiologic anisotropy and dispersion of atrial conduction is greatly enhanced by the electrophysiological changes induced by even a short burst of AF, becoming greatly altered by the appearance of diffuse fibrosis secondary to more sustained periods of this tachycardia.

The current understanding of induction and maintenance of AF is based on these fundamental clinical and experimental observations. The concept of triggers as fast bursts of automatic atrial tachycardia (AT) inducing atrial remodeling and altering the substrate to increase spontaneous discharges and perpetuate longer periods of AF has received considerable clinical support, and has served well in guiding modern ablative strategies.

The triggering of AF by AT had been reported long before a seminal observation localized the discharging focus to 1 of the PV and eliminated recurrence of AF by ablating the arrhythmogenic area.[4] This initial and the ensuing confirmatory reports helped establish the PVs and, more generally, the left atrium (LA) as the source of most AF triggers.

Having identified triggers and the effects of their repetitive discharges on atrial tissue, it remains to clarify the electrophysiological mechanism leading from a fast regular AT to a chaotic rhythm such as AF. There is general agreement that the irregular propagation of AF is greatly facilitated by the presence of localized areas of tissue anisotropy where a rapid single activation wave-front turns into fibrillatory conduction. Regions with variable conduction velocities and refractoriness due to heterogeneity in fiber orientation and thickness, such as the pectinate muscle, the crista terminalis (CT), and the posterior LA wall are incapable of maintaining 1 to 1 conduction at a high frequency of stimulation. In these circumstances, the uniform front of activation breaks into reentrant wavelets, causing AF. By inducing the changes previously described, any conditions that induce atrial remodeling, from bursts of rapid stimulation to disease-increasing atrial volume or pressure load, will increase the physiologic anisotropy present in normal atria.

There is, therefore, a shift in arrhythmia mechanism from regular, which is initiated and maintained on bursts of fast automatic AT, to a perpetuation of self-sustained chaotic tachycardia.

Although abnormal automaticity can explain the mechanism of triggers, the mechanism of degeneration and maintenance of AF is not fully understood.

There is general agreement that reentry is the basic mechanism of AF. This is not the anatomically determined reentry observed in atrial flutter

(AFL) in which physical boundaries govern the stable path of the arrhythmia. Instead, it is a functional reentry in which the reentrant path is not fixed but depends only on the conduction velocity and refractory period of the tissue and sufficient circuit dimensions.[5] Although in normal atria AF is usually self-terminated because the dimension of multiple functional reentry cannot be accommodated by the relative small size of the atria, changes such as reduction of refractoriness by reducing circuit size permit the coexistence of multiple reentrant circuits. Inhomogeneous conduction also favors the induction of reentry by creating areas of conduction block and delay that are fundamental in this arrhythmia mechanism.

It is still debated which model of reentry is the basis of AF. Whether leading circle or spiral wave best define the drivers maintaining AF, and what is the role of more organized continuously discharging automatic foci still persisting in AF, are still unresolved questions.[6,7]

Regardless of the type of functional reentry, AF is probably maintained by the continuous interactions of these numerous wavelets randomly propagating at high velocity. As they come into contact with refractory tissue or nonconducting obstacles, they break up into so-called daughter wavelets, continuing the meandering guided only by the availability of excitable tissue.

Determining the type of reentry is of marked clinical relevance because clarification of this issue will advance the understanding of AF and help guide the therapeutic approach to this arrhythmia.

Although triggers can most easily be diagnosed during prolonged periods of monitoring using Holter monitors or event recorders, and localized during invasive electrophysiology studies, the mechanism of AF cannot be identified by surface recordings and even intracardiac recordings are of limited use.

Partial human atrial mapping during AF has shown wave fronts propagating across both atria with variable degree of organization and cycle lengths. Attempts to classify the types of AF based on these observations did not elucidate the mechanism initiating or sustaining AF, and did not generate clinically relevant information. However, quantifying organization during AF has relevant clinical implications because a higher degree of structured activation portends, among other factors, a better response to pharmacologic or ablative procedures.[8]

Although a 12-lead ECG cannot provide information to quantify AF organization, different analysis of brief, continuous, electrocardiographic recordings of atrial electrograms can offer some insight on its structure and presence of focal activity maintaining AF.

ELECTROCARDIOGRAM TECHNIQUES IN THE DIAGNOSIS AND MANAGEMENT OF ATRIAL FIBRILLATION

The main role of electrocardiographic recording is to diagnose AF, either by using a 12-lead ECG (**Fig. 1**) or, in the case of paroxysmal AF (PAF), by implementing prolonged periods of monitoring using an ambulatory ECG (AECG) device. Currently, single-lead tracings can be obtained using small tools attached to a smartphone **Fig. 2**, allowing a low-cost continuous monitoring of patients with arrhythmias.

These 2 approaches are equally valid to confirm the presence of AF but they provide some specific understanding of the nature of triggers and arrhythmic substrate. Information provided by the ECG during AF is a limited but more complex analysis of the 12-lead tracing, and can offer further understanding of the mechanism of perpetuation of AF and its degree of organization. Finally, detailed observation of a P wave in SR can offer important prognostic data on the degree of electroanatomical remodeling before and after ablative procedures.

THE 12-LEAD ELECTROCARDIOGRAM

In most cases, the diagnosis of AF is extremely simple and is based on 2 easy electrocardiographic criteria:

1. Absence of a visible P wave on the 12-lead ECG
2. Irregularity of R-R intervals (see **Fig. 1**).

Although this diagnosis seems to be straightforward, several possible pitfalls must be pointed out. A low-voltage P wave, often related to the presence of numerous atrial scars, can make the detection of flutter wave difficult and, in the presence of irregular AV conduction, it is possible to confuse the 2 arrhythmias. Close observation of the tracings can help identify small but clearly reproducible atrial activity in more than 1 lead, usually the inferior ones. This is diagnostic of AFL because never it occurs in AF, in which more organized fibrillatory activity remains highly variable and is usually observed only in V1. Furthermore, the R-R interval in AFL, even when irregular, is regularly irregular and there is repetition of 2 or 3 varying fixed R-R intervals (**Fig. 3**).

Organization of AF, as previously discussed, refers to periods of high coherent activation of large portions of the atria that are possibly related to the emergence of a periodic dominant rotor. This phenomenon has been demonstrated in human epicardial recordings and correlated to the ECG

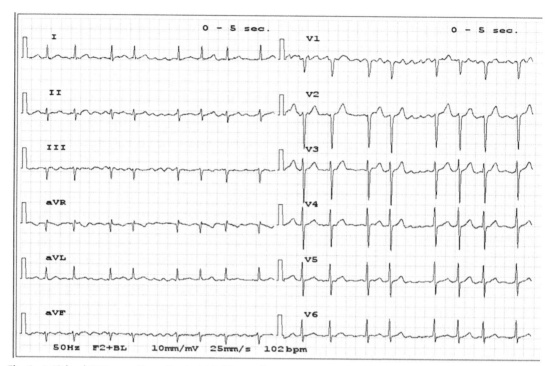

Fig. 1. A 12-lead ECG recording of typical AF. Absent discreet P wave and irregularly irregular R-R intervals are the hallmarks of the diagnosis. bpm, beats per minute.

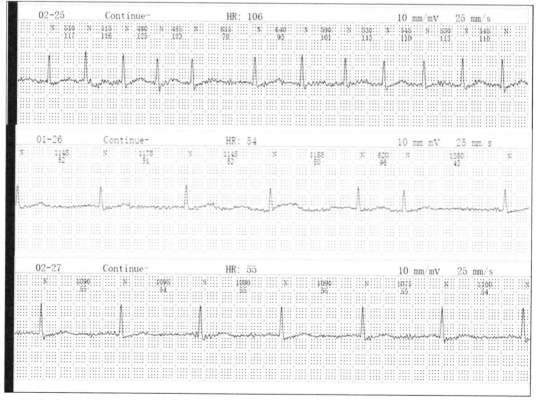

Fig. 2. Rhythm strips recorded and downloaded using a smartphone application. The tracing clearly shows periods of established AF (*top*) or accompanying APC (*middle*) and Simple SR (*bottom*).

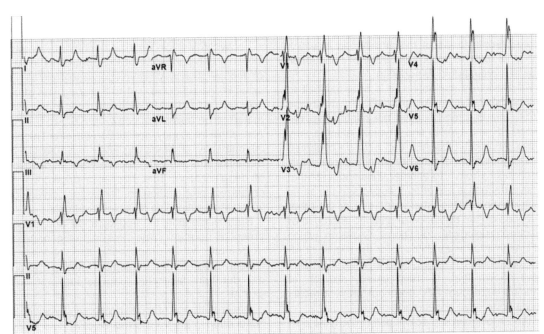

Fig. 3. The tracing shows a regular tachycardia with right bundle branch block (RBBB). aVR, augmented Vector Right; aVL, augmented Vector Left; aVF, augmented Vector Foot. There is no recognizable atrial activity in the limb leads but in V1 to V3 a small but definite P wave is present, in keeping with AFL. Also note the regularity of R-R interval.

appearance of AF. Some evidence also exists in human and animal studies correlating the degree of atrial remodeling with different AF types.

An electrocardiographic appearance of a more organized, coarse, type of AF (**Fig. 4**), corresponding to a V1 of greater than 0.12 mV, is observed more often in patients with better preserved

myocardial structure in which a substantial portion of either atria is uniformly activated.

Several studies have correlated the presence of organized activation mostly of the trabeculated right atrium (RA) with an increased voltage in V1 and, in the same lead, a reproducible F wave with a predominant polarity.

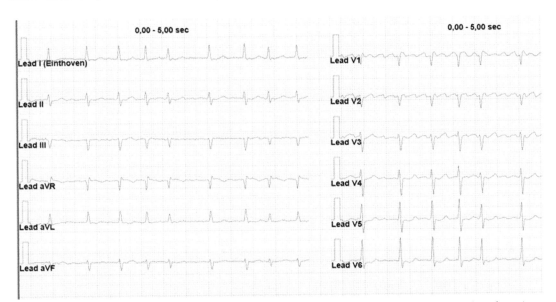

Fig. 4. A coarse AF. The F waves in V1 and V2 are more than 0.12 mV and, at times, seem to be of consistent morphology. Fibrillatory activity is present in the inferior leads and the R-R interval is irregularly irregular.

Instead, A fine AF (**Fig. 5**), defined by a V1 voltage of less than 0.11 mV, is characteristic of more chronic forms of this arrhythmia in which the atrial features mark anisotropy of conduction due to more marked remodeling.

As previously mentioned, it is often difficult to distinguish between AF and AFL on a 12-lead ECG. This is often because the relationship between AF and typical and atypical AFLs is very close. AF and typical AFL can both be observed in a large number of patients either independently or changing from 1 to another. This suggests that both arrhythmias are often 2 aspects of the same tachycardia and the emergence of 1 or the other depends on the presence of specific anatomic or electrophysiological conditions. Cases in which AFL seems to be unrelated to or the trigger of AF are uncommon. In fact, several clinical studies have shown that, in most cases, ablation of isthmus-dependent AFL does not prevent recurrence or de novo appearance of AF.

The 2 most relevant factors determining the predominance of 1 or the other of these 2 tachycardias are presence of a functional or anatomic line of block in the atria and arrhythmia cycle length. The line of block is usually represented by the CT in most isthmus-dependent flutters and, more rarely, accompanied by postsurgical incisional scars on the RA free wall. In the LA, where anatomic boundaries are not usually present,

post-AF ablation scars often create fixed borders to delimit the flutter reentrant pathway.

Tachycardia cycle length is the other parameter influencing organization of the arrhythmia in AFL or degeneration in AF. RA response to rapid stimulation is characterized by 1 to 1 propagation of the stimulus up to a certain stimulation frequency, estimated to be below a window from 6.5 to 6.7 Hz. Above this frequency, conduction wavefront blocks intermittently at branching sites near the CT or pectinate muscles with loss of consistent direction of depolarization. This induces a breakdown of organized propagation to fibrillatory conduction with degeneration into multiple wavefronts.

Both dispersion of repolarization and action potential duration play roles in the generation of complex wave propagation and, at least in animal studies, shortening of action potential duration facilitates degeneration of AFL into AF.

The importance of repolarization and velocity of conduction in the transformation of AF into AFL is highlighted by the effects of AADs, particularly those belonging to class I, during medical therapy for AF. These drugs promote conversion of AF to SR or, at times, into a slow flutter with a very wide QRS and a slow rate favoring 1 to 1 conduction (**Fig. 6**). The mechanism inducing this slow and incessant tachycardia is due to the block of sodium channels induced by class I AADs, which

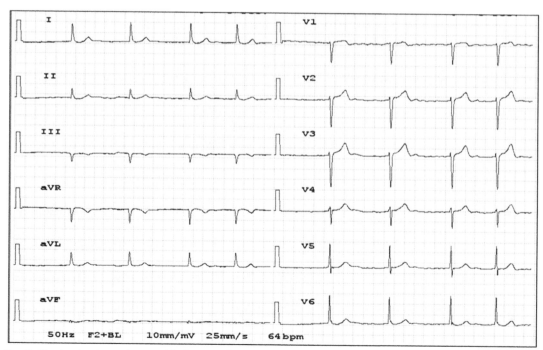

Fig. 5. The tracing is consistent with fine AF. The voltage of the F waves in V1 and V2 is less than 0.12 mV and fibrillatory activity is present in every lead. R-R interval is irregularly irregular.

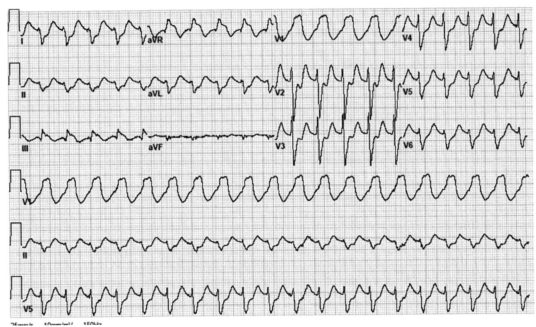

Fig. 6. This patient presented with this wide complex arrhythmia at the rate of 140 bpm. Propafenone had been started the weeks before for lone PAF. No atrial activity is clearly visible. Differential diagnosis includes ventricular tachycardia but the width of the QRS in a normal heart, the relatively slow rate, and the wide but typical RBBB in this patient make proarrhythmic AFL the most likely diagnosis.

decreases conduction velocity and prolongs the refractory period. Prolongation of both parameters increases the wavelength of existing reentrant circuits, leading to a formation of a single reentry that will terminate when its wavelength is longer than the available reentrant path. These electrophysiological changes induced by class I AADs can also produce propagation block, creating boundaries that can force a slow, single, reentrant circuit into a path delimited by areas of induced functional block. The irregular V response to AF is, therefore, transformed owing to this poor arrhythmic effect in a slower, hemodynamically, poorly tolerated AFL.

Initiation of AF can be documented serendipitously on 12-lead ECG and, more often, on prolonged monitoring. In these tracings it is also, at times, possible to document arrhythmic triggers of AF (**Fig. 7**) and the presence of AFL together with AF and to extrapolate the degree of dispersion of repolarization by observing the relationship between a sinus P and the atrial premature complex (APC) inducing AF (**Fig. 8**).

AMBULATORY ELECTROCARDIOGRAM

In view of the clinical implications associated with a diagnosis of AF, electrocardiographic evidence of this arrhythmia is the cornerstone of its management. Symptoms are often not specific or absent and episodes of AF can occur at any time during day or night.

Therefore, duration of ECG monitoring represents a crucial issue for the detection of PAF. The clinical role of AECG recording extends from clarifying the need for additional treatment to helping to reassure the patient, as well as predicting long-term prognosis. In addition, other arrhythmic triggers of AF or different causes of symptoms, such as AFT, AT, atrial ectopic, and ventricular beats, can be differentiated from AF episodes only by AECG monitoring. Duration and frequency of events vary greatly among patients with AF; therefore, the choice of AECG will affect the likelihood of capturing AF episodes, which will depend on the duration and continuity of recording. Reliance on symptoms alone (by patient or physician) may be misleading, both overestimating and underestimating the presence of AF. This has important implications for assessing treatment effects, including interventional ablation or patients with cryptogenic stroke.

Currently, new prolonged AECG recording systems have been developed that go beyond the standard 24-hour Holter monitor, including external AECG monitors (lasting 1–4 weeks) and implantable AECG monitors (lasting 2–3 years). A recent document, *ISHNE-HRS Expert Consensus*

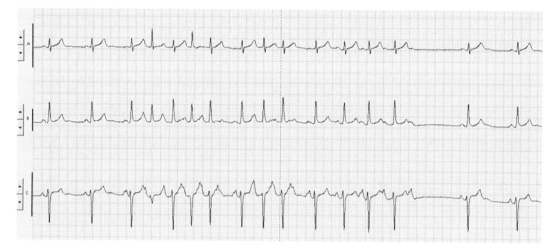

Fig. 7. Holter recorder showing SR interrupted by a burst of nonsustained atrial tachycardia with variable cycle length. This is often the trigger of AF. Although is not possible to localize the arrhythmic focus with this limited information, most the arrhythmic foci are found in the PVs.

Statement on Ambulatory ECG and External Cardiac Monitoring/Telemetry,[9-11] provided an extensive review on the technical aspects and clinical indications of contemporary AECG recording systems (**Table 1**). In general, 3 main recording modalities for prolonged AECG monitoring are now available: intermittent event recorders, external loop recorders (ELRs) or implantable loop recorders (ILRs), and continuous AECG recording.

Intermittent AECG recordings can be obtained by event recorders that memorize only few seconds of ECG tracing. Recently, event recorders have been implemented on smartphone-based systems, with the advantage of incorporating transtelephonic transmission capabilities. Event recorders are not suitable for the detection of silent PAF, although they can be useful to document or exclude the presence of PAF in case of symptoms (palpitations) or irregular pulse at clinic visit, or to

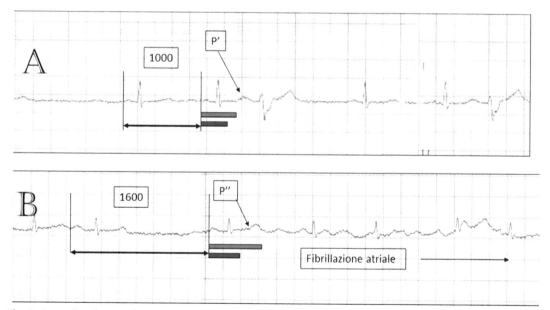

Fig. 8. Recording from Holter monitor showing SR and APCs occurring with different P-P intervals. In A the APC only resets the subsequent sinus beat, whereas in B it induces AF. This probably related to the occurrence of the premature beat at a time of maximum dispersion of repolarization favored by a longer preceding P-P interval (1600 milliseconds).

Table 1
Characteristics of ambulatory electrocardiogram monitoring systems

Definitions	Modalities of Recording	Duration	Type of Electrodes	Number of Leads	Clinical Indications
External event recorders Smartphone-based event recorders	Intermittent external event Transtelephonic transmission	Up to 30 s (multiple recordings)	Build-in, applied directly on the chest (or held by both hands)	1	• Rhythm monitoring for symptomatic arrhythmias (palpitations) • Scheduled screening for the detection of silent AF
Patch ECG monitors	Continuous external with or without wireless data transmission	Up to 14 d	Adhesive patches with built-in recording systems	1 or 2	• Rhythm monitoring for PAF, PSVT, VT, or pauses • Arrhythmic burden
External loop recorders	Intermittent external patient or autotriggered	4–8 wk	Adhesive disposable wired	1 or 2	• Rhythm monitoring (symptomatic and asymptomatic arrhythmias)
Holter monitors	Continuous multilead external	1. 1–7 d 2. 7–21 d	1. Adhesive disposable wired 2. Wireless embedded in vests or belts	1. 3–12 2. 1–3	• Rhythm monitoring • Arrhythmic burden • Risk stratification • Substrate characterization
Mobile cardiac outpatient telemetry	External real-time continuous cardiac tele-monitoring systems	Real-time streaming to call centers	1. Adhesive disposable wired 2. Wireless embedded in a patch, necklace pendant or a chest belt carrier	1. 1–3 2. 1	• Rhythm monitoring (see previous)
Implantable loop recorders	Intermittent (patient or autotriggered activation) with remote monitoring	Up to 3 y	Build-in	1	• Rhythm monitoring. symptomatic and asymptomatic arrhythmias (see previous)

Abbreviations: MCOT, Mobile cardiac outpatient telemetry; PSVT, Paroxysmal Supra-Ventricular Tachycardia; VT, Ventricular Tachycardia.

perform periodic controls in asymptomatic patients with suspected AF (**Figs. 9** and **10**).

Loop recording systems can be ELRs or ILRs, and can provide continuous ECG monitoring; however, they memorize only patient-activated or autotriggered ECG tracings, generally lasting 15 to 30 minutes. The stored ECG tracings can be analyzed offline or they can be transmitted by remote monitoring to dedicated centralized analysis centers. ELRs and ILRs can be used for the identification of both symptomatic and asymptomatic arrhythmias, including silent PAF, and are typically used in the diagnostic work-up of unexplained palpitations or syncope, or cryptogenic stroke (**Figs. 11–13**). Generally, loop recorders are based on 1-lead recording and

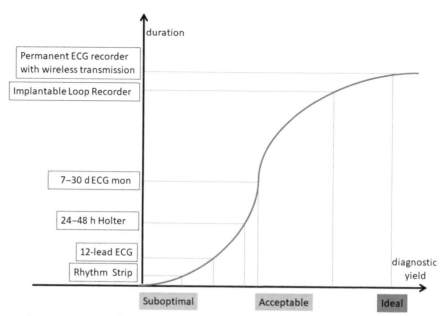

Fig. 9. Schematic representation of modalities of AECG recording as function of duration of monitoring, with a correspondent increase of the diagnostic yield. mon, monitoring.

cannot provide an accurate assessment of the arrhythmic burden because the autotriggered algorithms rarely provide a reliable detection of the offset of the arrhythmias. Generally, in event recorders and in ELRs or ILRs, the arrhythmia detection is based on R-R interval series and cycle length levels, although morphologic waveform analysis is not available.

Therefore, these tools can reliably identify supraventricular arrhythmias (paroxysmal supraventricular tachycardia and AF) or pauses, whereas detection of ventricular arrhythmias is generally less reliable, lacking reliable QRS morphologic analysis. Notably, the automatically detected AF episodes always need a manual validation because frequent premature supraventricular beats, ventricular beats, marked sinus arrhythmias, or (at times) artifacts are often misdiagnosed as episodes of PAF (**Fig. 14**).

Continuous AECG recordings, classically Holter monitoring, have now expanded from the original 24 hours to up to 30 days owing to new digital recorders with inexpensive large storage capacities that can record very long-term, continuous, high-quality AECG signals. The number of simultaneous recorded leads generally decreases with the recording duration, and 12-leads are currently available only for 24 to 48 hour recordings, 2 to 3 leads, for up to 7 day recordings, whereas longer (multiweek) recordings are usually based on 1 or 2 leads. Prolonged external continuous recordings are based on the classic wired adhesive electrode systems, which are inexpensive but often poorly tolerated during prolonged recording, or by more modern adhesive patches, more expensive but better tolerated, providing 1-lead recordings for up to 2 weeks. More recently, new vest or belt textile systems with embedded electrodes have been developed, providing good quality 2-lead to 3-lead continuous recordings. Prolonged continuous AECG systems generally require offline analysis, although a few most recent devices have the possibility of wireless transmission of selected stored ECG data to a remote receiving station, and can provide a reliable assessment of the arrhythmic burden, including AF duration and burden, because onset and offset of the episode can be precisely detected (**Fig. 15**). Monitoring devices for mobile cardiac outpatient telemetry are also available for high-risk cardiac patients, providing long-term continuous long-distance telemetric surveillance by online mobile telephonic transmission of ECG data to dedicated call centers.

The current definition of PAF has been set as a minimum of 30 seconds (often defined as an atrial high-rate episode with heart rate >190 beats per minute); however, the detection of those subclinical tachyarrhythmias is in reality quite erratic, particularly by intermittent recordings, and only continuous AECG recordings allow correct identification of such short events.

The duration and the modality of AECG recording also affect the likelihood of AF diagnosis, which depends on the frequency and the duration of events in the single patient. Short-

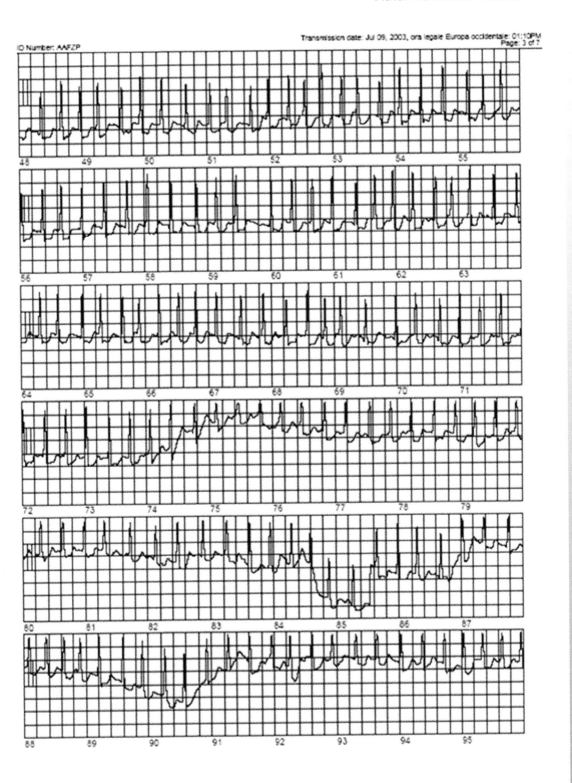

Fig. 10. Detection of symptomatic fast PAF by event monitor (Card Guard AG, CG 2206, Lifewatch, UK) in a patient with history of unexplained palpitations (female, 65 years).

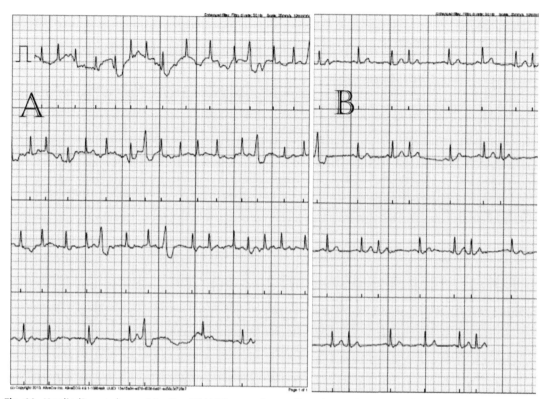

Fig. 11. Kardia (Smart phone, AliveCor, USA) 30-second recording obtained in a case of irregular pulse (in absence of symptoms) in a patient (male, 72 years, history of cryptogenic stroke). (*A*) An episode of PAF with spontaneous recovery of SR. (*B*) Sinus beat with frequent supraventricular beats and ventricular beats (VEBs).

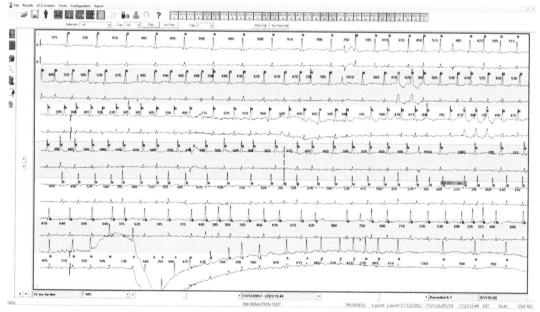

Fig. 12. Automatic detection of an asymptomatic atrial high-rate episode, duration about 60 seconds, by auto-triggering function by ELR (SpiderFlash, Livanova, Italy).

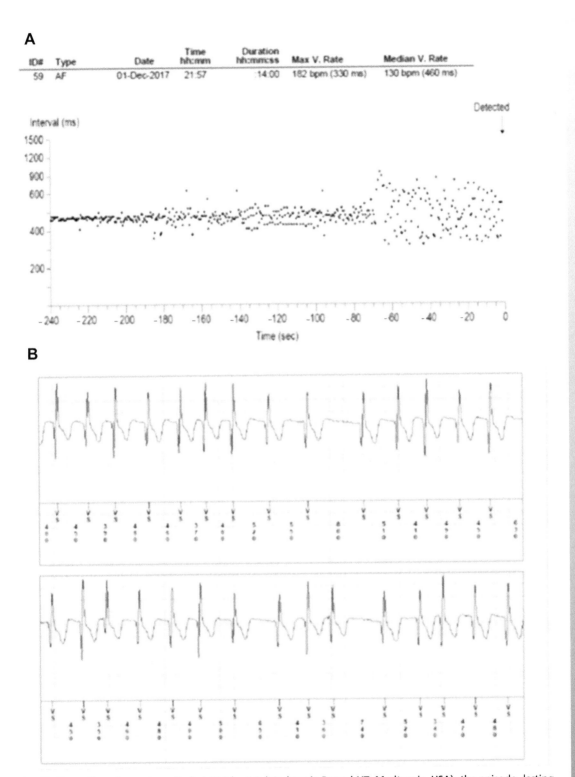

Fig. 13. Recording of symptomatic fast PAF by ILR (Medtronic Reveal XT, Medtronic, USA): the episode, lasting 14 minutes, was both automatically detected by the autotriggering function and activated manually by the patient as a symptom. (*A*) PAF episode. (*B*) ECG tracing automatically stored showing the PAF episode (the end of the episode was not recorded).

A   **B**

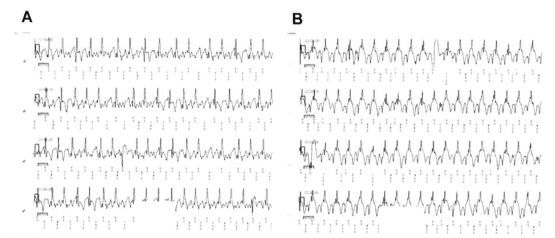

Fig. 14. Correct and incorrect detection of asymptomatic PAF by ILR (Medtronic LinQ, Medtronic, USA) in a patient (female, 75 years, history of cryptogenic stroke). (*A*) An episode of real PAF. (*B*) Sinus tachycardia with sporadic VEBs.

duration (24–72 hours) Holter recordings are best suited for patients with very frequent paroxysms of AF or persistent AF. For less frequent episodes, patient-activated event and loop recorders can be used for several weeks at a time. These devices are particularly useful for capturing ECG recordings during symptomatic events and clarify the arrhythmic basis for unexplained or ambiguous symptoms, especially if infrequent. Autotriggered devices have higher diagnostic yield than standard 24-hour Holter monitors and 30-day loop recorders. Although these monitors can detect the onset of an arrhythmia such as AF, their algorithms are not designed to include the offset of the arrhythmia. Thus, information about the burden of AF cannot be consistently ascertained. Patch monitors and Mobile cardiac outpatient telemetry (MCOT) are the most complete outpatient ECG recording, increasing the likelihood for detecting AF and they can provide accurate representation of AF burden for the duration of recording. Very prolonged recordings, by ILR, more expensive and minimally invasive, are recommended for selected cases.

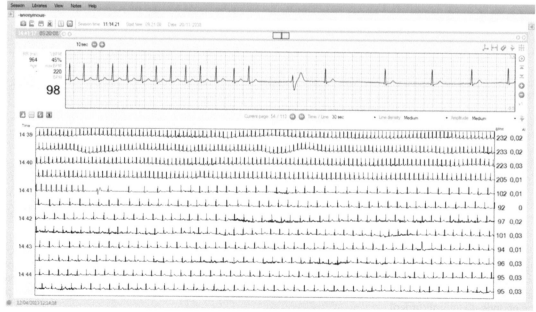

Fig. 15. Episode of PAF recorded by 30-day continuous monitoring (NUUBO 30, NUUBO, Spain). The total duration of the episode (16 minutes), including the offset, was recorded.

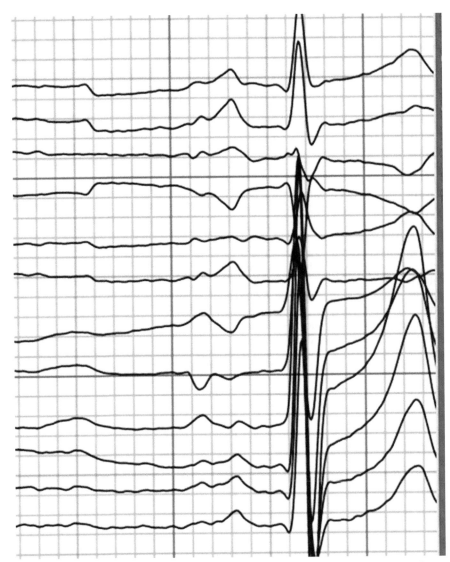

Fig. 16. Sinus rhythm with a notched broad (>110 milliseconds) P wave with terminal negative forces in V1. This finding is not specific for a single atrial pathologic condition but most likely represents the end result of extensive remodeling.

P WAVE MORPHOLOGY AND ATRIAL FIBRILLATION

The P wave in SR can show several abnormalities that seem to select patients at increased risk of developing AF or progressing from paroxysmal to persistent fibrillation. The ECG changes correlate with atrial remodeling and/or presence of conduction delays, possibly due to fibrosis.

The ECG criteria most predictive of these clinical events are alterations of P wave morphology, which supposedly reflect some of the anatomic or electrical changes induced by remodeling. This association is not always very strict and some P wave variations may be within normal limits or be attributed to diverse etiologic factors.

For example, a broad, notched P wave in lead II and a deep and broad negative P terminal force in lead V1 have classically been used as electrocardiographic criteria for left atrial enlargement (**Fig. 16**). The specificity of this feature is not very high because several pathologic conditions are associated with these findings: left atrial volume or pressure overload, an interatrial conduction defect, or a combination of these abnormalities. Patient with this P wave morphology are more likely to develop or already have a history of AF, suggesting that these ECG changes may reflect electrical or mechanical atrial remodeling. As in ventricular fibrillation, increasing dispersion of repolarization should parallel AF inducibility. Atrial repolarization is not measurable in standard ECG but P wave dispersion, measured as the difference between maximum and minimum P wave duration in any of the 12 leads, seems to be correlated with inhomogeneity of atrial excitation. Dispersion of excitation can be due to atrial structural alterations, conduction delays, or blocks or abnormal impulse propagation changes that are all central to the concept of remodeling.

In several studies, this index seems predictive of de novo development of PAF and progression from paroxysmal to persistent AF. Following observations made in patients with ventricular tachycardia, some investigators have studied prolonged P wave duration using signal average ECG techniques. The assumption behind these studies is that this method can enhance detection of conduction delay, especially if it occurs late in relatively small portions of the atria. Although this is probably true, the complexity of performing and interpreting an Signal averaged ECG compared with ECG reading has prevented this test from becoming a routine clinical investigation.

P WAVE CHANGES FOLLOWING ATRIAL FIBRILLATION CATHETER ABLATION

PV isolation (PVI), mostly achieved with radiofrequency or cryoenergy, is an increasingly common procedure in the therapy for drug-resistant AF. Notwithstanding its long-term superiority to AADs, PVI is associated, depending on the type of AF, with a recurrence rate of AF or AFL varying between 20% and 60%. The P wave postprocedure has been evaluated to identify possible predictors of recurrences.

The P wave duration following PVI should be correlated, among other factors, with the amount of LA tissue ablated. In particular, some investigators have speculated that activation of tissue inside the PVs contributes to the terminal portion of the P wave. A successful procedure is associated with complete PVI and, often, a wider circumferential ablation with more atrial tissue electrically disconnected and, therefore, a shorter P wave. Some studies have, in fact, shown that a reduction of P wave duration post-PVI is associated with a decreased number of AF recurrences postablation (**Fig. 17**).

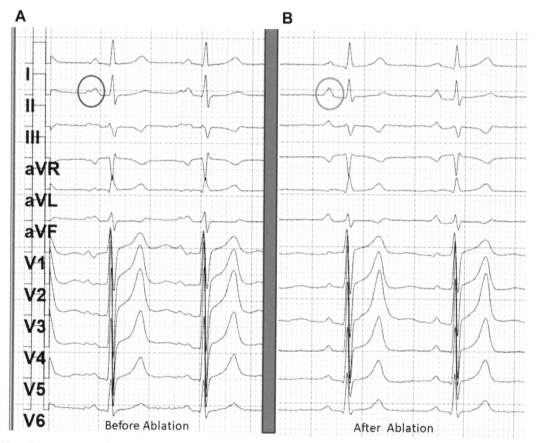

Fig. 17. P wave in SR before (*A*) and after (*B*) PVI for AF. Before ablation the P wave presented notching and a duration of 120 milliseconds. Following ablation the notching are less evident and P wave is 90 milliseconds.

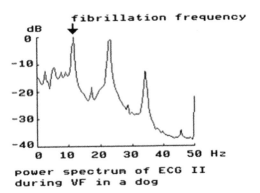

Fig. 18. Spectral analysis of an episode of AF. Dominant frequency is the highest frequency peak.

ELECTROCARDIOGRAM-DERIVED PARAMETERS TO ASSESS ATRIAL FIBRILLATION COMPLEXITY

The atrial remodeling, as previously mentioned, will induce progressive changes of ion channels function, overall cellular function, and cellular coupling, which enhances dispersion of refractoriness and propensity to spontaneous electrical activity. These modifications increase the tendency to develop and sustain AF once initiated. Furthermore, this inhomogeneous atrial structure creates obstacles to organized propagation by increasing the areas of conduction block.

Breakdown of conduction during AF will generate a higher number of coexisting fibrillation wavelets, increasing AF complexity. This phenomenon has been documented in animal and human studies using direct epicardial recordings demonstrating a direct relationship between degrees of complexity and duration of AF. The 12-lead ECG, as previously mentioned, does not reflect the organization of AF except for some inference based on the size of the F wave in V1. Other information can be extracted from the ECG using other

Equally, an absolute P wave duration above 150 milliseconds or abnormal indices of P wave dispersion seems to portend decreased success. Insufficient data are available to clarify whether this is due to a persistent connection of PVs, incomplete electrical remodeling, or an unfavorable hemodynamic situation with persistent elevated LA pressure and volume.

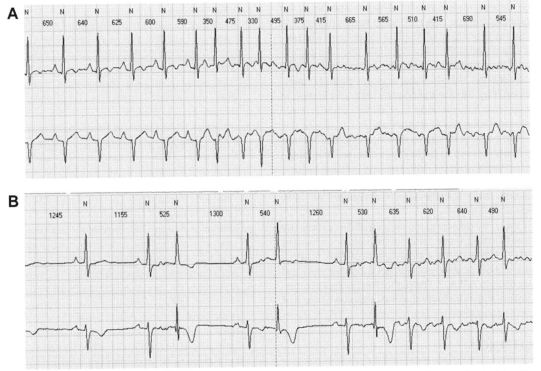

Fig. 19. Autonomic effects on the induction of AF. (*A*) Initiation of AF during an increased sympathetic drive. The arrhythmia is preceded by a period of sinus tachycardia and demonstrates a fast ventricular response. (*B*) Vagal induction of AF. Sinus bradycardia with frequent APCs and the ensuing AF has a slower ventricular rate. Both autonomic stimulations increase conduction and repolarization heterogeneity, facilitating AF induction.

analysis methods based mostly on frequency domain parameters.[12]

The frequency content of periods of single-lead or multilead recordings lasting at least 10 seconds can be evaluated using power spectral analysis, which can quantify the highest peak in the spectrum, also called dominant frequency (**Fig. 18**). The distribution of frequencies within the spectrum, the level of the dominant frequencies, and other parameters computed from the spectral analysis, correlate with the degree of organization of AF. In particular, with its marked variation of amplitude and morphology, dominant frequency analysis allows identification of a hidden order within an otherwise uninterpretable ECG recording of AF. The presence of discreet frequency peaks suggests that within the apparent disorganization of AF propagation there are periods of stable activation, corresponding in some animal studies, to slow meandering of rotors mostly localized in the LA posterior wall.[13]

Some investigators have, on the other hand, interpreted spectral peaks at specific frequencies as persistence of triggers inducing AF in the first place and continuing to discharge at fast regular rates. Support for this hypothesis has been garnered by observing, following PVI, residual ATs discharging at the same frequency, generating the spectral peaks already observed during AF. In a few cases, targeting with ablation the areas of dominant frequencies has led to termination of AF.

Spectral analysis of AF ECG is also useful to better characterize the behavior of AF and help to predict the arrhythmia response to several clinical interventions.[14] Both vagal and sympathetic stimulation (**Fig. 19**) are associated with a reduction in atrial refractory periods and an increase in atrial heterogeneity and AF induction.[15]

Furthermore, because slowing of fibrillatory rate has been shown to be highly predictive of spontaneous termination of PAF, spectral content associated with a low fibrillatory rate was able to identify patients with spontaneous termination AF with high accuracy.[16]

Finally, by reflecting the degree of AF complexity more faithfully, these parameters have been used to predict spontaneous cardioversion of PAF, maintenance of SR post-Direct Current Cardioversion and response to AADs.[17] The higher the degree of organization, the more favorable the outcome of each of these procedures.

REFERENCES

1. Schnabel RB, Yin X, Gona P, et al. 50 year trends in atrial fibrillation prevalence, incidence, risk factors, and mortality in the Framingham Heart Study: a cohort study. Lancet 2015;386(9989):154–62.

2. Wijffels MC, Kirchhof CJ, Dorland R, et al. Atrial fibrillation begets atrial fibrillation. A study in awake chronically instrumented goats. Circulation 1995; 92:1954–68.

3. Schotten U, Greiser M, Benke D, et al. Atrial fibrillation-induced atrial contractile dysfunction: a tachycardiomyopathy of a different sort. Cardiovasc Res 2002;53:192–201.

4. Haissaguerre M, Jais P, Shah DC, et al. Spontaneous initiation of atrial fibrillation by ectopic beats originating in the pulmonary veins. N Engl J Med 1998;339:659–66.

5. Rensma PL, Alleesie MA, Lammers WJ, et al. Length of excitation wave and susceptibility to reentrant atrial arrhythmias in normal conscious dogs. Circ Res 1988;62:395–410.

6. Jalife J, Berenfeld O, Mansour M. Mother rotors and fibrillatory conduction: a mechanism of atrial fibrillation. Cardiovasc Res 2002;54:204–16.

7. Haissaguerre M, Hocini M, Denis A, et al. Driver domains in persistent atrial fibrillation. Circulation 2014; 130:530–8.

8. Schuessler RB, Kawamoto T, Hand DE, et al. Simultaneous epicardial and endocardial activation sequence mapping in the isolated precursor canine right atrium. Circulation 1993;88:250–63, 1996;70:1105–11.

9. Kennedy HL. The history science and innovation of Holter technology. Ann Noninvasive Electrocardiol 2006;11:85–94.

10. ACC/AHA Guidelines for Ambulatory Electrocardiography. Executive summary and recommendations. Circulation 1999;100:886–93.

11. Steinberg JS, Varma N, Cygankiewicz I, et al. ISHNE-HRS expert consensus statement on ambulatory ECG and external cardiac monitoring/telemetry. Ann Noninvasive Electrocardiol 2017;22:e12447.

12. Rosenbaum DS, Cohen RJ. Frequency based measures of atrial fibrillation in man. IEEE Engineering in Medicine and Biology Magazine 1990;12(2):582–3.

13. Sanders P, Berenfeld O, Hocini M, et al. Spectral analysis identifies sites of high-frequency activity maintaining atrial fibrillation in humans. Circulation 2005;112:789–97.

14. Bollmann A, Husser D, Stridh M, et al. Frequency measures obtained from the surface electrocardiogram in atrial fibrillation research and clinical decision-making. J Cardiovasc Electrophysiol 2003;14:S154–61.

15. Prystowsky EN, Naccarelli GV, Jackman WM, et al. Enhanced parasympathetic tone shortens atrial refractoriness in man. Am J Cardiol 1983;51:96.

16. Nilsson F, Stridh M, Bollmann A, et al. Predicting spontaneous termination of atrial fibrillation using the surface ECG. Med Eng Phys 2006;28:802–8.

17. Bollmann A, Binias KH, Toepffer I, et al. Importance of left atrial diameter and atrial fibrillatory frequency for conversion of persistent atrial fibrillation with oral flecainide. Am J Cardiol 2002;90:1011–4.

Peculiar Electrocardiographic Aspects of Wide QRS Complex Tachycardia
When Differential Diagnosis Is Difficult

Roberto De Ponti, MD, FHRS[a],*, Jacopo Marazzato, MD[a],
Giuseppe Bagliani, MD[b,c], Alessandra Tondini, MD[d],
Stefano Donzelli, MD[d], Luigi Padeletti, MD[e,f]

KEYWORDS

- Wide QRS complex tachycardia • Ventricular tachycardia • Aberrant atrioventricular conduction
- Bundle branch reentry ventricular tachycardia • Antidromic atrioventricular reentrant tachycardia
- Hisian tachycardia

KEY POINTS

- Algorithms for discrimination between a supraventricular arrhythmia with aberrant conduction and a ventricular tachycardia are useful to guide electrocardiographic interpretation in case of wide QRS complex tachycardia.
- Ventricular tachycardia involving the specific conduction system can generate an electrocardiographic pattern that shares some aspects with supraventricular arrhythmias with aberrant conduction.
- Antidromic atrioventricular reentrant tachycardia involving accessory pathways with unique conduction properties may have an electrocardiographic aspect leading to a misdiagnosis of ventricular tachycardia.
- In complex clinical conditions, 2 arrhythmias sustained by different substrates may display a similar electrocardiographic pattern with a wide QRS complex.
- In case of supraventricular arrhythmia with aberrant conduction, antiarrhythmic drug therapy may modify the electrocardiographic pattern in a way that it resembles a ventricular arrhythmia.

INTRODUCTION

Wide QRS complex tachycardia (WCT) refers to a cardiac rhythm with a rate of more than 100 beats per minute and an increased duration ($\geq$120 ms) of the QRS complex that can be related to a ventricular origin, aberrant atrioventricular (AV) conduction, ventricular pacing, or ventricular preexcitation.[1] In clinical practice, this electrocardiographic pattern may be commonly

Disclosure: The authors have nothing to disclose.
[a] Department of Cardiology, School of Medicine, University of Insubria, Viale Borri, 57, Varese 21100, Italy;
[b] Arrhythmology Unit, Cardiology Department, Foligno General Hospital, Via Massimo Arcamone, Foligno, Perugia 06034, Italy; [c] Cardiovascular Disease Department, University of Perugia, Piazza Menghini 1, Perugia 06129, Italy; [d] Arrhythmology Unit, Cardiology Department, Terni Hospital, Piazzale Tristano da Joannuccio, 1, Terni 05100, Italy; [e] Heart and Vessels Department, University of Florence, Largo Brambilla, 3, Florence 50134, Italy; [f] Cardiology Department, IRCCS Multimedica, Via Milanese, 300, Sesto San Giovanni, Milan 20099, Italy
* Corresponding author.
E-mail address: roberto.deponti@uninsubria.it

Card Electrophysiol Clin 10 (2018) 317–332
https://doi.org/10.1016/j.ccep.2018.02.005
1877-9182/18/© 2018 Elsevier Inc. All rights reserved.

encountered and the correct differential diagnosis among these options is of the utmost importance for proper patient management. Above all, the presence of a ventricular tachycardia (VT) should be discriminated from a supraventricular rhythm. **Box 1** summarizes the electrocardiographic criteria that have been reported in detail by several authors[1–6] and can be adopted in a step-by-step approach to a WCT. Importantly, despite the high accuracy of these diagnostic algorithms, these criteria are not infallible and electrocardiographic interpretation in some cases remains particularly challenging. In fact, the diagnosis of some types of VT may be exceptionally difficult for the involvement of the distal AV conduction system, the persistence of a 1:1 ventriculoatrial

---

Box 1

Electrocardiographic criteria to discriminate between ventricular and supraventricular origin in wide QRS complex tachycardia

- Identification of atrial activity
- Relationship between atrial and ventricular activity
  - AV dissociation = VT
- Morphologic changes of the wide QRS complex during tachycardia
  - Capture and fusion beats = VT
  - Ashmann phenomenon (aberrant conduction related to variations of the preceding cardiac cycle length) = SVT
- Detailed morphologic analysis of the wide QRS complex
  - Brugada algorithm[5]
    - Absence of RS complex in all the precordial leads or negative/positive concordance → VT
    - Longest interval from R onset to S >100 ms in any precordial lead → VT
    - Further analysis of QRS complex morphology in V1, V2, and V6
      - RBBB or LBBB pattern (Sandler and Marriott criteria)[2]
        - Initial vector of the QRS complex identical to sinus rhythm → SVT
        - rSR' complex with S crossing isoelectric line → SVT
        - Triphasic QRS complex in V1 → SVT
      - RBBB pattern (Wellens criteria)[3]
        - QRS width >140 ms and left axis deviation → VT
        - QR, R, RSr' (with S not crossing the isoelectric line) in V1 → VT
        - R/S <1 or QS in V6 → VT
      - LBBB pattern (Kindwall criteria)[4]
        - R wave in V1 or V2 >30 ms → VT
        - Interval between QRS onset and nadir of the S wave in V1 or V2 >60 ms → VT
        - Notch on the downstroke of the S wave in V1 or V2 → VT
        - Any Q wave in V6 → VT
  - Vereckei algorithm[6]
    - Initial, dominant R wave in aVR → VT
    - Initial, non-dominant q or r in aVR greater than 40 ms → VT
    - Notch on the initial downstroke in aVR → VT
    - Amplitude of the last 40 ms of the QRS complex ≥ amplitude of the first 40 ms of the QRS complex in aVR → VT

Abbreviations: AV, atrioventricular; LBBB, left bundle branch block; RBBB, right bundle branch block; SVT, supraventricular tachycardia; VT, ventricular tachycardia; →, suggests diagnosis of.
   Data from Refs.[1–6]

conduction, and/or failure of some electrocardiographic criteria to distinguish these ventricular arrhythmias from a supraventricular one. Similarly, in some supraventricular tachycardias (SVT), the administration of antiarrhythmic drugs, severe electrolyte imbalance, or involvement of accessory AV pathways with peculiar conduction property may lead to a WCT with an electrocardiographic pattern that is very difficult to interpret. **Box 2** summarizes the most common causes possibly responsible for misinterpretation of a WCT. Therefore, in WCT, clinical aspects, such as a patient's history and presentation, should be considered, to adopt an integrated approach and avoid misinterpretation as much as possible.

The aim of this article is to present a series of cases with a peculiar electrocardiographic pattern during WCT to demonstrate that particular forms of arrhythmia or complex clinical contests may generate a challenging electrocardiographic pattern. Although rare, these forms should be always considered when a WCT of difficult interpretation is approached.

CASE 1. FASCICULAR VENTRICULAR TACHYCARDIA
Case Presentation

A 38-year-old man was admitted to the emergency department for palpitations, which had begun 2 hours before. The electrocardiogram (ECG) showed a WCT at 165 beats per minute with right bundle branch block morphology and marked left axis deviation configuring a left anterior hemiblock (**Fig. 1**). Intravenous beta-blocker

---

Box 2
Reasons of peculiar electrocardiographic pattern during wide QRS complex tachycardia

1. Antiarrhythmic drugs
2. Electrolyte imbalance
3. Acute myocardial inflammation
4. Particular forms of tachycardias involving or originating in the specific conduction system
   - Fascicular ventricular tachycardia
   - Bundle branch reentry ventricular tachycardia
   - Hisian tachycardia with distal conduction delay
5. Slow-conducting right or left atriofascicular or atrioventricular accessory pathways involved in antidromic atrioventricular reentrant tachycardia

---

administration failed to interrupt the arrhythmia. Sinus rhythm was restored by intravenous verapamil administration. No conduction defect during sinus rhythm was present and no structural heart disease was observed at transthoracic echocardiogram.

Electrocardiogram Interpretation

During tachycardia, the QRS complex is not greatly widened (140 ms) and its QRS morphology shares common aspects with aberrant conduction owing to right bundle branch block and left anterior hemiblock. After the QRS complex, negative P waves can be identified in leads II and aVF. However, P waves are present every second QRS complex, which is consistent with 2:1 ventriculoatrial block during a ventricular rhythm. This finding clearly rules out the supraventricular origin of the tachycardia and leads to the diagnosis of fascicular VT.

Clinical Considerations

Fascicular VT is an idiopathic form of verapamil-sensitive arrhythmia occurring predominantly in young males (between 15 and 40 years of age) with no structural heart disease.[7] The form related to the left posterior fascicle is by far the most frequent form, encountered in approximately 90% of cases, with a right bundle branch block morphology and left axis deviation; other forms in relation with left anterior fascicle and upper septal fascicle account for 10% of the cases.[8] The mechanism of the most common form is believed to be reentry involving the posterior fascicle of the left bundle branch and the Purkinje network,[9] although the reentry circuit is not well-understood, because the left ventricular myocardium may participate in the circuit, and the left posterior fascicle can be only passively activated.[10,11] Regardless of the pathophysiology, the anatomic location of the circuit generates a narrower QRS complex morphology, mimicking an SVT with aberrant conduction. The clinical context of a young healthy individual with tachycardia interruption by verapamil administration could be also misleading, considering that, opposite to what observed in the present case, there could be 1:1 ventriculoatrial conduction during tachycardia or the P wave cannot be easily identified. However, in the absence of any preexisting conduction disturbance in sinus rhythm, it is very unlikely that an SVT shows aberrant conduction for simultaneous functional conduction block over the right bundle branch and left anterior fascicle, especially if the arrhythmias has a relatively longer cycle length, as in the present case.

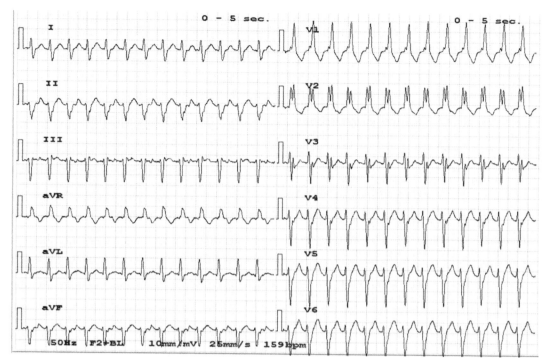

Fig. 1. Idiopathic left ventricular tachycardia involving the posterior fascicle.

CASE 2. RIGHT VENTRICULAR OUTFLOW TRACT TACHYCARDIA TERMINATED BY ADENOSINE

Case Presentation

A 73-year-old man was referred for recurrent palpitations during exercise. The presenting ECG showed sinus rhythm with normal morphology of the QRS complex and repetitive premature ventricular complexes with a left bundle branch block morphology, inferior axis deviation, and a longer coupling interval (**Fig. 2**). Transthoracic echocardiogram, as well as MRI, showed no structural heart disease. During exercise stress test, sustained WCT with the same morphology of the premature ventricular contractions was observed and persisted after effort stress test at a rate of 100 beats per minute (**Fig. 3**). An intravenous bolus of adenosine restored sinus rhythm. Coronary angiography was unremarkable.

Electrocardiogram Interpretation

During the sustained tachycardia, there is a stable 1:1 relationship between the atrial and ventricular activity with a P wave after the QRS complex, well evident as a notch in the peripheral leads. The QRS morphology is identical to the one of the premature ventricular complexes, except for an earlier transition in the precordial leads in the sustained form, which is likely to depend on

electrode positioning. Moreover, the detailed morphologic analysis of the QRS complex according to the criteria showed in **Box 1** clearly indicate the ventricular origin of the tachycardia. In fact, the patient was cured by catheter ablation of the ventricular focus in the right ventricular outflow tract.

Clinical Considerations

Right ventricular outflow tract tachycardia is a form of idiopathic ventricular arrhythmia and occurs more often in young people, both in males and females, although sometimes it can be present in the elderly. It has typically a benign course, but some cases with associated malignant ventricular arrhythmias have been reported when a short coupling interval of the premature ventricular contractions is present.[12] Most patients experience exercise-induced palpitations and the arrhythmia can be induced during effort stress test.[13] The adrenergic-dependent aspect of this arrhythmia has been documented. Although reentry and enhanced automaticity have been also postulated as potential mechanisms of this tachycardia,[14] cyclic adenosine monophosphate-mediated trigger activity is the most likely mechanism.[15] Adenosine injection, as well as other vagal stimulation maneuvers or verapamil administration, can terminate this and other forms of idiopathic VT[15–18] and in some cases this may lead to the misdiagnosis of SVT.[16] Therefore, these modalities of arrhythmia

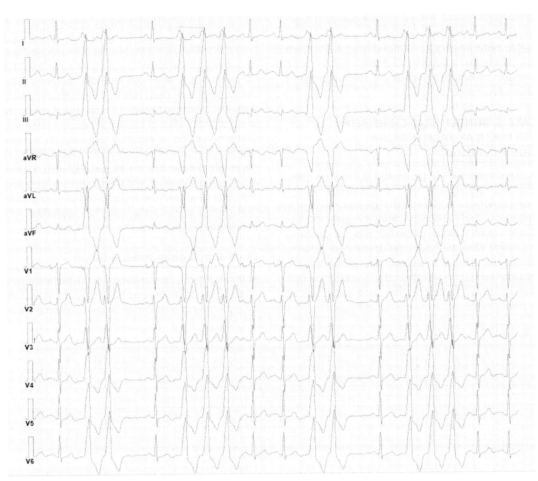

Fig. 2. Baseline electrocardiogram.

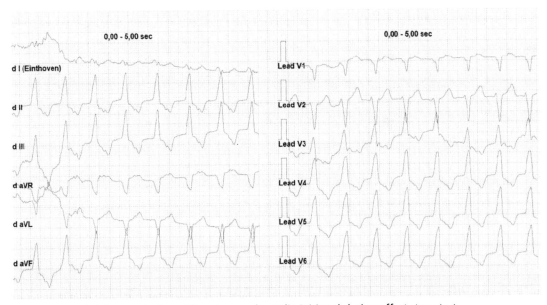

Fig. 3. Sustained right ventricular outflow tract tachycardia initiated during effort stress test.

termination should not be considered pathogno-monic of an SVT. Interestingly, some cases of idio-pathic right ventricular outflow tract tachycardia are adenosine insensitive and this may be due to somatic myocardial mutations involving the A_1 adenosine receptor.[19]

CASE 3. BUNDLE BRANCH REENTRY VENTRICULAR TACHYCARDIA
Case Presentation

A 77-year-old patient presented at the emergency room for poorly tolerated palpitations. Twenty years before, he suffered from anterior myocardial infarction and coronary angiography showed single-vessel disease of the left anterior descend-ing artery. Over the years, he developed ischemic cardiomyopathy with severely depressed left ven-tricular function and a left ventricular ejection frac-tion of 20%. Therefore, he underwent internal

cardioverter/defibrillation implantation for primary prevention. Subsequently, he did not attend regu-larly the follow-up visits. He did not take any anti-arrhythmic medication. Upon admittance, the ECG showed WCT with left bundle branch block morphology and heart rate of 175 beats per minute (**Fig. 4**A). Because the arrhythmia was poorly toler-ated, urgent external electrical cardioversion was performed in the emergency room, which restored sinus rhythm with first-degree AV block and com-plete left bundle branch block (**Fig. 4**B). Device interrogation showed that the cutoff rate for detec-tion was programmed higher than the ventricular rate during tachycardia and this explained why the device did not treat the arrhythmia.

Electrocardiogram Interpretation

At first sight, the interpretation of the tachycardia is challenging. If, on the one hand, the analysis of the

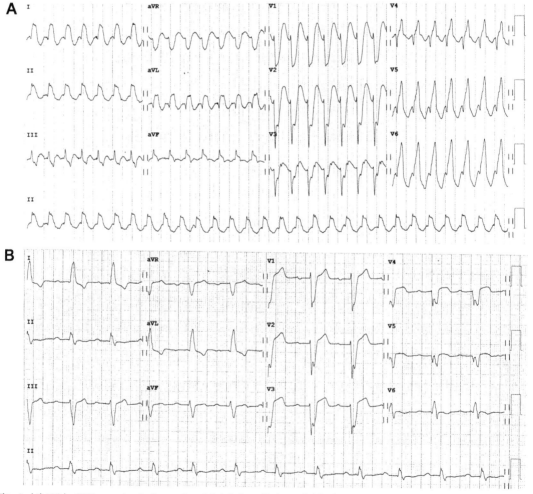

Fig. 4. (*A*) Wide QRS complex tachycardia with left bundle branch block morphology. (*B*) Sinus rhythm with first-degree atrioventricular conduction block and left bundle branch block.

right precordial leads according to the Brugada algorithm would suggest a supraventricular origin, the presence of a notch at the very end of the downstroke of the S wave in aVR would suggest a ventricular origin, according to the Vereckei algorithm. Compared with the ECG in sinus rhythm, the QRS axis is not superiorly deviated and the QRS complex is positive in the left precordial leads during tachycardia. However, the latter might depend on different electrode positioning after cardioversion. Moreover, notches just after the end of the QRS complex, observed only in lead V3 could be misinterpreted as retrogradely conducted P waves. Based on clinical considerations, a WCT with a left bundle branch block morphology, similar but not identical to the QRS morphology in sinus rhythm, in a patient with severe structural heart disease is highly suspicious for bundle branch reentry VT. Moreover, the combination of a first-degree AV block and left bundle branch block in sinus rhythm may be indicative of a long H-V interval, a marker of conduction delay over the AV conduction system distal to the His bundle. This pattern further favors the hypothesis that there could be the substrate for a reentry circuit involving the 2 bundle branches and able to sustain this tachycardia. During hospital stay, the patient underwent electrophysiologic study. The H-V interval measured 72 ms and programmed S2S3 ventricular stimulation reproducibly induced the clinical tachycardia that, based on electrophysiologic criteria, was diagnosed as bundle branch reentry VT and adequately treated.

Clinical Consideration

Bundle branch reentry VT is an infrequent form of arrhythmia, generally observed in patients with nonischemic cardiomyopathy[20] exhibiting left bundle branch block in sinus rhythm, although it can be observed also in patients with ischemic cardiomyopathy or without an evident structural heart disease.[21,22] Generally, it has a fast ventricular rate and it is thought to be the cause of sudden cardiac death in patients with structural heart disease, if they do not receive an implantable cardioverter/defibrillator.[22] It may be not induced by programmed ventricular stimulation, even by using specific protocols with long–short–long coupling intervals.[23] When the reentry is sustained retrogradely by the left bundle branch and antegradely by the right, activation of the ventricular myocardium begins at the terminus of the right bundle branch and therefore the QRS morphology mimics that of a supraventricular rhythm with aberrant conduction, although functional or anatomic reasons could be responsible for a slightly different QRS morphology. In this case, as well as in other cases encountered in clinical practice, the tachycardia cycle length was relatively longer, probably related to the marked conduction delay in the distal AV conduction system and not to the effect of antiarrhythmic drugs that the patient did not receive. Peculiarly, the tachycardia was easily inducible by programmed electrical stimulation, confirming the diagnostic hypothesis based on clinical considerations.

CASE 4. HISIAN TACHYCARDIA WITH WIDE QRS COMPLEX OWING TO PREEXISTING RIGHT BUNDLE BRANCH BLOCK AND LEFT ANTERIOR HEMIBLOCK
Case Presentation

A 67-year-old patient was referred for congestive heart failure and recurrent atrial arrhythmia. He suffered from hypertension and ischemic cardiomyopathy owing to an old anterior myocardial infarction with severely depressed left ventricular function (ejection fraction of 25%) with moderate mitral regurgitation. Before referral he underwent coronary angiography with evidence of chronic occlusion of the left anterior descending artery. Upon admittance, he received continuous electrocardiographic monitoring, which showed sinus rhythm with first-degree AV block, right bundle branch block, and left anterior hemiblock (**Fig. 5**). During subsequent monitoring, sinus rhythm alternated with atrial fibrillation with a ventricular rate of about 100 beats per minute (**Fig. 6**A). A slightly different electrocardiographic pattern was also evident (**Fig. 6**B).

Electrocardiogram Interpretation

Although the patient never had syncope, a major AV conduction disturbance is present. Moreover, a bifid, low-voltage, and longer P wave in sinus rhythm is consistent with a marked atrial conduction delay and atrial enlargement and, therefore, it is not surprising that this patient had paroxysmal recurrent atrial fibrillation with a QRS complex identical to the one in sinus rhythm. **Fig. 6**B shows an irregular ventricular rhythm as during atrial fibrillation, with the same morphology of the QRS complex, considering that during continuous monitoring there could be modifications of the electrode or body position. However, in this tracing, no atrial fibrillatory activity is evident and dissociated P waves can be noted. Although this rhythm and sinus rhythm alternate, the patient underwent electrophysiologic study. During sinus rhythm, the H-V interval measured 75 ms, confirming critical conduction delay of the distal AV conduction system. Moreover, the rhythm showed in

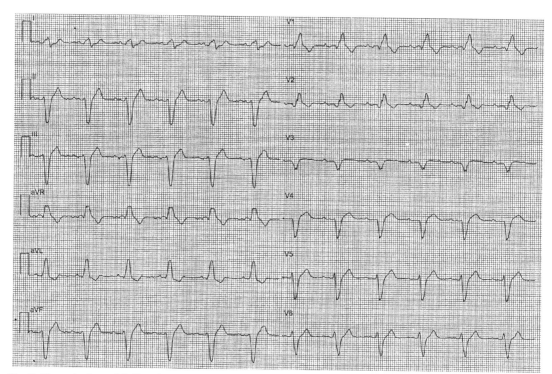

Fig. 5. Sinus rhythm with first degree atrioventricular block, right bundle branch block, and left anterior hemiblock. A markedly prolonged P wave is evident in each lead.

Fig. 6B was diagnosed as an iterative Hisian tachycardia (H-V interval during tachycardia of 90 ms) with an irregular cycle length and dissociated sinus activity. The patient received an implantable cardioverter/defibrillator capable of cardiac resynchronization therapy. Induction of AV conduction block by ablation completely prevented recurrence of the Hisian tachycardia and allowed regular biventricular pacing.

Clinical Considerations

Hisian ectopy/tachycardia is an uncommon rhythm disorder and only sporadically reported in previous published reports.[24,25] To reach the diagnosis, it is of the utmost importance to exclude both the atrial and the ventricular origin of the tachycardia. As previously reported,[24] the main features include the lack of atrial activation preceding the His bundle potential and the close similarity of the QRS complex to the one recorded during sinus rhythm. Moreover, the finding of a reversed activation sequence of the His bundle during ectopy compared with that during sinus rhythm is another criterion to confirm the diagnosis. Although a narrow morphology of the QRS is usually reported,[24,25] in this case the widened QRS complex morphology is due to a preexistent distal conduction defect. Opposite to

what has been described for a ventricular rhythm originating close to the specific conduction system, in this case the combination of the severe disturbance of the distal AV conduction and higher rate during tachycardia could be responsible for mild H-V prolongation (15 ms) compared with sinus rhythm, although decremental conduction is not characteristic of the normal distal AV system.

CASE 5. ANTIDROMIC ATRIOVENTRICULAR REENTRANT TACHYCARDIA INVOLVING A RIGHT-SIDED ATRIOFASCICULAR ACCESSORY PATHWAY
Case Presentation

A 25-year-old man presented at the emergency room for a prolonged episode of palpitation. His prior history was unremarkable for cardiovascular diseases: he only had short-lasting sporadic self-terminating episodes of palpitation and his echocardiogram and Holter monitoring did not show structural heart disease or significant arrhythmias. Upon hospital admittance, the ECG shown in **Fig. 7**A was recorded: a regular tachycardia at 165 beats per minute with a left bundle branch block morphology is evident. A rapid intravenous bolus of adenosine interrupted the tachycardia and restored sinus rhythm (**Fig. 7**B).

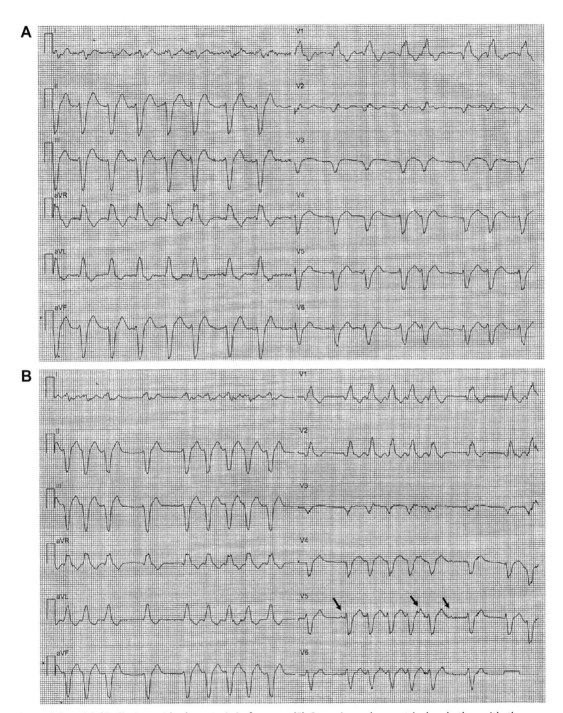

Fig. 6. (*A*) Atrial fibrillation with characteristic f waves. (*B*) Same irregular ventricular rhythm with the same morphology of the QRS complex (except for V2), but with dissociated P waves (*arrows*).

Electrocardiogram Interpretation

The analysis of WCT suggests an SVT with aberrant conduction owing to left bundle branch block. In particular, according to the criteria in **Box 1**, the absence of AV dissociation or capture/fusion beats and the morphology of the QRS complex in the right precordial leads with short-lasting r wave, and absence of notching in the downstroke of the S wave in V2-V3 strongly favor this hypothesis. Moreover, a short P-R interval and no sign of preexcitation suggest the presence of a fast AV

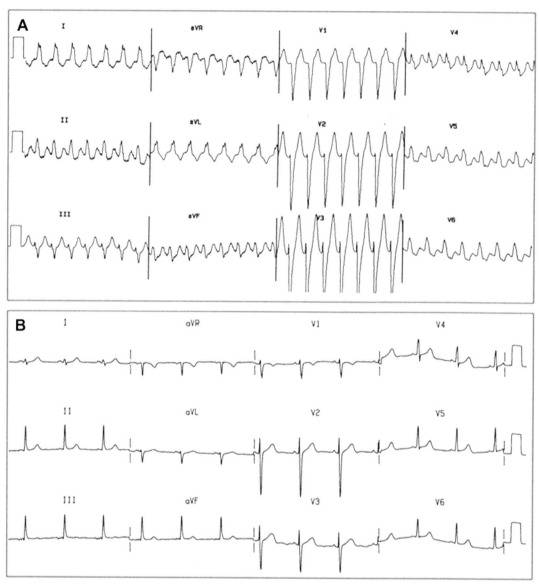

Fig. 7. Twelve-lead electrocardiogram during the clinical arrhythmia (*A*) and sinus rhythm (*B*).

nodal pathway, further in favor of AV nodal reentry tachycardia. However, it remains unclear why a young, healthy individual would exhibit a left bundle branch block during a relatively slow tachycardia. The patient underwent electrophysiologic study and an atriofascicular accessory pathway located in the anterolateral region of the tricuspid annulus exhibiting only slow and decremental antegrade conduction was diagnosed. During programmed ventricular stimulation an antidromic AV reentrant tachycardia was reproducibly induced with a QRS morphology identical to the one of the spontaneous episode. **Fig. 8**A schematically represents the tachycardia circuit. The accessory pathway was successfully ablated by radiofrequency energy and the patient was permanently cured.

Clinical Considerations

Right-sided atriofascicular accessory pathways with antegrade slow and decremental conduction, also known as "pseudo-Mahaim" or "Mahaim-type" fibers have been very well described in the literature more than 20 years ago.[26–28] They are characterized by a nodelike structure at their atrial insertion, a long course in the right ventricle, distal insertion that fuses with the right bundle branch, and almost exclusive antegrade decremental conduction.[29,30] The eponym of "Mahaim"

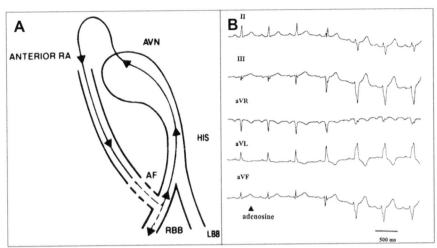

Fig. 8. (*A*) Circuit of the antidromic atrioventricular reentrant tachycardia involving antegrade conduction over a right atriofascicular accessory pathway. (*B*) Adenosine injection during sinus rhythm in a patient with atriofascicular accessory pathway. Adenosine prolongs normal atrioventricular conduction and does not affect conduction over the accessory pathway, which generates a wider QRS complex associated with a long P-R interval. This confirms the presence of slow conduction over these fibers. AF, atriofascicular pathway; AVN, atrioventricular node; RA, right atrium; LBB, left bundle block; RBB, right bundle block.

is incorrectly used to name this accessory pathways.[29] Their distal insertion at the terminus of the right bundle branch is responsible during antidromic AV reentrant tachycardia for a morphology of the QRS complex very difficult to differentiate from the one of an SVT with aberrant conduction owing to left bundle branch block.[31] It could be important to identify these cases in advance of an electrophysiologic procedure, because their presence is associated with longer procedures, lower success, and higher recurrence rate.[27] One possible noninvasive method to unmask conduction over this accessory pathway is a rapid intravenous bolus of adenosine, which prolongs normal AV conduction and has minimal or no effect on conduction over these fibers (**Fig. 8B**).

CASE 6. ANTIDROMIC ATRIOVENTRICULAR REENTRANT TACHYCARDIA INVOLVING A LEFT-SIDED SLOW-CONDUCTING ATRIOVENTRICULAR ACCESSORY PATHWAY
Case Presentation

A 39-year-old patient was admitted to the emergency room for a prolonged episode of palpitation. This was his first episode and it initiated during his daily normal activity as a teacher 6 hours before and was well-tolerated. His prior history was unremarkable. Upon admittance, the ECG showed a WCT of at 180 beats per minute with a right bundle branch block morphology (**Fig. 9**). Termination of the tachycardia was attempted by the cardiologist on duty by intravenous bolus injection of

adenosine and resulted in sinus rhythm restoration (**Fig. 10**). The ECG in sinus rhythm, subsequently recorded, showed incomplete right bundle branch block (**Fig. 11**). The transthoracic echocardiogram showed no structural heart disease.

Electrocardiogram Interpretation

The ECG during tachycardia shows no sign of AV dissociations or capture/fusion beats. Moreover, although incomplete right bundle branch block is present during sinus rhythm, the QRS complex morphology during WCT is atypical for right bundle branch block and this is against aberrant conduction. Considering that termination of VT by adenosine is possible (see case 2) and that 1:1 ventriculoatrial conduction is likely to occur during VT in a young patient, the most probable hypothesis is a ventricular origin of this arrhythmia, from the inferior wall of the left ventricle, possibly related to the posterior fascicle, which further justify sensitivity to adenosine. The small r waves in the inferior leads followed by S waves suggest an endocardial origin.[32,33] Moreover, the absence of any sign of ventricular preexcitation under the effect of adenosine just after tachycardia termination definitely rules out the presence of a slow conducting AV accessory pathway (see case 5). The patient underwent electrophysiologic study that, unexpectedly, showed the presence of a slow conducting AV accessory pathway, located in the posterolateral region of the mitral ring. Incremental and programmed atrial stimulation easily

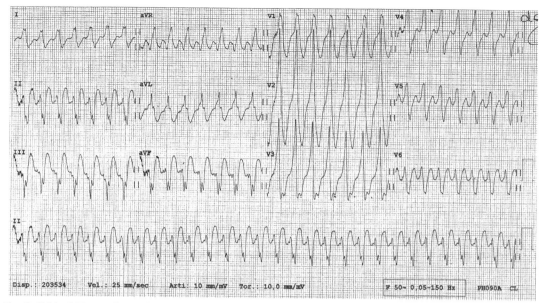

Fig. 9. Wide QRS complex tachycardia with right bundle branch block morphology.

and reproducibly induced the clinical tachycardia. The accessory pathway was ablated during coronary sinus pacing using the transseptal approach.

Clinical Considerations

Left AV accessory pathways exhibiting slow and/ or decremental conduction, although rare, have been previously described.[34,35] The peculiarity of this case is the complete absence of ventricular preexcitation during adenosine injection. Possibly, the increased adrenergic tone related to the long-lasting tachycardia did not allow prolongation of the antegrade AV conduction (the first P-Q interval in sinus rhythm measures 160 ms) and the dose administered (6 mg) was just enough to block the retrograde conduction over the AV node and terminate the tachycardia. This case highlights

the key role of an invasive electrophysiology procedure for correct diagnosis and patient management when a WCT is of difficult interpretation on surface ECG.

CASE 7. TYPICAL ATRIAL FLUTTER WITH 1:1 ABERRANT ATRIOVENTRICULAR CONDUCTION ON FLECAINIDE
Case Presentation

A 56-year-old woman was referred for electrophysiologic evaluation after an episode of WCT with fast ventricular rate (**Fig. 12**). From 2 years earlier, she was on flecainide 100 mg twice a day for paroxysmal atrial fibrillation. While on flecainide, the patient experienced a single sustained episode of 2:1 typical atrial flutter with atrial cycle length of 240 ms. Sinus rhythm was restored by

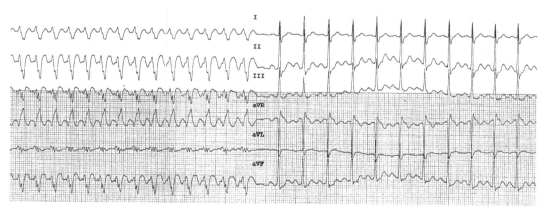

Fig. 10. Tachycardia termination by intravenous bolus of adenosine.

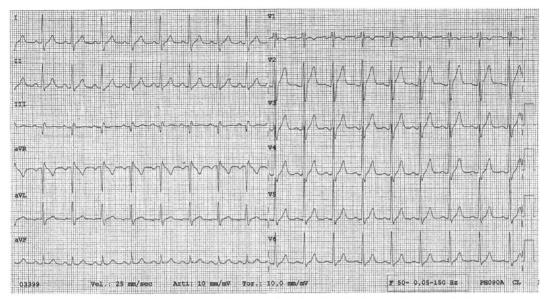

Fig. 11. Electrocardiogram in sinus rhythm with incomplete right bundle branch block morphology.

electrical cardioversion, flecainide was continued, and no beta-blocker prescribed by the attending physician. The patient reported neither symptoms of cardiac origin nor previous syncope during her whole lifetime. Echocardiogram and cardiac magnetic resonance showed no structural heart disease. Coronary angiography was unremarkable. A ventricular origin of the arrhythmia was suspected.

Electrocardiogram Interpretation

This ECG interpretation is challenging. AV dissociation cannot be assessed, because distinct P waves are not clearly seen. The notch that appears before each QRS complex in the inferior leads could be misinterpreted as a P wave. However, they are part of the QRS complex T wave, which is quite prolonged in this case, equaling the tachycardia cycle length (240 ms) and resembling a ventricular flutter. Both the negative QRS complex morphology in all the precordial leads and the north–west axis deviation would suggest a ventricular origin of the tachycardia. However, the onset of each ventricular complex does not show slurred morphology, notches in the downstroke of S waves are not observed, and the nadir of each S wave in the precordial leads is not synchronous, which would favor a supraventricular origin of the tachycardia. Conversely, the careful analysis of the aVR lead shows an almost positive QRS complex that, according to the Vereckei algorithm, favors a ventricular origin. The patient underwent electrophysiologic study and no ventricular arrhythmia was induced by aggressive stimulation

protocols. Similarly, no atrial arrhythmia was inducible, although the antegrade Wenckebach point was 220 ms with no aberrant conduction. Based on the observation that the cycle length of the WCT and the one of typical atrial flutter were the same, it was assumed that the WCT could have been typical atrial flutter with a 1:1 AV conduction and left bundle branch block, favored by flecainide. Therefore, ablation of the cavotricuspid isthmus was performed and bidirectional conduction block achieved. Afterward, over 8 years of follow-up the patient did not experience any recurrence of the WCT, even when flecainide was administered again. Two years after the index procedure, the patient underwent successful pulmonary vein ablation for recurrent drug-refractory atrial fibrillation.

Clinical Considerations

Although spontaneous 1:1 AV conduction of typical atrial flutter merely related to markedly increased sympathetic tone is possible, there are 2 main conditions that can favor this phenomenon. The first may occur in the presence of a fast-conducting AV accessory pathway, and the second can be more frequently observed in relation to administration of intracardiac antiarrhythmic drugs, which can slow the arrhythmia cycle length with no effect on AV node conduction and facilitate 1:1 AV conduction possibly with aberrancy.[36,37] Interestingly, in this case, aberrant conduction associated with antiarrhythmic drug therapy generated a very widened QRS complex with significant alteration of the aberrant pattern owing to left bundle branch block.

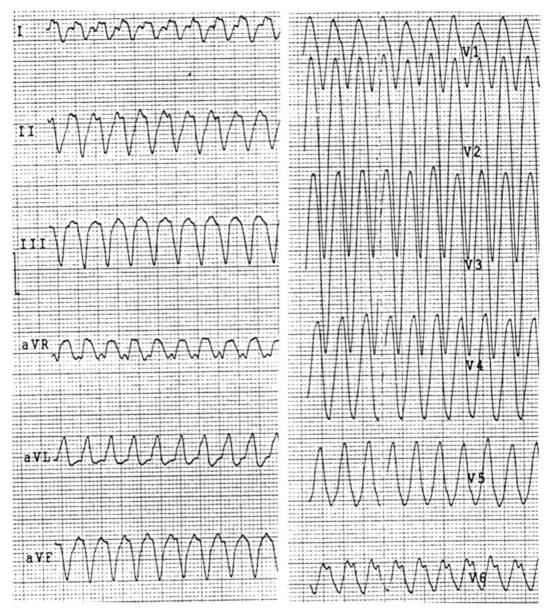

Fig. 12. Wide QRS complex tachycardia with left bundle branch block morphology owing to aberrant conduction during 1:1 typical atrial flutter.

Therefore, in patients receiving intracardiac antiarrhythmic drugs for atrial fibrillation, supraventricular origin of a WCT should be excluded to prevent pointless and potentially harmful indication for ICD implantation with possible multiple inappropriate shocks.[36] Provided that in these cases the ECG interpretation of a WCT could be particularly challenging for the influence of the drug on ECG pattern during aberrant conduction, a careful evaluation of the clinical context could provide some useful hints for patient management. In the present case, the evidence to treat typical atrial flutter by ablation was

quite weak. However, the diagnosis could be made ex juvantibus in a long-term follow-up and this process had clear clinical implications for this patient. Finally, flecainide should be avoided in patients with both atrial fibrillation and flutter, unless the latter arrhythmia is successfully ablated.

SUMMARY

Algorithms for detailed electrocardiographic analysis[1–6] are very useful to guide the interpretation of WCT. Discrimination between supraventricular and ventricular origin of some electrocardio-graphic pattern remains difficult. A comprehensive approach combining clinical aspects and invasive electrophysiologic data is instrumental for a correct diagnosis and proper treatment.

REFERENCES

1. De Ponti R, Bagliani G, Padeletti L, et al. General approach to a wide QRS complex. Card Electrophysiol Clin 2017;9:461–85.
2. Sandler IA, Mariott HJ. The differential morphology of anomalous ventricular complexes of RBBB type in lead V5; ventricular ectopy versus aberration. Circulation 1965;31:551–6.
3. Wellens HJ, Bar FW, Lie KI. The value of the electrocardiogram in the differential diagnosis of a tachycardia with a widened QRS complex. Am J Med 1978;64:27–33.
4. Kindwall KE, Brown J, Josephson ME. Electrocardiographic criteria for ventricular tachycardia in wide complex left bundle branch block morphology tachycardia. Am J Cardiol 1988;61:1279–83.
5. Brugada P, Brugada J, Mont L, et al. A new approach to the differential diagnosis of a regular tachycardia with a wide QRS complex. Circulation 1991;83:1649–59.
6. Vereckei A, Duray G, Szenasi G, et al. New algorithm using only lead aVR for differential diagnosis of wide QRS complex tachycardia. Heart Rhythm 2008;5: 89–98.
7. Zipes DP, Foster PR, Troup PJ, et al. Atrial induction of ventricular tachycardia: reentry versus triggered automaticity. Am J Cardiol 1979;44:1–8.
8. Belhassen B, Rotmensch HH, Laniado S. Response of recurrent sustained ventricular tachycardia to verapamil. Br Heart J 1981;46:679–82.
9. Nakagawa H, Beckman KJ, McClelland JH, et al. Radiofrequency catheter ablation of idiopathic left ventricular tachycardia guided by a Purkinje potential. Circulation 1993;88:2607–17.
10. Morishima I, Nogami A, Tsuboi H, et al. Negative participation of the left posterior fascicle in the reentry circuit of verapamil-sensitive idiopathic left ventricular tachycardia. J Cardiovasc Electrophysiol 2012;23:556–9.
11. Maeda S, Yokoyama Y, Nogami A, et al. First case of left posterior fascicle in a bystander circuit of idiopathic left ventricular tachycardia. Can J Cardiol 2014;30:1460.e11-3.
12. Viskin S, Rosso R, Rogowski O, et al. The short-coupled variant of right outflow ventricular tachycardia: a not-so benign form of ventricular tachycardia? J Cardiovasc Electrophysiol 2005; 16:912–6.
13. Gill JS, Prasad K, Blaszyk K, et al. Initiating sequences in exercise induced idiopathic ventricular tachycardia of left bundle branch-like morphology. Pacing Clin Electrophysiol 1998;21: 1873–80.
14. Kobayashi Y, Yazawa T, Adachi T, et al. Ventricular arrhythmias with left bundle branch block pattern and inferior axis: assessment of their mechanisms on the basis of the response to ATP, Nicorandil and verapamil. Jpn Circ J 2000;64:835–41.
15. Lerman BB, Belardinelli L, West GA, et al. Adenosine-sensitive ventricular tachycardia: evidence suggesting cyclic AMP mediated triggered activity. Circulation 1986;74:270–80.
16. Kassotis J, Slesinger T, Festic E, et al. Adenosine-sensitive wide-complex tachycardia: an uncommon variant of idiopathic fascicular ventricular tachycardia. Angiology 2003;54:369–72.
17. Ozer S, Allen S, Schaffer MS. Adenosine- and verapamil-sensitive ventricular tachycardia in the newborn. Pacing Clin Electrophysiol 2001;24: 898–901.
18. Kabunga P, Lipton J, Sy RW. Adenosine-sensitive ventricular tachycardia arising from the middle cardiac vein. Heart Lung Circ 2015;24:838–9.
19. Cheung JW, Ip JE, Yarlagadda RK, et al. Adenosine-insensitive right ventricular tachycardia: novel variant of idiopathic outflow tract tachycardia. Heart Rhythm 2014;11:1770–8.
20. Delacretaz E, Stevenson WG, Ellison KE, et al. Mapping and radiofrequency catheter ablation of the three types of sustained monomorphic ventricular tachycardia in nonischemic heart disease. J Cardiovasc Electrophysiol 2000;11:11–7.
21. Lopera G, Stevenson WG, Soejima K, et al. Identification and ablation of the three types of ventricular tachycardia involving the His-Purkinje system in patients with heart disease. J Cardiovasc Electrophysiol 2004;15:52–8.
22. Mazur A, Kusniec J, Strasberg B. Bundle branch reentrant ventricular tachycardia. Indian Pacing Electrophysiol J 2005;5:86–95.
23. Caceres J, Jazayeri M, McKinnie J, et al. Sustained bundle branch reentry as a mechanism of clinical tachycardia. Circulation 1989;79:256–70.
24. Choi KJ, Shah DC, Jais P, et al. Successful ablation of Hisian ectopy identified by a reversed his bundle activation sequence. J Interv Card Electrophysiol 2002;6:183–6.
25. Eizmendi I, Almendral J, Hadid C, et al. Successful catheter cryoablation of Hisian ectopy using 2 new diagnostic criteria based on unipolar and bipolar recordings of the his electrogram. J Cardiovasc Electrophysiol 2012;23:325–9.
26. McClelland JH, Wang X, Beckman KJ, et al. Radiofrequency catheter ablation of right atriofascicular (Mahaim) accessory pathways guided by accessory pathway activation potential. Circulation 1994;89: 2655–66.

27. Cappato R, Schluter M, Weiss C, et al. Catheter-induced mechanical conduction block of right accessory fibers with Mahaim-type preexcitation to guide radiofrequency ablation. Circulation 1994;90:282–90.

28. Haissaguerre M, Cauchemez B, Marcus F, et al. Characteristics of the ventricular insertion sites of accessory pathways with antegrade decremental conduction properties. Circulation 1995;91:1077–85.

29. De Ponti R, Salerno-Uriarte JA. "Mahaim" fasciculoventricular fibers: rare variant of ventricular preexcitation or subtle clinical problem? Heart Rhythm 2005;2:7–9.

30. Gandhavadi M, Sternick EB, Jackman WM, et al. Characterization of the distal insertion if the atriofascicular accessory pathways and mechanisms of the QRS patterns in atriofascicular antidromic tachycardia. Heart Rhythm 2013;10:1385–92.

31. Sternick EB, Cruz FE, Timmermans C, et al. Electrocardiogram during tachycardia in patients with antegrade conduction over a Mahaim fiber: old criteria revisited. Heart Rhythm 2004;1:406–13.

32. Berruezo A, Mont L, Nava S, et al. Electrocardiographic recognition of the epicardial origin of ventricular tachycardias. Circulation 2004;109:1842–7.

33. Vallès E, Bazan V, Marchlinski FE. ECG criteria to identify epicardial ventricular tachycardia in non ischemic cardiomyopathy. Circ Arrhythm Electrophysiol 2010;3:63–71.

34. Johnson CT, Brooks C, Jaramillo J, et al. A left free-wall, decrementally conducting, atrioventricular (Mahaim) fiber: diagnosis at electrophysiological study and radiofrequency catheter ablation guided by direct recording of the Mahaim potential. Pacing Clin Electrophysiol 1997;20:2486–8.

35. Francia P, Pittalis MC, Ali H, et al. Electrophysiological study and catheter ablation of a Mahaim fibre located at the mitral annulus-aorta junction. J Interv Card Electrophysiol 2008;23:153–7.

36. Turitto G, Akhrass P, Leonardi M, et al. Atrial flutter with spontaneous 1:1 atrioventricular conduction in adults: an uncommon but frequently missed cause for syncope/presyncope. Pacing Clin Electrophysiol 2009;32:82–90.

37. Taylor R, Gandhi MM, Lloyd G. Tachycardia due to atrial flutter with rapid 1:1 conduction following treatment of atrial fibrillation with flecainide. BMJ 2010;340:b4684.

Localization of Ventricular Arrhythmias for Catheter Ablation
The Role of Surface Electrocardiogram

Domenico Giovanni Della Rocca, MD[a],*,
Carola Gianni, MD, PhD[a], Sanghamitra Mohanty, MD[a],
Chintan Trivedi, MD, MPH[a], Luigi Di Biase, MD, PhD[a,b,c,d],
Andrea Natale, MD, FACC, FHRS[a,b,e,f,g,h]

KEYWORDS

- Ventricular arrhythmias • Site of origin • Electrocardiography • Catheter ablation
- Ventricular tachycardia • Idiopathic ventricular arrhythmias • Structural heart disease

KEY POINTS

- Preprocedural analysis of 12-lead Electrocardiogram (ECG) of a clinical arrhythmia is of pivotal importance to predict the site of origin either in case of idiopathic ventricular arrhythmias (VAs) or in patients with structural heart disease (SHD).
- The main mechanism underlying idiopathic VAs is generally an abnormal and rapid activation of a focal area of normal myocardium.
- VAs in SHD generally result from a scar-related reentry mechanism.
- ECG analysis might help tailoring the ablation strategy to optimize procedural duration, increase the probability of success, and recognize and prevent risks and complications.

INTRODUCTION

Over the past few decades, significant advances have been made in the diagnosis and management of ventricular tachycardia (VT). Antiarrhythmic drug therapy (eg, amiodarone and β-blockers) may significantly reduce the risk of ventricular arrhythmias (VAs) but carries a significant risk of side effects, which frequently lead to drug discontinuation.[1] Implantable cardioverter defibrillators (ICDs) are the mainstay of treatment of primary and secondary prevention of sudden cardiac death (SCD).[2,3] ICD therapies,

Disclosures: Dr L. Di Biase is a consultant for Biosense Webster, Boston Scientific, Stereotaxis, and St. Jude Medical and has received speaker honoraria from Medtronic, AtriCure, EPiEP, and Biotronik. Dr A. Natale has received speaker honoraria from Boston Scientific, Biosense Webster, St. Jude Medical, Biotronik, and Medtronic and is a consultant for Biosense Webster, St. Jude Medical, and Janssen. All other authors have reported that they have no relationships relevant to the contents of this article to disclose.
[a] Texas Cardiac Arrhythmia Institute, St. David's Medical Center, Austin, TX, USA; [b] Department of Biomedical Engineering, University of Texas, Austin, TX, USA; [c] Montefiore Medical Center, Albert Einstein College of Medicine, Bronx, NY, USA; [d] Department of Clinical and Experimental Medicine, University of Foggia, Foggia, Italy; [e] Interventional Electrophysiology, Scripps Clinic, La Jolla, CA, USA; [f] MetroHealth Medical Center, Case Western Reserve University School of Medicine, Cleveland, OH, USA; [g] Division of Cardiology, Stanford University, Stanford, CA, USA; [h] Electrophysiology and Arrhythmia Services, California Pacific Medical Center, San Francisco, CA, USA
* Corresponding author. Texas Cardiac Arrhythmia Institute, St. David's Medical Center, Suite 720, 3000 North I-35, Austin, TX 78705.
E-mail address: domenicodellarocca@hotmail.it

cardiacEP.theclinics.com

Abbreviations	
AMC	Aortomitral continuity
ASOV	Aortic sinuses of Valsalva
AV	Atrioventricular
BBR	Bundle branch reentry
ECG	electrocardiogram
ICD	Implantable cardioverter defibrillator
LBBB	Left bundle branch block
LCC	Left coronary cusp
LV	Left ventricular
MA	Mitral annulus
MDI	Maximum deflection index
MI	Myocardial infarction
NCC	Noncoronary cusp
OT	Outflow tract
PA	Pulmonary artery
PPM	Papillary muscle
RBBB	Right bundle branch block
RCC	Right coronary cusp
RV	Right ventricular
SCD	Sudden cardiac death
SHD	Structural heart disease
SOO	Site of origin
TA	Tricuspid annulus
VA	Ventricular arrhythmia
VT	Ventricular tachycardia

either antitachycardia pacing and/or shock, can effectively terminate potentially life-threatening VAs.[2,3] In selected patients, a combined approach based on antiarrhythmic drug therapy and ICD implantation may reduce the incidence of VAs and improve survival. In addition to antiarrhythmic drug side effects, however, recurrent ICD therapies may correlate with worsening quality-of-life scores and increase mortality rates.[4] Catheter ablation has emerged as an effective treatment of recurrent VTs, either idiopathic or secondary to structural heart disease (SHD). Idiopathic VTs account for approximately 10% of patients with documented VTs and occur in the absence of cardiac structural abnormalities or ion channellopathies.[5] In this case, specific anatomic structures (eg, ventricular outflow tracts [OTs], atrioventricular [AV] annuli, and papillary muscles [PPMs]) are involved in the development of arrhythmias. Catheter ablation of idiopathic VTs is an effective procedure, whose success rate ranges between 80% and 100%[6–8] and is relatively safe; nevertheless, anatomic obstacles (eg, coronary arteries, AV conduction system, and epicardial fat pads) might make the procedure more challenging in some cases.

In a majority of patients with recurrent episodes of sustained VT, it is possible to identify a structural arrhythmogenic substrate, which can be the result of cardiomyocyte replacement and scar formation. VT ablation has been demonstrated to be superior to antiarrhythmic drugs in patients suffering from VAs due to SHD; additionally, substrate modification seems superior to standard ablation in reducing the risk of VA recurrences and all-cause mortality.[9,10]

Preprocedural analysis of 12-lead ECG of the clinical VA is of pivotal importance to predict the arrhythmia site of origin (SOO) either in cases of idiopathic VAs or in patients with SHD. Although ECG interpretation might be complicated by factors like chest wall deformity, metabolic and drug effects, and presence and distribution of scar, a detailed analysis of 12-lead ECG can be a valuable mapping tool and provide useful information in localizing the VA SOO. This might help tailor the ablation strategy to optimize procedural duration, increase the probability of success, and recognize and prevent risks and complications. The aim of this article is to review the ECG features of both idiopathic and scar-related VAs and discuss their potential implications for optimizing the ablation strategy.

LOCALIZATION OF IDIOPATHIC VENTRICULAR ARRHYTHMIAS: GENERAL CONSIDERATIONS
Anatomic Considerations

OT VAs are the most common form of idiopathic VAs, accounting for approximately 10% of all VAs. The OT has a complex anatomy, and its understanding is crucial to be able to interpret correctly the 12-lead ECG. The OT centers on the 2 semilunar valves, pulmonary valve and aortic valve, and includes the right ventricular OT (RVOT), the pulmonary artery (PA), the para-Hisian region, the left ventricular OT (LVOT), the mitral annulus (MA), aortic root/sinuses of Valsalva (ASOV), and the left ventricular (LV) epicardium above (LV summit). The RVOT is a conical structure bordered superiorly by the pulmonic valve and inferiorly by the right ventricular (RV) inflow tract and the top of the tricuspid valve. The RVOT can be divided into 3 segments: proximal, mid, and distal. The proximal segment lies to the right of the LVOT, beginning at the superior margin of the tricuspid annulus (TA). The mid and distal segments lie anterior and leftwards to the aortic root, wrapping around the LVOT. The posteroseptal aspect of the RVOT is adjacent to the right coronary cusp (RCC); the anteroseptal aspect is adjacent to the LV epicardium and the left anterior descending coronary and anterior to the RCC and a portion of the left coronary cusp (LCC). The lateral aspect of the RVOT is the RV free wall. The pulmonary valve lies above the ventricular septum. In young patients, the valve is parallel to the aortic valve, which is perpendicular to the mitral valve; in older patients, the aortic valve is frequently more vertical and parallel to the mitral valve. As a general rule, the pulmonary valve is 1 cm to 2 cm above and to the left of the aortic valve. The aortic root is defined inferiorly by the attachment of the aortic leaflets and superiorly by the sinotubular junction of the aorta. Histologic examination of the pulmonary valve shows adventitial extensions of the ventricular myocardium in 90% of cases; those myocardial fibers are frequently the source of focal activity triggering VAs arising from the RVOT. Fibers of ventricular myocardium can be similarly observed at the base of both left aortic and right aortic coronary sinuses.[11,12] Conversely, the non-coronary cusp (NCC) is made of fibrous tissue; as a result, VAs originating from the coronary cusps are significantly more common than those originating from the NCC. As discussed previously, the RCC and a portion of the LCC are closely related to the septal aspect of the RVOT; this explains similar 12-lead ECG features shared by VAs arising from those regions. The more inferior and posterior locations of the aortic valve compared with the pulmonary valve, however, result in subtle ECG differences, which may help localize the correct VA SOO.

General ECG Considerations

The main mechanism underlying idiopathic VAs is generally an abnormal and rapid activation of a focal area of normal myocardium. Typical and repetitive ECG patterns can be documented on 12-lead ECG as a result of the rapid activation of the same focal area triggering the arrhythmia. Conversely, VAs in SHD generally result from a scar-related reentry mechanism. As a general rule, VAs arising from the LV show a right bundle branch block (RBBB)-like configuration because the LV is activated before the RV; for similar reasons, VAs exiting from the RV have a left bundle branch block (LBBB)-like morphology. VTs arising on or adjacent (<1 cm paraseptal) to the LV septum may display an LBBB-like morphology, especially in patients with SHD, as a result of a more rapid spread of the activation wavefront to a less diseased RV.

In cases of a septal origin, VAs generally display a narrower QRS complex owing to a synchronous activation of the ventricles. A positive precordial concordance is observed in cases of VAs arising from basal sites, whereas VAs from apical sites have negative precordial concordance.

Specifically, (1) the transition of RBBB VTs (first lead with a predominant S wave) becomes progressively earlier as the SOO moves from the base toward the apex of the LV and (2) the transition of LBBB VTs (first lead with a predominant R wave) becomes progressively late as the SOO moves from the basal septal area toward the RV free wall.

The QRS axis in the frontal plane is (1) inferior in cases of VAs originating from the superior aspect of the ventricles (predominant R wave in leads II, III, and aVF); (2) superior in cases of VAs originating from the inferior aspect of the ventricles (predominant S wave in leads II, III, and aVF); (3) right in cases of VAs originating from the LV free wall (predominant S wave in I and aVL); and (4) left in cases of VAs originating from the septum (predominant R wave in I and aVL).

Even though these general rules better apply for idiopathic VAs, they also can be used in the presence of SHD, such as in the presence of significant scarring, which might reduce the accuracy of ECG diagnosis. Myocardial scar can form an electrical barrier represented by areas of slow conduction, which alters the contour of the QRS. As a result, the QRS complex during VAs has a lower amplitude, a wider duration, and fragmentation compared with that of a patient without SHD arising from a similar location. As discussed previously, the main mechanism underlying the development of VAs in patients with SHD is a scar-related reentry. In contrast to patients with idiopathic VAs, the 12-lead ECG morphology of a scar-related VA depends on the area of normal myocardium adjacent to the exit site of the reentrant circuit. The diastolic isthmus, such as the region of slow conduction where mid-diastolic potentials are recorded during VT, as well as the suitable target site for ablation, does not always correspond to the exit site at the scar border. Because the QRS onset on 12-lead ECG reflects the area of normal myocardium adjacent to VT exit site and the slow conducting isthmus may precede the electrical activation of this area, the target site for ablation might have a limited effect on surface ECG. Thus, 12-lead VT ECG may direct attention to a region that does not coincide with the ideal ablation target site but in close proximity to that. For scar-related VAs, another important factor limiting the precision of 12-lead ECG as a localizing tool is the size and distribution of myocardial scar; a large scar can have a significant impact on the overall 12-lead ECG morphology in both reentrant and focal VAs.

ECG FEATURES OF IDIOPATHIC VENTRICULAR ARRHYTHMIAS ARISING FROM THE RIGHT VENTRICLE
Right Ventricular Outflow Tract Ventricular Arrhythmias

Idiopathic RVOT VTs are the most common forms of idiopathic VTs, accounting for approximately

70% to 80% of all idiopathic VTs and 10% of all VTs seen for further evaluation in clinical practice.[5] The RVOT is in close proximity to the PA and the para-Hisian region. VTs arising from the OT are generally monomorphic and have an LBBB configuration. The frontal plane QRS axis is inferiorly directed. ECG shows deeply negative PS complexes in leads aVL and aVR. As discussed previously, the anteroseptal aspect is the RVOT is adjacent to the left anterior descending coronary and anterior to the RCC and a portion of the LCC; the posteroseptal aspect is closely related to the RCC. Pace and activation mapping studies have shown some common features in ECG location of RVOT VT (**Table 1**).

- Septal sites generally have narrower LBBB morphology with earlier precordial transition (positive QRS by V_3 or earlier), with larger amplitudes in inferior leads (**Fig. 1**).[13] Conversely, VTs arising from the RVOT free wall tend to have broader LBBB morphology with later precordial transition ($\geq V_4$) and notching in the inferior leads (**Figs. 2** and **3**).[13] It is pivotal, however, to keep in mind that, regardless of the site (free wall or septal sites), conduction velocities in idiopathic VAs are more rapid than in the presence of SHD; as a result, a significantly wide QRS complex duration is uncommon and should drive the diagnosis toward a scar-related form of VA.
- Anterior sites have either isoelectric or negative, frequently multiphasic forces in limb lead I[14] (see **Figs. 2** and **3**). A positive QRS

complex in lead I is observed in RVOT VAs arising from posterior sites, as a result of a leftward initial vector[13] (see **Fig. 1**).

- A majority of RVOT VT foci arise from the top of the RVOT, within 1 cm to 2 cm from the pulmonary valve. Foci lying within this segment typically produce a negative QS pattern in aVL,[15] whereas foci lying at the base of the RVOT, potentially adjacent to the His bundle, produce isoelectric or positive forces in lead aVL.[16]

Para-Hisian Ventricular Arrhythmias

Septal para-Hisian foci generally display shorter QRS complex duration in the inferior leads, lower R-wave amplitude in leads III and aVF, negative QS pattern in V_1, and larger R-wave amplitude in leads V_5, V_6, and I[17] (**Fig. 4**). The precordial transition occurs in lead V_2–V_3. QRS complex duration in leads II, III and aVF is generally narrower that in RVOT VAs. QRS morphology of para-Hisian VAs may overlap with VAs arising in the LVOT (discussed later), given the close proximity of the aortic root.[16]

Tricuspid Annulus Ventricular Arrhythmias

TA VAs account for approximately 8% of idiopathic VAs; VAs arising from the septal aspect of the TA are 3 times more frequent than those from the TA free wall.[18] Given the close proximity of the para-Hisian region, the base of the RVOT, and the NCC, there is significant overlap among VAs arising from these regions and TA VAs, especially those

Table 1
ECG patterns of idiopathic ventricular arrhythmias arising from the right ventricle

Location of Ventricular Arrhythmia	Bundle Branch Block	Axis	Precordial Transition	I	V1	V6	Other Features
RVOT							
Anteroseptal	LBBB	Inferior	$\leq V_3$	rS	rS	R	Negative, isoelectric, or multiphasic I
Posterior, free wall	LBBB	Inferior	$\geq V_3$	R	rS	R	Positive I; broad late notched inferior leads
Para-Hisian	LBBB	Inferior	$> V_3$	R	QS	R	Isoelectric or positive aVL; large R amplitude in I, V_5, V_6; taller inferior R
TA							
Septal	LBBB	Inferior	$< V_3$	R/r	QS	R	Positive, isoelectric, or multiphasic aVL
Free wall	LBBB	Variable	V_4–V_5	R/r	rS	R	Notching in limb leads
PA	LBBB	Inferior	$> V_3$	rS/QS	rS/QS	R	Q-wave amplitude aVL/aVR ratio >1

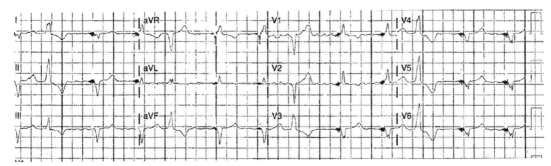

Fig. 1. PVC originating from the posterior RVOT.

originating from the anteroseptal aspect of the TA.[18] Foci lying within the TA typically display LBBB configuration with inferior axis and monophasic positive or multiphasic forces in lead aVL, which are generally of low amplitude. In addition to these ECG features, TA VAs arising from the free wall of the valve ring can show notching in limb leads, similarly to those from the RVOT free wall. Foci lying in the posterolateral portion of the TA show discordant forces in the inferior leads; those forces depend on how inferiorly the focus arises.[18]

Pulmonary Artery Ventricular Arrhythmias

Myocardial extensions into the PA beyond the ventriculoarterial junction are relatively common (approximately 15%–20%) and may involve the adventitia as well as the epicardial surface.[19] Those fibers of ventricular myocardium may function as the arrhythmogenic substrate for VAs arising from the PA. PA VAs generally arise 0.5 cm to 2.1 cm cranial to the ventriculoarterial junction; as a result, foci lying within the PA display ECG features similar to those of the RVOT. Compared with them, PA VAs generally display taller R waves in the inferior leads.[20] The pulmonary trunk lies more leftward than the infundibulum; as a result, the ECG during PA VAs may display an earlier precordial transition. The transitional zone generally occurs from V_4 in both PA and RVOT VAs but also can be observed in V_2 or V_3 (**Fig. 5**). In patients with PA VAs, the amplitude of R wave is generally lower in V_2 and the R/S amplitude ratio on the

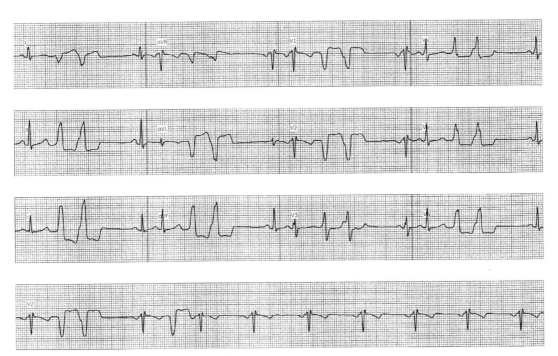

Fig. 2. PVC originating from the anterior right RVOT.

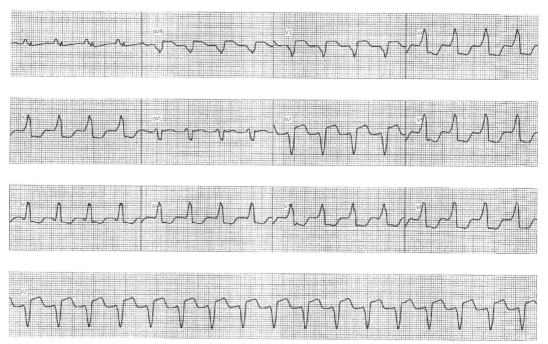

Fig. 3. VT originating from the lower RVOT.

same lead is significantly larger compared with that of patients with RVOT VAs. Additionally, PA VAs tend to display deeper QS complexes in aVL that in aVR and the average Q-wave amplitude aVL/aVR ratio is greater than 1 and significantly larger than that in RVOT VAs.[21]

Ventricular Arrhythmias Arising from the Right Ventricular Papillary Muscles

VAs originating from the RV PPMs can display an RBBB or LBBB morphology, with the QRS frontal axis either inferior or superior depending on the

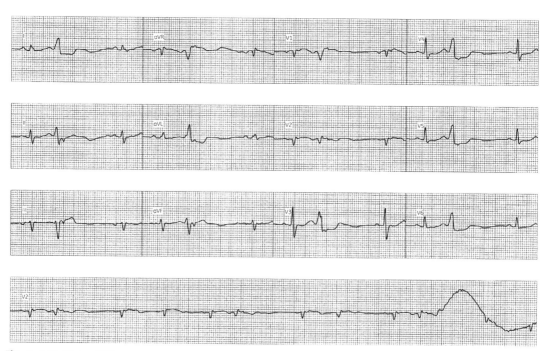

Fig. 4. Para-Hisian PVC.

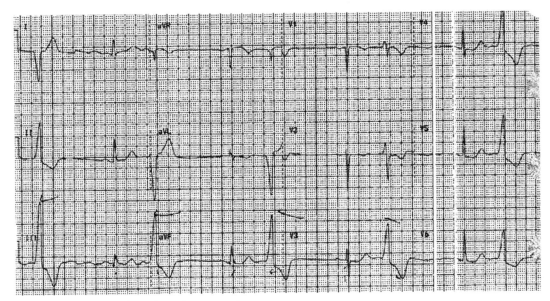

Fig. 5. PVC originating from the pulmonary valve cusp.

PPM of origin.[22] Foci lying from the anterior or posterior PPM generally display LBBB morphology with a later transitional zone (>V$_4$) and a superior or inferior axis, respectively; those from the septal PPM usually display an RBBB morphology and a superior axis (**Fig. 6**). A notch in the precordial leads is a common finding of most PPM VAs. Lead V$_1$ frequently has an rS or QS morphology.

ECG FEATURES OF IDIOPATHIC VENTRICULAR ARRHYTHMIAS ARISING FROM THE LEFT VENTRICLE
Left Ventricular Outflow Tract Ventricular Arrhythmias

Approximately 20% to 30% of idiopathic VTs arise from the LV and 15% to 25% of those from the OT originate from the LVOT.[22–25] LVOT sites of origin

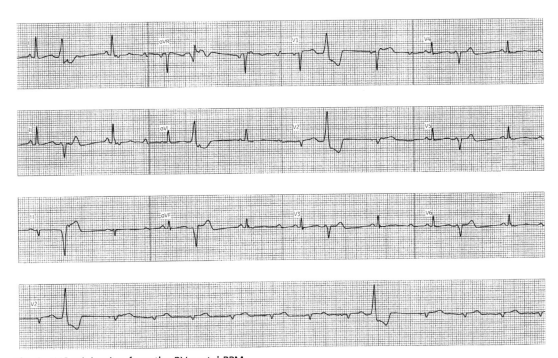

Fig. 6. PVC originating from the RV septal PPM.

Table 2
ECG patterns of idiopathic ventricular arrhythmias arising from the left ventricle

Location of Ventricular Arrhythmia	Bundle Branch Block	Axis	Precordial Transition	I	V1	V6	Other Features
LVOT							
Supravalvular							
LCC	LBBB	Inferior	≤V2	rS	rS, RS	R	QS or RS in lead I; notched M or W in V1
RCC	LBBB	Inferior	≤V3	R	rS, RS	R	Broad R in V2
LCC/RCC junction	LBBB	Inferior	V3	R/Rsr'	qrS	R	Notched on the downward deflection or W pattern in V1
Infravalvular							
AMC	RBBB	Inferior	Positive concordance	R/Rs	qR	R	No S in V6
Septal–para-Hisian	LBBB	Left inferior	Early	Rs	QS, Qr	Rs	QS amplitude lead II/III ratio >1
Anterior interventricular vein/ great cardiac vein junction	LBBB	Inferior	Early	rS	rS, QS	R	Precordial pattern break; MDI >0.55
MA							
Anterolateral	RBBB	Inferior	Early	QS/rS	R	Rs	Wider QRS; late inferior lead notching
Posterior	RBBB	Superior	Early	Rs	R	Rs	Absence of inferior lead notching
PPM							
Posteromedial	RBBB	Superior	Variable	R	rsR'	RS	Late R to S precordial transition
Anterolateral	RBBB	Inferior	<V1	S	rsR'	RS	qR/qr pattern in lead aVR; rS pattern in V6
Crux	LBBB	Left superior	Early	Rs	Variable	R	MDI >0.55; pseudo-delta wave; slurred intrinsicoid deflection
Fascicular							
Left posterior	RBBB	Left superior	Early	Q	rsR'	RS	Loss of late precordial R waves with more apical exits
Left anterior	RBBB	Right	None	Q	rsR'	RS	Similar to posterior ones with the exception of the axis
Upper septal	LBBB	Normal/right	V3	Rs	rS	Rs	Narrow QRS complex

of idiopathic VAs can be classified as supraventricular, infravalvular, and epicardial (**Table 2**).

Supravalvular (general considerations)

The most common SOO of VAs from the supravalvular area of LVOT is the LCC, followed by the RCC and the NCC (uncommon). Arrhythmias from these structures are the result of foci arising from ventricular myocardial extensions into the ASOV and beyond the ventriculoarterial junction.[19] Typically, the 12-lead ECG exhibits LBBB morphology with inferior axis, an early precordial transition, taller R waves in V_1 and V_2 and in the inferior leads, an S wave in lead I, and no S waves in V_5 and V_6. In these leads, an R-wave duration greater than 50% of the total QRS duration and an R/S ratio of more than 30% have been shown to strongly predict an origin of VA from the coronary cusps, especially from the LCC.[7]

- LCC: pace mapping studies have shown that VAs arising from the LCC have a typical multiphasic notched patter in V_1 and a W-shaped pattern, as a result of trans-septal activation after initial PV activation from the LCC[26,27] (**Fig. 7**). Lead I generally has a prevalence of negative forces (QS or rS)
- RCC: pace mapping from the RCC produces an early precordial transition as for LCC arrhythmias but with a broader R wave in V_2 and a longer QRS duration. Lead I displays positive forces compared with LCC arrhythmias, but this finding is variable and depends on location and orientation of the aortic annulus (**Fig. 8**).[26] The LBBB pattern seen in VAs from the RCC has a broad small R wave with precordial transition most frequently in V_3.[27]
- LCC/RCC junction: VAs arising from the LCC/RCC junction have been described by Yamada and collaborators.[28] They share with LCC VAs a multiphasic notched V_1 pattern and display a precordial transition in lead V_3 and a QS morphology in lead V_1 with notching on the downward deflection[29] (**Fig. 9**).

Infravalvular

- Aortomitral continuity (AMC): the AMC is a mainly fibrous structure located between aortic and mitral valve annuli. Although it is a prevalently fibrous structure, histologic examination has shown cells that share morphologic and functional features with the cells of the AV junction.[30] Those cells are thought to trigger atrial as well as some idiopathic VAs. Depending on some anatomic factors, mainly the extent of the left fibrous trigon, VAs arising from the AMC show a qR pattern in V_1 or an RBBB pattern with positive precordial concordance and no S waves in V_6 (**Fig. 10**).
- Septal–para-Hisian sites (discussed previously).

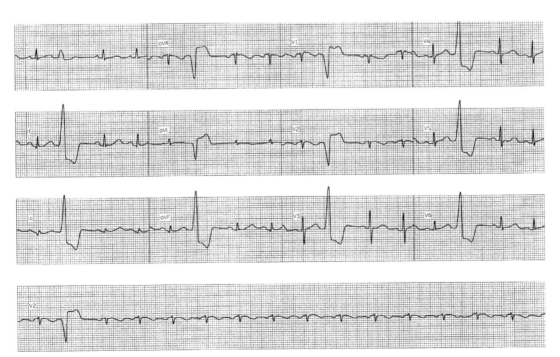

Fig. 7. PVC originating from the LCC.

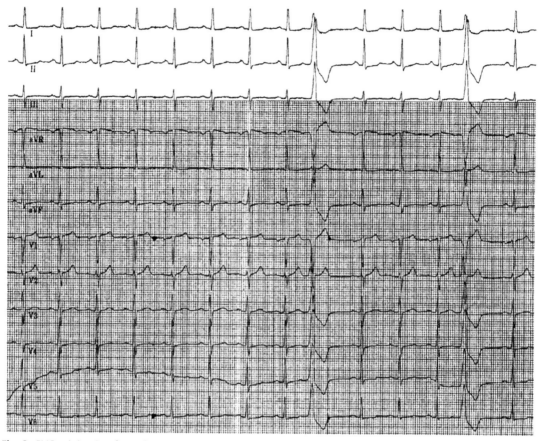

Fig. 8. PVC originating from the RCC.

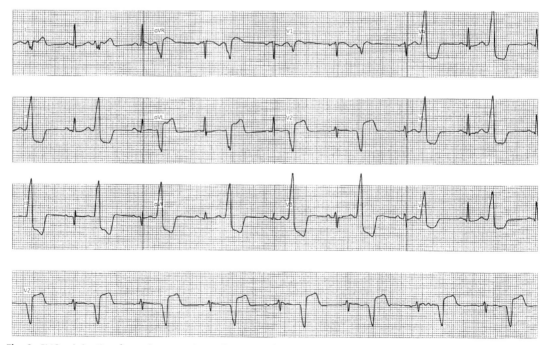

Fig. 9. PVC originating from the commissure between the RCC and LCC.

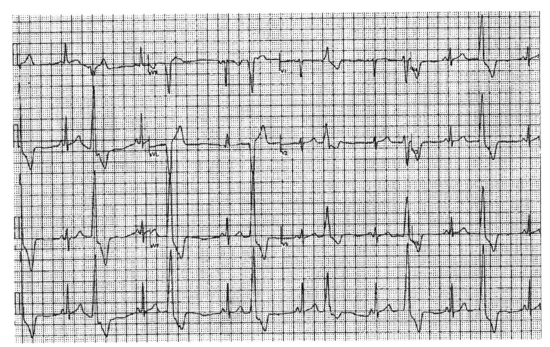

Fig. 10. PVC originating from the AMC.

Left ventricular summit and epicardial

VAs from the LV summit and the epicardium region arise from perivascular myocardial tissue associated with the junction of the great cardiac vein and the anterior interventricular vein. Other sites, however, may harbor foci triggering VAs.[31] Those arrhythmias generally show an LBBB morphology with inferior frontal axis and precordial transition in lead V_3 with S wave in $V_2 > V_1$ (**Fig. 11**). Because their origin is far from the His-Purkinje system, the

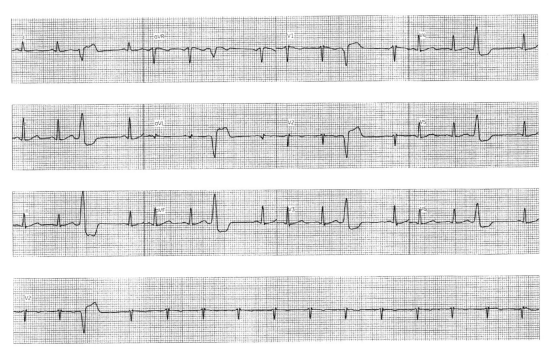

Fig. 11. PVC originating from the LV summit.

intrinsicoid deflection is frequently delayed. A small r wave, and rarely an R wave, is a common feature of VAs arising from the AMC, the LCC, the great cardiac vein, and the anterior interventricular vein. The Q-wave amplitude aVL/aVR ratio, however, is significantly higher in epicardial VTs. The maximum deflection index (MDI), such as the ratio between the shortest time to maximal positive or negative deflection in any precordial lead and the QRS duration, is a useful tool to discriminate between epicardial foci and other OT VAs. An MDI greater than 0.55 seems to accurately predict an epicardial origin.[31] Based on 5 criteria (an RBBB pattern, the transition zone, the R-wave amplitude ratio in leads III to II, the Q wave amplitude ratio in leads aVL and aVR, and the S wave in lead V_6), Yamada and colleagues[32] demonstrated that VAs showing an RBBB pattern, an earlier precordial transition, a Q-wave amplitude ration in aVL/aVR greater than 1.1, and S waves in V_5 and V_6 are likely epicardial and successfully targeted within the great cardiac vein or the anterior interventricular vein.

Mitral Annulus Ventricular Arrhythmias

The MA is located posteriorly within the LV and can harbor arrhythmogenic foci, arising more frequently from anterolateral sites rather than posteromedial ones. Typically, anterolateral MA VAs have an RBBB pattern with inferior axis. The RBBB pattern frequently displays a late notching in the inferior leads. The precordial transition is early, with concordant positive QRS pattern in leads V_2 through V_4.[33] Late notching in the inferior leads or an S wave in lead I, which are common in cases of VAs from the anterolateral and posterior sites, may be absent in anterior and posteroseptal MA VAs. Compared with septal sites, anterolateral and lateral sites also exhibit a wider QRS complex and predominantly negative forces in lead I.[13] Some algorithms have been developed to help identify the SOO of MA VTs.[33,34]

Papillary Muscle Ventricular Arrhythmias

Arrhythmias arising from the LV PPMs display an RBBB pattern, refractoriness to verapamil and Na^+ channel blockers, inducibility with exertion, lack of inducibility with programmed ventricular or atrial stimulation, and requirement of high radiofrequency power for a successful ablation. PPM VAs are usually repetitive premature ventricular complexes rather than sustained VTs. Foci from the anterolateral PPM exhibit an RBBB pattern with right inferior axis (**Fig. 12**). The mean QRS duration is 168 ms.[35] A qR or qr pattern in aVR and an rS pattern in lead V_6 with an R/S ratio less than 1 can help differentiate an anterolateral PPM site from other LV sites. Compared with an anterolateral PPM VA, VAs arising from the inferoseptal PPM have an RBBB with right or left superior axis (**Fig. 13**). The duration of the QRS complex is approximately 160 ms.[36] An R/S ratio

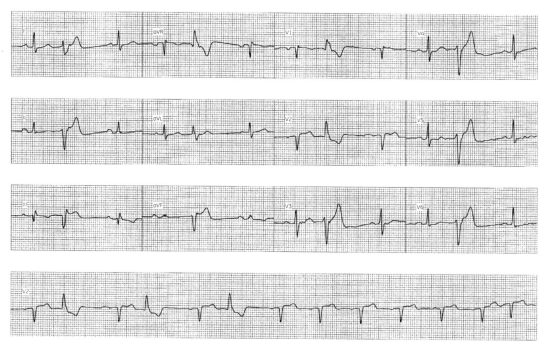

Fig. 12. PVC originating from the LV anterolateral PPM.

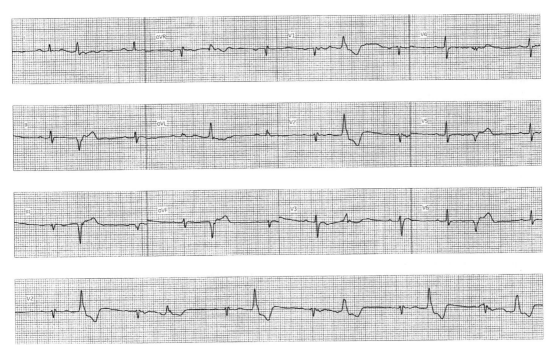

Fig. 13. PVC originating from the LV inferoseptal PPM.

less than 1 in lead V_6 is useful to differentiate this site from other LV sites. In addition, monophasic R and qR pattern are generally found in lead I.

Ventricular Arrhythmias from the Crux

The crux is an epicardial site of the heart, close to the junction of the middle cardiac vein and the coronary sinus. VAs arising from this site display an LBBB morphology with left superior axis. The precordial transition is early, generally at or before V_2. The MDI is greater than 0.55. A pseudodelta wave greater than or equal to 34 ms and an intrinsicoid deflection time in lead V_2 greater than or equal to 85 ms are typical findings.[37]

Fascicular Ventricular Tachycardia (Verapamil-Sensitive Ventricular Tachycardia)

Fascicular VT (verapamil-sensitive) is an idiopathic arrhythmia due to reentry, involving altered Purkinje fibers on the LV septal side.

Left posterior fascicular ventricular tachycardia
Left posterior fascicular VT is the most common form of fascicular VT. The reentry circuit involves the left posterior fascicle with an exit at the inferoapical LV septum. Left posterior fascicular VT has an RBBB morphology with left superior axis and RS complexes in V_5 and V_6.[38,39] A loss of late precordial waves is observed on the occurrence of a more apical exit.

Left anterior fascicular ventricular tachycardia
Left anterior fascicular ventricular tachycardias arrhythmias exhibit an RBBB configuration with right axis deviation. The reentry circuit involves the left anterior fascicle.

Upper septal fascicular ventricular tachycardia
The upper septal fascicular form of VT is uncommon and has a narrow QRS complex with normal or rightward axis deviation. The reentry circuit involves the left bundle branch.

IDIOPATHIC VENTRICULAR ARRHYTHMIAS: ECG FEATURES FOR DIFFERENTIAL DIAGNOSIS
Differential ECG Diagnosis Between Ventricular Arrhythmias of Left/Right Origin

Although an S wave in lead I can be present in other sites, this ECG finding is helpful to differentiate an LV focus. Another useful tool for differential diagnosis of OT VAs is R/S ratio in lead V_3.[15] An R/S ratio less than 1 has been associated with foci from the RVOT; conversely, if the R/S ratio is greater than or equal to 1 and the initial R-wave amplitude in leads V_1 and V_2 the focus is likely located in the LVOT. Another finding in LVOT arrhythmias is that the R-wave precordial transition is similar or earlier than that during sinus rhythm and is later in an RVOT VA.

RVOT VAs share also some ECG features with those arising from the ASOV. A longer R-wave duration index (>0.5) and a higher R/S-wave amplitude index (>0.3) in leads V_1 and V_2 are common in VAs originating from the ASOV.[7]

Differential ECG Diagnosis Between Ventricular Arrhythmias of Epicardial/Endocardial Origin

Approximately 15% of VAs arising from the OT have an epicardial origin. Epicardial ablation can require an access through the coronary venous system and mainly targets the great cardiac vein, the junction of the great cardiac vein, and the middle cardiac vein. The most common site of epicardial ventricular foci is the region located between the junction of the great cardiac vein and the anterior interventricular vein, which is referred to as the LV summit, and represents the most superior aspect of the LV. The apex of the LV summit is defined by the bifurcation of the left anterior descending and the circumflex coronary arteries. Barruezo and colleagues[37] have described 3 ECG criteria for predicting an epicardial origin of VAs in patients with failed endocardial ablation.

The 3 criteria are (1) the presence of a pseudo-delta wave greater than or equal to 34 ms in any precordial leads during VTs with an RBBB pattern; (2) a delayed intrinsicoid deflection in V_2, such as a time from QRS complex onset to the peak of the R wave greater than or equal to 85 ms; and (3) the shortest RS interval, such as the time from the first ventricular deflection to the nadir of the first S wave in any precordial leads greater than or equal to 120 ms.

The MDI, discussed previously, such as the ratio between the shortest time to maximal positive or negative deflection in any precordial lead and the QRS duration, is a useful tool to discriminate between epicardial foci and other OT VAs. An MDI greater than 0.55 seems to accurately predict an epicardial origin.[31]

Another common finding during epicardial VTs is the presence of precordial pattern break, such as a regression/progression of the precordial R waves (abrupt loss of R wave in V_2 and subsequent resumption from V_3 to V_6).[28]

ECG FEATURES OF VENTRICULAR ARRHYTHMIAS IN PATIENTS WITH STRUCTURAL HEART DISEASE
Ventricular Arrhythmias due to Ischemic Heart Disease/Prior Myocardial Infarction

The most common cause of VAs is a prior extensive myocardial infarction (MI). A majority of VAs owing to ischemic cardiomyopathy result from a reentry mechanism, generally within endocardial circuits. VAs arising from the LV free wall display an RBBB configuration whereas left septal/paraseptal ones have an LBBB pattern. VT exit sites are located within or at the periphery of the infarcted myocardium; as a result, knowledge of

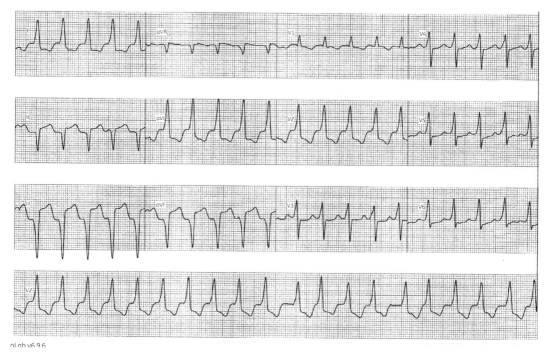

Fig. 14. Inferoseptal basal VT in a patient with a prior MI.

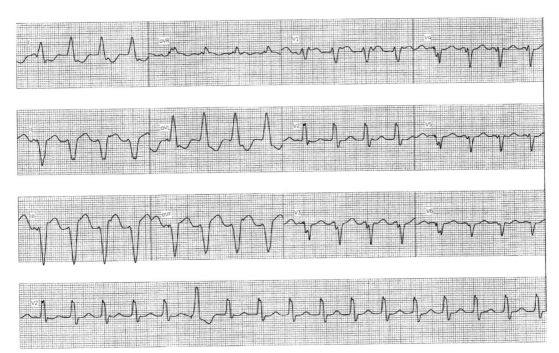

Fig. 15. Inferoseptal apical VT in a patient with a prior MI.

the scar location is helpful in driving localization of the exit sites.

1. With inferior infarction, reentrant VTs have generally a basal exit and precordial R waves are generally preserved. A lateral basal exit displays an RBBB pattern, right superior frontal axis, and positive precordial concordance. Higher exit sites tend to determine more inferior frontal axes. Compared with a lateral basal exit, a septal basal one leads to an LBBB pattern with left axis deviation (**Fig. 14**). An

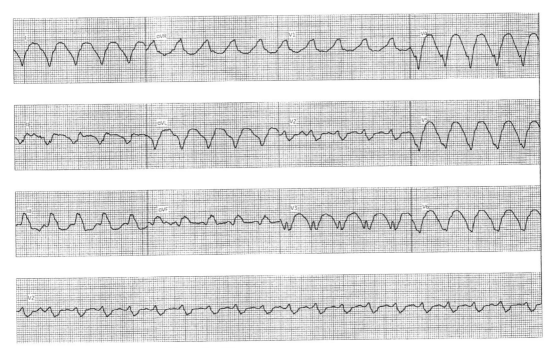

Fig. 16. Apical VT in a patient with a prior MI.

apical exit displays QS complexes from V_4 to V_6 (**Figs. 15** and **16**). The mitral isthmus tachycardia is a form of inferior infarction-related VT, characterized by a slow zone of diastolic activation abutting MA.[40] The arrhythmia can exhibit an LBBB morphology with left superior axis if the exit is on the inferior slow zone or an RBBB with right superior axis in cases of a parietal free wall exit.

2. An anterior MI is generally characterized by a large scar, which makes ECG localization more difficult. Typically, an LBBB configuration with left axis deviation is related to inferoapicoseptal exits and a negative precordial concordance with QS complexes from V_4 to V_6 is related to an apical exit. Septal sites have LBBB left superior axis morphology (**Fig. 17**) and lateral sites have LBBB right superior axis (**Fig. 18**).

3. Postinfarction VTs arising from the PPMs have an RBBB pattern and late R to S transition.[41] A superior axis is seen in cases of inferoseptal PPM origin, whereas VTs arising from the anterolateral PPM display an inferior axis. Similar morphologies have been described for idiopathic PPM VTs.

Hybrid morphologies can be seen in cases of VTs in patients with multiple scar areas. Several algorithms have been developed in the effort to localize exit sites of VTs.[42–45]

Ventricular Arrhythmias due to Nonischemic Cardiomyopathy

Idiopathic dilated cardiomyopathy

VTs in the contest of an idiopathic dilated cardiomyopathy are secondary to myocardial scarring, which has frequently a basal location and a mid-myocardial and epicardial distribution. In the early stages of the disease, myocardial scar has a basal distribution and large precordial leads can be observed during tachycardia. In the late stages, poor R-wave progression is a sign of extensive scarring and severe heart failure. As a result of the multifocal distribution of the scar, notching and fragmentation of the QRS complex are common findings as well as a significantly wide QRS complex (**Figs. 19** and **20**). These findings are also due to a significant disease in the His-Purkinje system.

A common cause of VTs in patients with idiopathic dilated cardiomyopathy is bundle branch reentry (BBR). BBR can occur in patients with significant disease of the His-Purkinje system, leading to the development of LBBB on the sinus rhythm ECG. Reentry within the His-Purkinje system may cause spontaneous VT in up to 30% of those patients. BBR can display either an LBBB pattern similar to that during sinus rhythm or an RBBB morphology with left anterior or posterior fascicular block (**Fig. 21**). An uncommon form of BBR is intrafascicular reentry, which displays

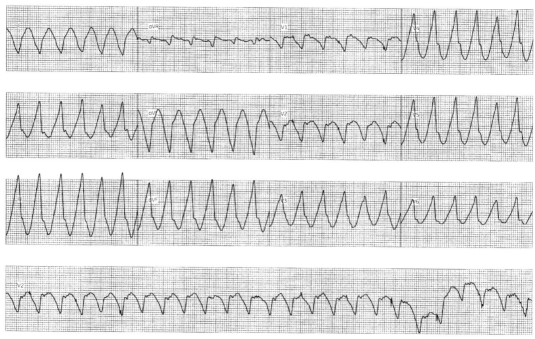

Fig. 17. Anteroseptal basal VT in a patient with a prior MI.

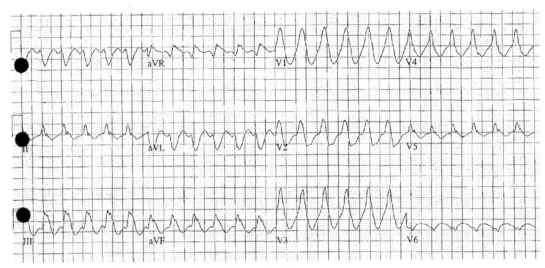

Fig. 18. Anterolateral basal VT in a patient with a prior MI.

several bundle branch block patterns and QRS complex durations.

Arrhythmogenic right ventricular cardiomyopathy

As a result of the most common involvement of the RV, VTs in patients with arrhythmogenic RV cardiomyopathy frequently display an LBBB pattern in lead V_1 (**Fig. 22**). Epicardial approaches are frequently needed. A leftward superior axis is seen in cases of exit sites from the inferior-inferolateral basal region (in close proximity to the tricuspid valve), whereas an inferior axis results from an exit from the OT region. Due to severe scarring, QRS complexes can be significantly wide. Patients with biventricular involvement can show an RBBB pattern in V_1. Multiple VT morphologies are also common and help differentiate arrhythmogenic RV cardiomyopathy VTs from RVOT or other idiopathic VTs.

Sarcoidosis

Patients with sarcoid cardiomyopathy may display several noncharacteristic VT morphologies. An LBBB VT pattern with delayed downstroke QS complex in lead V_1, however, is the most common finding, as a result of the RV involvement. Biventricular involvement is frequently associated to an RBBB VT morphology.

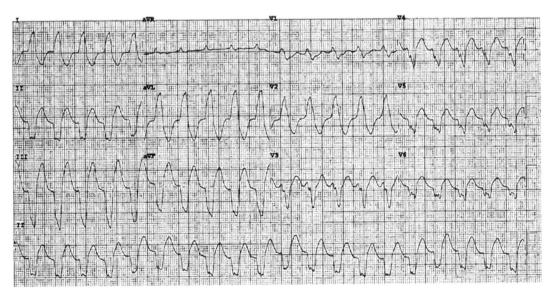

Fig. 19. LV VT in a patient with nonischemic cardiomyopathy.

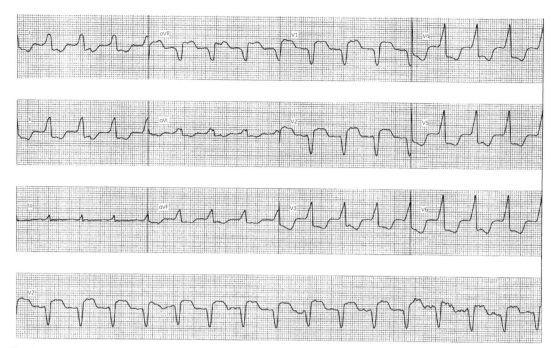

Fig. 20. RV VT in a patient with nonischemic cardiomyopathy.

Chagas cardiomyopathy

Patients with Chagas cardiomyopathy may display a typical RBBB VT pattern with rightward axis, as a result of the main involvement of the inferolateral basal and apical LV. An RV disease may determine an LBBB VT morphology.

Hypertrophic cardiomyopathy

The most common exit site is from the apical region. VTs frequently have small R waves or QS complexes in precordial leads, a superior axis, and either an LBBB or an RBBB pattern (**Fig. 23**).

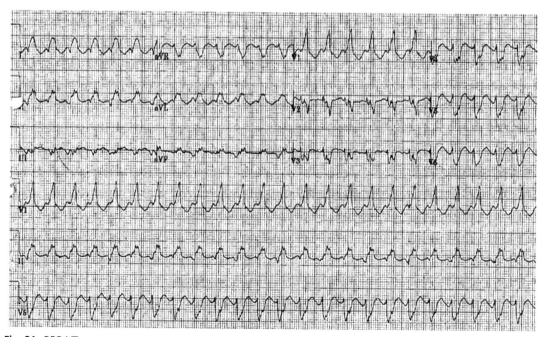

Fig. 21. BBR VT.

A

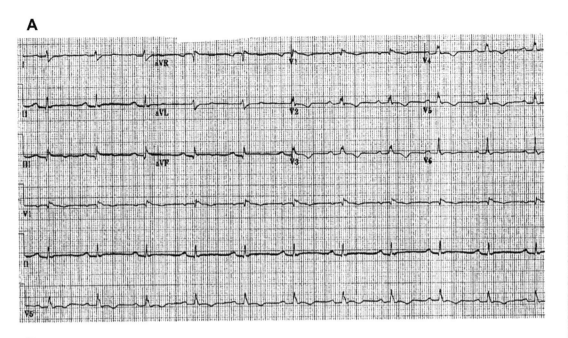

B

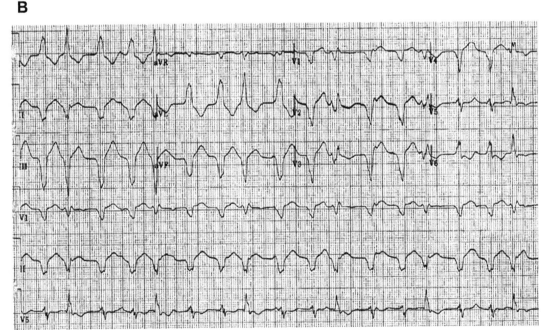

Fig. 22. (*A*) Baseline ECG and (*B*) VT in a patient with arrhythmogenic RV cardiomyopathy.

Epicardial Ventricular Tachycardia due to Structural Heart Disease

Several ECG characteristics have been studied to predict the need of epicardial approach on the bases of VT morphology. These criteria can be classified into 2 categories, based on interval/duration or QRS contour/morphology.

Interval/duration criteria (only for LV VTs with RBBB pattern):

1. Pseudodelta wave greater than or equal to 34 ms in any precordial leads during VTs with an RBBB pattern[37]
2. Delayed intrinsicoid deflection in V_2, such as a time from QRS complex onset to the peak of the R wave greater than or equal to 85 ms[37]
3. Shortest RS complex interval greater than or equal to 121 ms[37]

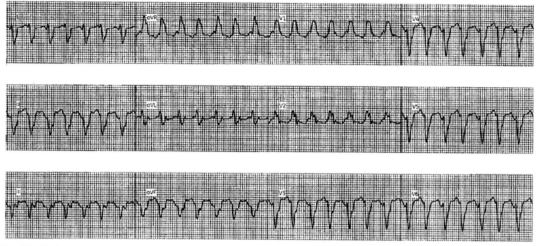

Fig. 23. VT in a patient with hypertrophic cardiomyopathy.

4. QRS duration greater than or equal to 200 ms in any lead[37]
5. MDI greater than or equal to 0.55.[31]

Contour/morphology criteria:

1. Initial q wave in lead I followed by an r wave (especially for RBBB VTs with inferior axis and LVVV VTs from the anterior RV)
2. QS in lead V2 in LBBB VTs (which correlates with an anterior RV exit site)
3. Initial q wave in inferior leads followed by an r wave (which correlates with an inferobasal RV exit site)

SUMMARY

The surface ECG is a valuable mapping tool in patients with idiopathic and scar-related VAs. Its use might help tailoring the ablation strategy to optimize procedural duration, increase the probability of success, and prevent complications.

REFERENCES

1. Connolly SJ, Dorian P, Roberts RS, et al. Comparison of beta-blockers, amiodarone plus beta-blockers, or sotalol for prevention of shocks from implantable cardioverter defibrillators: the OPTIC Study: a randomized trial. JAMA 2006; 295(2):165–71.
2. Bardy GH, Lee KL, Mark DB, et al. Amiodarone or an implantable cardioverter-defibrillator for congestive heart failure. N Engl J Med 2005;352(3):225–37.
3. Connolly SJ, Hallstrom AP, Cappato R, et al. Meta-analysis of the implantable cardioverter defibrillator secondary prevention trials. AVID, CASH and CIDS studies. Antiarrhythmics vs Implantable Defibrillator study. Cardiac Arrest Study Hamburg. Canadian Implantable Defibrillator Study. Eur Heart J 2000; 21(24):2071–8.
4. Qian Z, Zhang Z, Guo J, et al. Association of implantable cardioverter defibrillator therapy with all-cause mortality-a systematic review and meta-analysis. Pacing Clin Electrophysiol 2016;39(1): 81–8.
5. Joshi S, Wilber DJ. Ablation of idiopathic right ventricular outflow tract tachycardia: current perspectives. J Cardiovasc Electrophysiol 2005;16(Suppl 1):S52–8.
6. Kanagaratnam L, Tomassoni G, Schweikert R, et al. Ventricular tachycardias arising from the aortic sinus of valsalva: an under-recognized variant of left outflow tract ventricular tachycardia. J Am Coll Cardiol 2001;37(5):1408–14.
7. Ouyang F, Fotuhi P, Ho SY, et al. Repetitive monomorphic ventricular tachycardia originating from the aortic sinus cusp: electrocardiographic characterization for guiding catheter ablation. J Am Coll Cardiol 2002;39(3):500–8.
8. Lerman BB. Mechanism, diagnosis, and treatment of outflow tract tachycardia. Nat Rev Cardiol 2015; 12(10):597–608.
9. Sapp JL, Wells GA, Parkash R, et al. Ventricular tachycardia ablation versus escalation of antiarrhythmic drugs. N Engl J Med 2016;375(2):111–21.
10. Briceño DF, Romero J, Villablanca PA, et al. Long-term outcomes of different ablation strategies for ventricular tachycardia in patients with structural heart disease: systematic review and meta-analysis. Europace 2017. https://doi.org/10.1093/europace/eux109.
11. Anderson RH. Clinical anatomy of the aortic root. Heart 2000;84:670–3.
12. Sutton JP, Ho SY, Anderson RH. The forgotten interleaflet triangles: a review of the surgical anatomy of the aortic valve. Ann Thorac Surg 1995;59:419–27.

13. Dixit S, Gerstenfeld EP, Callans DJ, et al. Electrocardiographic patterns of superior right ventricular outflow tract tachycardias: distinguishing septal and free-wall sites of origin. J Cardiovasc Electrophysiol 2003;14:1–7.

14. Jadonath RL, Schwartzman DS, Preminger MW, et al. Utility of the 12-lead electrocardiogram in localizing the origin of right ventricular outflow tract tachycardia. Am Heart J 1995;130:1107–13.

15. Kamakura S, Shimizu W, Matsuo K, et al. Localization of optimal ablation site of idiopathic ventricular tachycardia from right and left ventricular outflow tract by body surface ECG. Circulation 1998;98:1525–33.

16. Yamada T, McElderry HT, Doppalapudi H, et al. Catheter ablation of ventricular arrhythmias originating in the vicinity of the His bundle: significance of mapping the aortic sinus cusp. Heart Rhythm 2008;5:37–42.

17. Yamauchi Y, Aonuma K, Takahashi A, et al. Electrocardiographic characteristics of repetitive monomorphic right ventricular tachycardia originating near the His-bundle. J Cardiovasc Electrophysiol 2005;16:1041–8.

18. Tada H, Tadokoro K, Ito S, et al. Idiopathic ventricular arrhythmias originating from the tricuspid annulus: prevalence, electrocardiographic characteristics, and results of radiofrequency catheter ablation. Heart Rhythm 2007;4:7–16.

19. Hasdemir C, Aktas S, Govsa F, et al. Demonstration of ventricular myocardial extensions into the pulmonary artery and aorta beyond the ventriculo-arterial junction. Pacing Clin Electrophysiol 2007;30:534–9.

20. Tada H, Tadokoro K, Miyaji K, et al. Idiopathic ventricular arrhythmias arising from the pulmonary artery: prevalence, characteristics, and topography of the arrhythmia origin. Heart Rhythm 2008;5:419–26.

21. Sekiguchi Y, Aonuma K, Takahashi A, et al. Electrocardiographic and electrophysiologic characteristics of ventricular tachycardia originating within the pulmonary artery. J Am Coll Cardiol 2005;45:887–95.

22. Santoro F, Di Biase L, Hranitzky P, et al. Ventricular tachycardia originating from the septal papillary muscle of the right ventricle: electrocardiographic and electrophysiological characteristics. J Cardiovasc Electrophysiol 2015;26:145–50.

23. Lerman BB, Stein KM, Markowitz SM. Mechanisms of idiopathic left ventricular tachycardia. J Cardiovasc Electrophysiol 1997;8:571–83.

24. Callans DJ, Menz V, Schwartzman D, et al. Repetitive monomorphic tachycardia from the left ventricular outflow tract: electrocardiographic patterns consistent with a left ventricular site of origin. J Am Coll Cardiol 1997;29:1023–7.

25. Hachiya H, Aonuma K, Yamauchi Y, et al. How to diagnose, locate, and ablate coronary cusp ventricular tachycardia. J Cardiovasc Electrophysiol 2002;13:551–6.

26. Bala R, Marchlinski FE. Electrocardiographic recognition and ablation of outflow tract ventricular tachycardia. Heart Rhythm 2007;4:366–70.

27. Lin D, Ilkhanoff L, Gerstenfeld E, et al. Twelve-lead electrocardiographic characteristics of the aortic cusp region guided by intracardiac echocardiography and electroanatomic mapping. Heart Rhythm 2008;5:663–9.

28. Yamada T, Yoshida N, Murakami Y, et al. Electrocardiographic characteristics of ventricular arrhythmias originnating from the junction of the left and right coronary sinuses of Valsalva in the aorta: the activation pattern as a rationale for the electrocardiographic characteristics. Heart Rhythm 2008;5:184–92.

29. Bala R, Garcia F, Hutchinson M, et al. Electrocardiographic and electrophysiologic features of ventricular arrhythmias originating from the right/left coronary cusp commissure. Heart Rhythm 2010;7:312–22.

30. Kumagai K, Fukuda K, Wakayama Y, et al. Electrocardiographic characteristics of the variants of idiopathic left ventricular outflow tract ventricular tachyarrhythmias. J Cardiovasc Electrophysiol 2008;19:495–501.

31. Daniels DV, Lu YY, Morton JB, et al. Idiopathic epicardial left ventricular tachycardia originating remote from the sinus of Valsalva: electrophysiological characteristics, catheter ablation, and identification from the 12-lead electrocardiogram. Circulation 2006;113:1659–66.

32. Yamada T, McElderry H, Doppalapudi H, et al. Idiopathic ventricular arrhythmias originating from the left ventricular summit: anatomic concepts relevant to ablation. Circ Arrhythm Electrophysiol 2010;3:616–23.

33. Tada H, Ito S, Naito S, et al. Idiopathic ventricular arrhythmia arising from the mitral annulus: a distinct subgroup of idiopathic ventricular arrhythmias. J Am Coll Cardiol 2005;45:877–86.

34. Kumagai K, Yamauchi Y, Takahashi A, et al. Idiopathic left ventricular tachycardia originating from the mitral annulus. J Cardiovasc Electrophysiol 2005;16:1029–36.

35. Yamada T, Mcelderry HT, Okada T, et al. Idiopathic focal ventricular arrhythmias originating from the anterior papillary muscle in the left ventricle. J Cardiovasc Electrophysiol 2009;20:866–72.

36. Doppalapudi H, Yamada T, McElderry HT, et al. Ventricular tachycardia originating from the posterior papillary muscle in the left ventricle. Circ Arrhythm Electrophysiol 2008;1:23–9.

37. Berruezo A, Mont L, Nava S, et al. Electrocardiographic recognition of the epicardial origin of ventricular tachycardias. Circulation 2004;109: 1842–7.

38. Nogami A, Naito S, Tada H, et al. Demonstration of diastolic and presystolic Purkinje potentials as critical potentials in a macroreentry circuit of verapamil-sensitive idiopathic left ventricular tachycardia. J Am Coll Cardiol 2000;36:811–23.

39. Betensky BP, Park RE, Marchlinski FE, et al. The V2 transition ratio: a new electrocardiographic criterion for distinguishing left from right ventricular outflow tract tachycardia origin. J Am Coll Cardiol 2011;57: 2255–62.

40. Wilber DJ, Kopp DE, Glascock DN, et al. Catheter ablation of the mitral isthmus for ventricular tachycardia associated with inferior infarction. Circulation 1995;92:3481–9.

41. Bogun F, Desjardins B, Crawford T, et al. Postinfarction ventricular arrhythmias originating in papillary muscles. J Am Coll Cardiol 2008;51: 1794–802.

42. Miller JM, Marchlinski FE, Buxton AE, et al. Relationship between the 12-lead electrocardiogram during ventricular tachycardia and endocardial site of origin in patients with coronary artery disease. Circulation 1988;77(4):759–66.

43. Kuchar DL, Ruskin JN, Garan H. Electrocardiographic localization of the site of origin of ventricular tachycardia in patients with prior myocardial infarction. J Am Coll Cardiol 1989;13(4):893–903.

44. Segal OR, Chow AW, Wong T, et al. A novel algorithm for determining endocardial VT exit site from 12-lead surface ECG characteristics in human, infarct-related ventricular tachycardia. J Cardiovasc Electrophysiol 2007;18(2):161–8.

45. Yokokawa M, Liu TY, Yoshida K, et al. Automated analysis of the 12-lead electrocardiogram to identify the exit site of postinfarction ventricular tachycardia. Heart Rhythm 2012;9(3):330–4.

J-Wave Syndromes
Electrocardiographic and Clinical Aspects

Silvia G. Priori, MD, PhD[a,b,*], Carlo Napolitano, MD, PhD[a]

KEYWORDS

- Inherited arrhythmogenic diseases • Sudden death • Genetics • Electrocardiography
- Risk assessment

KEY POINTS

- The term J-wave syndromes incorporates 2 arrhythmogenic conditions, Brugada syndrome and early repolarization syndrome, characterized by terminal QRS and ST segment abnormalities and by increased risk of cardiac events.
- Brugada syndrome and early repolarization syndrome share similarities in terms of pathophysiology, genetic background, and clinical presentation.
- Risk stratification and clinical management of early repolarization are still ill defined, and the current knowledge does not allow delineation of clear guidelines for clinical management, except for the few subjects who have already experienced an aborted sudden death.
- Only a minority of Brugada syndrome and early repolarization cases are caused by single genetic defects. Oligogenic inheritance has been hypothesized.
- With the exception of quinidine that can be useful in specific instances of Brugada syndrome, no pharmacologic therapies are available; therefore, implantable cardioverter-defibrillator is to be considered as the only option for high-risk subjects.

DEFINITIONS

The term "J wave" (or Osborn wave) was introduced to describe a positive J-point deflection at the end of the QRS complex.[1] In 1953, Osborn first associated this electrocardiogram (ECG) pattern, defined as "current of injury" (from which the "J" originates), with the onset of arrhythmias and ventricular fibrillation (VF) during hypothermia.[1]

In more recent years, the term "J-wave syndromes" was proposed as a unifying definition for 2 clinical entities, namely Brugada syndrome (BrS) and early repolarization syndrome (ERS).[2,3] Their common manifestation is the presence of electrocardiographic abnormalities involving the terminal part of the QRS complex at the transition point with the ST segment, that is, the J point in the normal ECG. The available data support the idea that BrS and ERS share common arrhythmic substrates consisting of increased transmural dispersion of action potential (AP) duration and slow conduction. AP dispersion generates pathologic J-point elevation, the so-called J waves (Fig. 1), which are similar to those described by Osborn. Slow conduction further contributes to the arrhythmogenic substrate.

PATTERN VERSUS SYNDROME

Several investigators proposed a distinction between J waves (the ECG pattern) and J-wave syndromes, that is, the ECG pattern plus a series

Disclosure: The authors have nothing to disclose.
[a] Molecular Cardiology, ICS Maugeri, IRCCS, Pavia, Italy; [b] Department of Molecular Medicine, University of Pavia, Pavia, Italy
* Corresponding author. Molecular Cardiology, ICS Maugeri, IRCCS, Via Maugeri 10/10A, Pavia 27100, Italy.
E-mail address: silvia.priori@icsmaugeri.it

Card Electrophysiol Clin 10 (2018) 355–369
https://doi.org/10.1016/j.ccep.2018.02.009
1877-9182/18/© 2018 Elsevier Inc. All rights reserved.

cardiacEP.theclinics.com

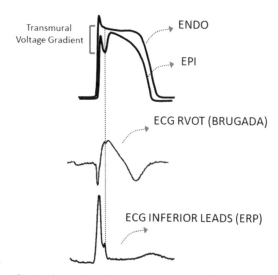

Fig. 1. Electrophysiological mechanisms of J waves. The upper panel depicts the genesis of the voltage gradient due to the prominent I_{To} generating a quick phase 1 repolarization only in the epicardial AP. These transmural differences of AP generate BrS pattern when present in the RVOT and ERP pattern when present in inferior leads. ENDO, endocardial action potential; EPI, epicardial action potential.

of clinical signs and/or symptoms contributing to justify the term "syndrome."[2,4] The distinction between "ECG pattern" and "syndrome" was initially introduced in 2005[4] when it was suggested that Brugada "syndrome" could be diagnosed in the presence of a Brugada ECG pattern plus at least one additional criterion, including ventricular arrhythmias, inducibility at programmed electrical stimulation (PES), syncope, family history of sudden cardiac death (SCD). This approach was conceived to facilitate the identification of the subset of patients with full-blown disease and higher risk. Nevertheless, the evidence that SCD can be the first manifestation of the disease in previously asymptomatic subjects with no family history called for caution before dismissing the presence of a risk of events in subjects with a "pattern" but not a "syndrome."[5,6]

Accordingly, the criteria enabling the diagnosis of BrS have been modified and summarized in the so-called Shanghai criteria.[2] The Shanghai criteria for BrS are less stringent as compared with those suggested in 2005. Indeed, the presence of a spontaneous type 1 ECG is now considered sufficient to diagnose "probable/definite" BrS.

A similar distinction between "pattern" and "syndrome" has been proposed for early repolarization. An ERS should be diagnosed in the presence of an early repolarization pattern (ERP)[2] and additional criteria: unexplained cardiac arrest, suspected arrhythmic syncope, dynamic J-point changes, short-coupled premature ventricular contractions (PVCs), family history of unexplained SCD. However, the classification problem that initially emerged for BrS versus Brugada pattern is even more evident for ERP given the incompletely defined ECG and clinical criteria enabling dissection of an "arrhythmogenic ERP" from the frequently observed benign pattern (see later discussion). Shanghai criteria for ERS have not been validated with experimental or prospective clinical studies, and caution should be taken before a systematic implementation of this concept.

In the following discussion, the authors outline the ECG presentation and clinical features of J-wave syndromes keeping in mind that a distinction between "pattern" and "syndrome" may be arbitrary.

CELLULAR MECHANISMS

Experimental studies investigating the electrophysiologic mechanisms of J wave were carried out since the late 1980s.[7] The working hypothesis, obtained in canine myocardium wedge models, was based on the presence of transmural differences of AP shape and duration generated by a differential expression of the transient outward current, I_{To}.[7,8] The presence of transmural dispersion of repolarization defines the so-called repolarization hypothesis. I_{To} is physiologically more expressed in the ventricular epicardium where it modulates the AP shape so to induce a fast phase 1 repolarization (notch) followed by a "dome"; APs in the endocardium have a small phase 1 notch (less I_{To}) and a longer plateau phase (see **Fig. 1**). In pathologic conditions, the notch and the following dome are abnormally amplified, leading to an overall shortening of AP in the epicardium. The consequent excessive increase of transmural AP dispersion can generate arrhythmias (see later discussion). Of note, I_{To} is not the only determinant of pathologic J waves as shown by genetic studies demonstrating mutations in multiple genes for BrS and ERS (**Table 1**). Both conditions can be due to reduced inward currents, such as sodium and calcium currents[2,9] or increased ATP-dependent potassium current.[2,10] Therefore, it appears that the arrhythmogenic substrate is actually created by an imbalance between depolarizing and repolarizing current in the early phase of cardiac AP.

The reason for the existence of different phenotypes, namely BrS end ERS, having similar cellular and genetic pathophysiology has been the object

Table 1
Genes associated with Brugada syndrome and early repolarization syndrome

Gene	BrS	ERS	Protein	Functional Defect
SCN5A	✔	✔	Cardiac sodium channel alpha subunit (Nav1.5)	Loss of function, reduced Na^+ current
GPD1-L	✔	—	Glycerol-6-phosphate-dehydrogenase	Loss of function, reduced Na+ current
CACNA1c	✔	✔	L-type calcium channel alpha subunit (Cav1.2)	Loss of function, reduced Ca^{2+} current
CACNB2	✔	✔	L-type calcium channel beta-2 subunit	Loss of function, reduced Ca^{2+} current
SCN1B	✔	—	Cardiac sodium channel beta1 subunit	Loss of function, reduced Na^+ current
KCNE3	✔	—	Transient outward current beta subunit-transient outward current	Gain of function, increased K^+ Ito current
SCN3B	✔	—	Cardiac sodium channel beta-3 subunit	Loss of function, reduced Na^+ current
KCNH2	✔	—	Rapid component of the cardiac delayed rectifier current	Increased repolarizing current (gain of function)
KCNJ8	✔	✔	Acetylcholine-dependent potassium current	Incomplete closing of the ATP-sensitive potassium channels
CACNA2D1	✔	—	L-type calcium channel delta 2 subunit	Loss of function, reduced Ca^{2+} current
RANGRF	✔	—	RAN protein GTP releasing factor	Unknown (possible effect on sodium current)
KCNE5	✔	—	Potassium channel beta 5 subunit-transient outward current	Gain of function, increased K^+ Ito current
KCND3	✔	—	SHAL potassium channel isoform 3-transient outward current	Gain of function, increased K^+ Ito current
HCN4	✔	—	Hyperpolarization activated potassium channel (If)	No functional studies available
SLMAP	✔	—	Sarcolemmal membrane–associated protein	Reduced Na^+ current (impaired NaV 1.5 trafficking)
TRPM4	✔	—	Calcium-activated cationic channel subfamily M isoform 4	Reduced sodium current
SCN2B	✔	—	Cardiac sodium channel Beta 2 subunit	Loss of function, reduced Na^+ current
SCN10A	✔	✔	Voltage-gated sodium channel alpha subunit 10	Reduced NaV1.8 current
MOG1	✔	—	Guanine nucleotide release factor, control of NaV1.5 trafficking	Loss of function, reduced Na^+ current
PKP2	✔	—	Plakophilin 2–desmosomal protein	Reduced adhesion, ARVC/BRS overlap phenotype
ABCC9	✔	✔	SUR2A (sulfonylurea receptor subunit 2 A)	Gain of function, increased outward current

of experimental studies. It has been proposed that the dispersion of AP leading to J waves can be transmural (epicardium vs endocardium) but also "transversal" between the myocardial regions where the dome is lost in the epicardium and regions at which it is maintained.[11] The regional depolarization/repolarization imbalance leading to different AP shape and duration in the epicardium is the current hypothesis for the generation of a pathologic J wave in the right ventricular outflow tract (RVOT; BrS) or in the inferior/lateral wall (ERS).[2] Despite this theoretic explanation, there is still no definite experimental support in whole heart models.

The transmural AP dispersion is not the only abnormality identified in J-wave syndromes. Other investigators have reported impaired electrical conduction, which is the basis of the "depolarization hypothesis" initially advocated to explain BrS[12] after the identification of a reduced conduction velocity in the RVOT.[12] More recently, ECG mapping studies showed the presence of both repolarization (transmural dispersion) and depolarization (reduced conduction velocity) defects.[13] On the other hand, in ERP, a reduced conduction velocity was found using a Langendorff-perfused heart model.[9] In this study, the administration of a sodium channel blocker in a coronary artery branch serving the inferior wall induced a slowing of electrical conduction and the appearance of the inferior ERP pattern. The presence of increased late potential at nighttime in patients with ventricular fibrillation and ERP further supports the presence of a depolarization abnormality.[14]

Thus, the available evidence suggests that BrS and ERS are generated by similar combinations of abnormal depolarization and repolarization.[15] However, the lack of reliable animal models for both conditions has so far prevented gathering the final experimental proof of this hypothesis.

Arrhythmogenic Mechanism in the Presence of Pathologic J Waves

The most accredited hypothesis for the genesis of arrhythmias is the presence of an exaggerated transmural AP dispersion leading to an ectopic activity defined as "phase 2 reentry."[16] Phase 2 reentry occurs when the epicardial AP dome electronically propagates to nearby regions, giving rise to a closely coupled extrasystole (**Fig. 2**). Further propagation of this ectopic activity can generate sustained arrhythmias. In pharmacologic models of BrS and ERS, phase 2 reentry has been induced using potassium channel openers, calcium channel blockers, and sodium channel blockers with or without acetylcholine to simulate vagal stimulation[16–19]; on the contrary, 4-aminopyridine and quinidine that block I_{To} are able to reduce the epicardial AP notch and to exert an antiarrhythmic affect.[16,17] No direct proof of the presence of a phase 2 reentry in humans has been collected so far, but the evidence of increased J-point elevation in the sinus beat preceding ventricular ectopies in

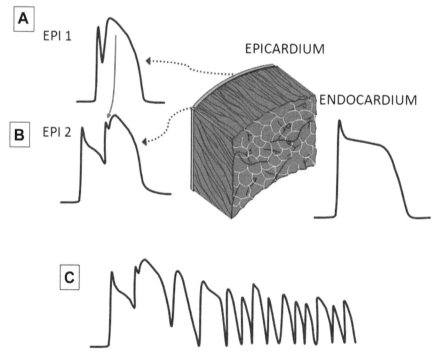

Fig. 2. Mechanisms of phase 2 reentry. The endocardial AP has a small phase 1 and a wide plateau. The dome-shaped and shorter duration of the epicardial AP (*A*) generates J wave and can give rise to arrhythmias. When the dome is pathologically increased (eg, for the presence of a genetic mutation, vagal stimulation, drugs), it can be propagated to a nearby epicardial site (*B*) originating an ectopic beat and (*C*) sustained arrhythmias. This phase 2 reentry can become sustained because of the presence of conduction defect and discontinuous electrical conduction.

BrS patients has been taken as an indirect suggestion of increased AP dispersion immediately before cardiac arrhythmia.[20]

Localized conduction delay can also have a key arrhythmogenic role. The slowing of wavelength can exacerbate anisotropy and discontinuous conduction. In these conditions, conduction block, reentry, and wave breaks are promoted and make an ectopic activity generated by a phase 2 reentry to become sustained.[12] Slow conduction areas have been demonstrated with endocardiac end epicardial mapping in BrS patients.

Autonomic Modulation of J Waves

Autonomic tone can noticeably modulate the disease expressivity of both BrS and ERS. The initial suggestion for an autonomic modulation dates back to 1996 when Miyazaki and colleagues[21] showed that intravenous isoproterenol reduced ≥ 0.1 mV ST segment elevation, while intracoronary acetylcholine or intravenous edrophonium augmented it. This observation was accompanied by the clinical findings that in BrS the onset of cardiac events is predominantly at rest or during sleep, whereas the ECG abnormalities become less severe during exercise and increase during recovery.[22] Overall, it was suggested that vagal stimulation can be proarrhythmic in BrS. Other studies addressing heart rate variability suggested the presence of increased vagal activity before the episodes of VF.[23] A similar vagal-mediated worsening was reported in patients with ERS and ventricular fibrillation.[14,24] Shinohara and colleagues[25] identified increased baroreflex sensitivity (but not heart rate variability) in patients with both BrS and ERS. Mizumaki and colleagues[24] also showed increased high-frequency component at power spectrum analysis of heart rate variability (marker of increased parasympathetic tone) in patients in inferior J wave and ventricular fibrillation. Although parasympathetic activation worsens ECG manifestations and may represent an arrhythmogenic trigger in BrS and ERS, there is evidence that the sympathetic component of the autonomic system can be antiarrhythmic in both conditions.[26,27] Overall, the available evidence points to fact that autonomic tone modulates in a similar fashion the arrhythmogenic substrate of BrS and ERS.

BRUGADA SYNDROME

BrS in an arrhythmogenic condition was described for the first time in 1992[28] and was characterized by J-point elevation in leads V1-V2, often associated with incomplete or complete right bundle branch block and increased risk of arrhythmic events.[28,29]

Electrocardiographic Aspects

BrS can be diagnosed in the presence of a "type 1 ECG," consisting of a J-point elevation ≥ 2 mm with descending ST segment and negative T wave in the right precordial leads V1 and V2 (see **Fig. 1**). Two additional ECG patterns, type 2 and type 3, are associated with possible BrS, but they are nondiagnostic and require the execution of a provocative test with the intravenous administration of sodium channel blockers (flecainide 2 mg/kg up to 150 mg or ajmaline 1 mg/kg) to unmask a diagnostic type 1. The current guidelines[29] suggest recording the right precordial leads (V1 and V2) in the third and second intercostal space to improve detection of the electrical signal coming from the RVOT. The rationale for this approach comes from a series of studies that have specifically addressed the localization of the electrophysiological abnormalities occurring in BrS.

The right ventricular outflow tract of the Brugada patients

In the clinical setting, the electrocardiographic evidence of abnormal J waves in the right precordial leads suggested the presence of electrophysiological defects occurring in the RVOT. As pointed out earlier, wedge preparations[30] showed transmural dispersion of repolarization in experimental BrS models, and several lines of evidence concur to highlight the presence of specific abnormalities of the RVOT of BrS patients. Body surface ECG mapping identified both ST elevation (possibly corresponding to transmural dispersion) and slow conduction in the RVOT region.[31]

Electroanatomical mapping studies consistently found abnormal electrical signals in RVOT.[32-35] The activation time of the right ventricle was found to be almost twice as long as that of the controls, and isochrones in the anterolateral RVOT were slower with a conduction delay of approximately 40 ms and with an activation time during sinus rhythm of greater than 100 ms, coinciding with the peak of J-point elevation on the surface ECG.[35] Other investigators showed the presence of low-voltage and fragmented QRS in the same area.[31] Finally, catheter ablation of the slow conduction zone and low voltage area modified Brugada ECG pattern and suppressed VF.[36,37]

The reasons for localized RVOT abnormalities in BrS are not yet understood, and a comprehensive picture putting together conduction abnormalities and transmural AP duration abnormalities is not yet available. Nonetheless, the mapping studies have consistently highlighted the presence of conduction defect and fractionated electrograms in the RVOT, supporting the important role of a depolarization abnormality in the pathogenesis of the disease.

Clinical Aspects

Epidemiology and natural history

Given the incomplete knowledge of the genetic causes of BrS, the prevalence can be only indirectly estimated based on the frequency of the ECG pattern in the general population. This approach has limitations because of the transient nature of the ECG manifestations,[38] and the possibility of false positives. In addition, the ECG criteria for the disease have changed,[29] creating further uncertainties. Accordingly, the available data portray very different figures between 1:1000 and 1:10,000.[27]

BrS manifests with syncope caused by self-terminating polymorphic ventricular tachycardia (VT) and/or cardiac arrest usually occurring at rest. The BrS has a male predominance (8:1 male:female), and the average age of sudden death is 40 years with a peak in the third and fourth decades of life, although arrhythmic events can occur at any age. Fever and exposure to specific drugs can exacerbate the ECG abnormalities and trigger events.[39] Data from the international registries suggest a cardiac arrest/sudden death rate between 1% and 3%.[38,40,41] More recent data, collected in an unselected group of BrS probands only (n = 289), which should have higher rates of events by definition, substantially confirm this figure with a 1% yearly incidence of cardiac arrest over an observation period of 10 years.[42] Overall, the figure on the rate of events in BrS seems now reasonably settled, and it is in sharp departure from the initial figures[43–45] that portrayed much worrisome figures (likely because of selection bias) with greater than 8% yearly event rate. Furthermore, risk stratification procedures (see later discussion) can identify the large subset of BrS patients with a very low risk of events that do not need antiarrhythmic treatments.

Genetics

Genetic discoveries in BrS are portraying an increasingly complex picture. Currently, there are at least 21 genes (see **Table 1**) and 3 susceptibility loci identified (see later discussion). After the initial successful discovery of SCN5A mutations by Chen and colleagues[46] in 1998 and despite many genotyping studies done in the last 20 years, most BrS patients remain genetically undetermined. Although SCN5A mutations are identified in a relevant percentage of cases (20%), all the remaining genetic loci account only for a small proportion of cases (5%–10% at the most).[39]

This picture has not substantially changed in the last few years even if several new genes have been added to the list.

Other investigators attempted to increase the yield of genetic testing by assessing the presence of copy number variation and large genomic rearrangements not detectable with the standard sequencing techniques. Unfortunately also in this case, the overall yield remains poor as demonstrated by Mademont-Soler and colleagues,[47] who identified only one large SCN5A deletion out of 220 patients screened.

It is important to observe that the BrS genes have been mostly identified through candidate gene screening. Indeed despite the disease is still considered monogenic, it often presents in sporadic cases or in families with unclear inheritance pattern.[39] Thus, it is very difficult to demonstrate an association of a genetic locus or candidate mutation with the phenotype using cosegregation analysis (ie, the typical approach of linkage studies used for the identification of the major genes causing inherited arrhythmias). Candidate gene screening is a weaker methodology because it bears higher probability of false discoveries. Next-generation sequencing screening projects in BrS probands should rely on the capability of excluding the presence of the candidate variant in control subjects. However, control cohorts should include well-phenotyped subjects accounting for the fact that ECG abnormalities may be concealed. Even when complemented with functional expression studies, candidate gene screening may bring about false positives.[48] Accordingly, retrospective analysis showed that some of variants previously associated with BrS are probably benign innocent bystanders.[49]

The low prevalence of familiar BrS cases can also question the paradigm of the "monogenicity" of the disease. This concept is supported by literature findings suggesting an oligogenic inheritance. There are examples in the literature of the fact that common variants such as the H558R single-nucleotide polymorphism on the SCN5A gene can modulate the expressivity of a BrS-associated mutation[50] or that the same genetic defect can have different consequences when presenting different SCN5A splicing variants.[51] More recent genome-wide analysis provides further support to this hypothesis with the identification of a set of common variants in HEY2, SCN5A, and SCN10A genes. The variants occurring at these "BrS susceptibility loci" significantly increase the probability of expressing the BrS phenotype with an odds ratio (OR) from 1.84 to 21.48 depending on the number of concomitant variants (from 2 and up to 6).[52]

In summary, after 20 years of research, the genetic basis of BrS remains incomplete. Genetic testing is considered clinically relevant for familial screening when a definitive pathogenic mutation is identified and to better delineate the long-term follow-up when in the presence of variants potentially associated with overlap phenotypes like SCN5A and progressive conduction defect or sinus node dysfunction (SND).

Risk stratification and clinical management

In 2002, the authors published the first study proposing a risk-stratification scheme for BrS.[53] The data collected in a cohort of 200 consecutive unselected subjects demonstrated that the combined presence of a spontaneous type 1 ECG and a history of syncope was the strongest predictor (hazard ratio [HR], 6.4, 95% confidence interval [CI], 1.9–21.2) of the occurrence of cardiac arrest/sudden death. This concept, subsequently confirmed in several studies, is still the fulcrum of risk stratification for BrS.[27] However, the need of a refined risk stratification is evident when considering the asymptomatic subjects with spontaneous type 1 ECG.[54] These subjects were considered at intermediate risk in the authors' 2002 study.[53]

As a consequence, several additional risk markers have been proposed (**Fig. 3**): inducibility of VT/VF during PES,[44,55] QRS fragmentation,[40,56] SND,[57] family history of SCD,[57,58] late potentials,[59,60] T-wave alternans,[61] T_{peak}-T_{end} dispersion,[60] the temporal and spatial burden of ST elevation during 24-hour ambulatory ECG monitoring,[62] heart rate variability/complexity.[63,64]

Among these risk markers, inducibility of VT/VF during PES is the best investigated. After several years of conflicting evidence,[65] recent meta-analyses have contributed to shed light on this intricate issue. Among such studies, Sroubek and colleagues[55] included more than 1300 patients from 8 studies. Of note and at variance with others, the strength of the study by Sroubek and colleagues is the analysis of individual-level data collected in a merged database thanks to an international collaboration. Overall, the results showed an increased risk of events (HR 2.66; 95% CI 1.44–4.92) among asymptomatic subjects with spontaneous type 1 ECG who were inducible with ≤2 extra stimuli with 200 ms as the shortest coupling interval. Thus, inducibility with a "soft" protocol can be reasonably considered to guide implantable cardioverter-defibrillator (ICD) implantation in BrS patients with "intermediate" risk. Of note, however, noninducible subjects had approximately 1% per year incidence of events. Thus, the negative predictive accuracy of PES is limited, and the lack of inducibility cannot be taken as a robust indication for a low risk of events.

Other attempts of including additional risk markers in multiparametric schemes had limited success so far. A meta-analysis of prospective studies (27 studies, 4494 patients) analyzed 6 risk factors: family history of SCD, syncope, inducible ventricular arrhythmias, spontaneous type 1 ECG, male sex, and SCN5A mutation.[58] Only the known risk factors (inducible ventricular arrhythmias, spontaneous type 1 ECG) plus a family history of SCD in a first-degree family member were independently associated with outcome. Another attempt of combining multiple risk factors to improve the identification of subjects at risk of events was carried out by Sieira and colleagues,[57] who assessed several variables, including clinical history and family history of SCD at presentation, SND, conduction parameters, inducibility at PES,

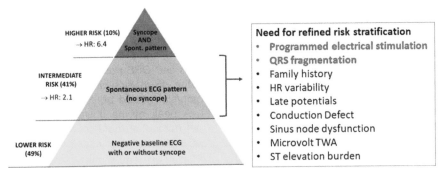

Fig. 3. Risk stratification in BrS. The 3 major risk groups identified in the early 2000s are shown, including the HR for cardiac events (lower risk group as reference category); the percentage of population included in each group is reported in brackets. The intermediate risk group represents approximately 49% of the population and requires further risk stratification. The right panel reports all the proposed risk stratifiers. Only PES and QRS fragmentation have been confirmed in independent studies but so far have not been included in a formal comprehensive risk stratification scheme (see text). (*Adapted from* Priori SG, Napolitano C, Gasparini M, et al. Natural history of Brugada syndrome: insights for risk stratification and management. Circulation 2002;105(11):1345; with permission.)

history of atrial fibrillation. A model with significant variables at multivariate analysis included gender (male), presentation with syncope or aborted SCD, SND, proband status, early familial SCD <35 years in first-degree relatives; spontaneous type I had 90% predictive accuracy. Each predictor was quantified using its HR, and a scoring system was defined. However, the study included 400 subjects, and the 6 categories created by the scoring scheme were small (25–35 subjects) with few events (5–8 events per group), thus shedding uncertainties on the reproducibility in larger cohorts.

Overall risk stratification in BrS remains challenging, and over the last decade, only minor advancements have been made to improve the clinical management scheme developed 2000 almost two decades ago based on the presence of spontaneous type 1 pattern and history of symptoms. The authors have learned that inducibility of VT/VF may identify a subset at higher risk, but that the lack of inducibility does necessarily set a benign condition. The additional risk markers that have been proposed in the attempt of reaching a higher granularity were identified in single, often unconfirmed, studies and cannot be used with confidence in the clinical setting at present.

Clinical management and therapy

The treatment of BrS is largely based on lifestyle modifications and ICD.[27] All patients with a clinical diagnosis of BrS should avoid drugs that can unmask or worsen the ECG pattern (www.brugadadrugs.org) (class I). Fever is also a recognized trigger for arrhythmias. Patients should be instructed accordingly. Recording an ECG during fever may support a correct definition of the clinical picture by detecting "natural" susceptibility.

Quinidine may prevent arrhythmia inducibility at PES and may prevent the occurrence of cardiac arrhythmias at follow-up.[66] Quinidine may be useful to prevent recurrences of cardiac arrest in patients who already received an ICD, and a clinical trial is ongoing for primary prevention in asymptomatic patients (NIH ID: NCT00789165). Albeit encouraging, these results are to be considered as preliminary, and at present, quinidine is indicated only for the treatment of electrical storms (class IIa) or in patients with contraindications for ICD (class IIa).[27] Epicardial catheter ablation of fragmented potentials and slow conduction in RVOT has been proposed.[33] This approach can be currently considered for the treatment of patients with arrhythmic storm and to reduce the chance of multiple ICD shocks (class IIb indication). Other studies are now assessing catheter ablation for routine treatment of BrS[37]; however,

the observation time after the procedure is still limited and the analysis of long-term complications is unavailable. Importantly, recurrence of cardiac events has been observed with both quinidine and catheter ablation.[31,67]

EARLY REPOLARIZATION SYNDROME

The term "early repolarization" refers to a J-point elevation and terminal QRS abnormalities that may be relatively high in prevalence in the population. In the last decade, it has been suggested that ERP may be associated with an increased risk of VF, and thus, the term "early repolarization syndrome" was adopted. Several studies investigated ways to distinguish benign ERP from the malignant type, based on its electrocardiographic appearance.

Electrocardiographic Aspects

ERP was initially noted in young healthy individuals more than 70 years ago and was considered a benign "juvenile ST pattern."[68,69] The earlier studies have overlooked a precise definition of the J-wave morphology. Therefore, they could have included heterogeneous subjects with different substrates. In recent years, the inclusion criteria have gradually shifted away from the initial focus on ST-segment elevation toward the abnormalities of the terminal QRS (notching or slurring) and J wave. This concept of the gradual modification of ECG criteria emerges clear from the analysis of the consensus papers on ERP.

In 2009, the American Heart Association (AHA)/ American College of Cardiology (ACC)/Heart Rhythm Society (HRS) consensus document on ECG interpretation[70] identified the ECG pattern with "J-point elevation and rapidly upsloping or normal ST segment" as "a normal variant." The 2015 Experts' consensus paper on ERP[71] has explicitly removed ascending ST-segment elevation without QRS notching and/or slurring (**Fig. 4**A), and ERP was defined in the presence of (1) an end-QRS notch (**Fig. 4**B): or slur (**Fig. 4**C) on the downslope of a prominent R wave. The notch/slur should be entirely above the baseline. (2) A peak of the J wave (notched or slurred) ≥0.1 mV in 2 or more contiguous leads of the 12-lead ECG, excluding leads V1 to V3 (to avoid confusion with BrS diagnosis). (3) QRS duration less than 120 milliseconds.

In 2016, the AHA published a scientific statement on ERP that introduced different ECG criteria.[72] Two ECG features were considered harbingers of arrhythmic risk because of their higher prevalence among patients with idiopathic VF: (1) J waves in the inferior leads; (2) horizontal/descending pattern of ST segment after the J point. Although the

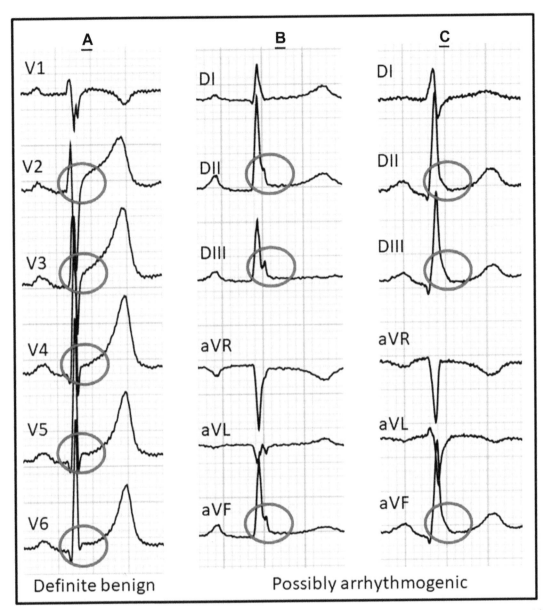

Fig. 4. J-wave pattern in ERP. (*A*) J-point elevation with upsloping ST segment in precordia leads is now considered a benign pattern. Notch (*B*) or slurred (*C*), especially if >0.2 mV, is considered potentially arrhythmogenic even if clear management strategies are not yet available.

investigators of the AHA document acknowledged the fact that most of the Aborted Cardiac Arrest/SCD patients with ERP present with ≥2-mm elevation, the large degree of overlap of ST elevation between cases and controls prevented a clear definition of the "critical" amplitude of the J wave that constitutes an arrhythmogenic condition. In April 2017, the Asian Pacific Heart Rhythm Association (APHRS), European Heart Rhythm Association (EHRA), Sociedad Latinoamericana de Estimulación Cardíaca y Electrofisiología (SOLAECE) consensus document provided another update on the ECG criteria for ERP, including the following: (1) the amplitude (≥0.2 mV), which was considered less stringently in the 2016 document; (2) the number of leads (≥2 inferior and/or lateral ECG leads with horizontal/descending ST segment); and the presence of (3) the dynamic changes of J-point elevation (≥0.1 mV).

There is now consensus that an upsloping ST segment after the J point, especially in the lateral leads, should be regarded as a benign ECG presentation, whereas the horizontal/descending ST segment has potential clinical meaning.

Clinical Aspects

Initial studies

As previously observed, ERP has been described as a benign ECG manifestation presenting with higher prevalence in young subjects and considered as such for several decades.[73,74] In 2003, Klatsky and colleagues[74] reported an analysis of 2234 ECGs of individuals undergoing health evaluation and reported higher prevalence of the pattern among men, especially if Black, Hispanic, and of younger age (<40 years). No increased risk of death was found in individuals with ERP pattern. High prevalence has been also observed in male athletes[75] with a clear age-related penetrance peaking at 15 to 20 years in lateral leads.[76]

Studies in idiopathic ventricular fibrillation patients

A sharp departure from the paradigm of the benignity of ERP was provided in 2008 when Haïssaguerre and colleagues[77] showed ERP in 31% of SCD cases as compared with 5% of controls suggesting its causal link. Interestingly, in the same paper, Haïssaguerre and colleagues were also able to map the origin of ventricular ectopies that initiated arrhythmias to sites concordant with the localization of repolarization abnormalities. Subsequent studies appeared to confirm this finding with higher prevalence of ERP in survivors of idiopathic ventricular fibrillation (IVF) ranging from 15% to 70% of cases.[78–80] More recently, Siebermair and colleagues[81] investigated the correlation between ERP and the propensity to develop life-threatening ventricular arrhythmias, identifying ERP as the only predictor of arrhythmia recurrence in a cohort of 35 IVF survivors followed for 9 years (HR 3.9, 95% CI 1.4–11.0; $P = .01$).

Population studies and early repolarization pattern morphology

The prevalence of ERP in the general population is in the range of 1% to 30%, and it appears to be influenced by age, gender, and the specific features of the enrolled cohort (eg, being athletes). Overall, the incidence tends to be lower than that reported in IVF patients.[74,77,82,83] Tikkanen and colleagues[75] first reported an increased incidence of SCD among 10,864 subjects with ERP (relative risk 2.92) of Finnish origin, after a very long follow-up of 30 ± 11 years. Interestingly, the same group showed J wave with horizontal/descending ST segments conferred a higher risk of sudden death (HR 1.43; 95% CI 1.05–1.94) than ERP with upsloping ST segments.[83] The relevance of considering J-wave morphology is further supported by the fact that when all patients are analyzed irrespective of the J-wave shape, as in the large study on greater than 15,000 subjects of Olson and colleagues,[84] there is no significant increase risk of events in the presence of ERP. In a recent meta-analysis by Cheng and colleagues,[85] 16 studies on 334,524 subjects were included. In an absolute risk increase of 140 SCD per 100,000 person-years, ERP was estimated to be the cause of 7.3% of SCD in the general population (95% CI 1.9–15.2). The relative risk of SCD in the presence of ERP ranged from 1.33 (95% CI 1.13–1.57, $P = .005$) in population studies to 4.25 (95% CI 1.84–9.81) in case-control studies.

In summary, a signal of increased risk of arrhythmic events associated with ERP is evident in population studies; however, the reported prevalence of ERP (up to 30%) is higher than the actual incidence of events reported in the same studies (3%–5%), suggesting that an alternative possibility would be that of considering ERP as a risk marker more than an autonomous clinical entity.

Early repolarization pattern as a risk modifier

Along this line of reasoning, several studies tried to quantify the relative risk increase of death in patients with other diagnoses, spanning from acquired conditions, such as coronary artery disease, to inherited arrhythmogenic diseases, such as long QT syndrome (LQTS). In 2012, Naruse and colleagues[86] reported ERP as an independent predictor (together with Killip class) of occurrence of VF within 48 hours after the onset of an acute myocardial infarction with an OR of 3.77. This observation was confirmed in other cohorts.[86–88] A recent meta-analysis[89] of the studies of ERP in acute and chronic coronary artery disease included a total of 19 papers on 7268 patients and showed a 5-fold increase in the risk of SCD and ventricular arrhythmias in patients with ERP compared with those without ERP.[89]

Other investigators have assessed the predictive role of ERP-inherited arrhythmogenic diseases. Laksman and colleagues[90] found an independent association of a ≥2-mm J-point elevation (with QRS slurring or notching) with the occurrence of a combined endpoint of syncope, documented polymorphic VT, and resuscitated cardiac arrest in LQTS patients (n = 113; OR 5.97). Tülümen and colleagues[91] found increased incidence of ERP in a small group of patients (n = 51) with catecholaminergic polymorphic VT with syncopal events (78%) as compared with asymptomatic events (39% $P = .005$). Georgopoulos and colleagues[92] addressed the role of ERP in BrS in a meta-analysis of 5 studies and 1375 patients showing an increased risk of arrhythmia (OR 3.29, 95% CI: 2.06–5.26). Interestingly, when considering spatially diffuse ERP (inferior and lateral), the OR for arrhythmic events was even higher (OR 4.87, 95% CI: 2.64–9.01). In consideration of the fact that BrS subjects (by definition) have pathologic J wave in anterior leads (V1 and V2), this very high-risk subgroup actually includes subjects with "global" J-wave abnormalities in inferior, lateral, and anterior leads. Finally, a possible association between ERP and short QT syndrome (SQTS) has been suggested by Haïssaguerre and colleagues[77] and by Watanabe and colleagues,[93] who showed the presence of ERP in 88% SQTS with associated OR of 5.64 (95% CI 1.97–16.15) for arrhythmic events as compared with SQTS with no ERP. These observations motivated the authors to assess the prevalence of ERP in their cohort of 73 SQTS patients: they found that ERP was present in 29% of cases and was not associated with an increased risk of experiencing life-threatening arrhythmias.[3]

Genetics

In agreement with the proposed pathogenesis of J wave, it is reasonable to expect that ERP-causing genes would be at least partially overlapping with those causing BrS (see **Table 1**). Candidate gene screenings have contributed to the identification of 7 loci: mutations have been identified in ATP-dependent potassium current (KCNJ8 and ABCC9), in the calcium channel (CACAN1c, CACNB2b, CACNA2D1), and in the sodium channel (SCN5A, SCN10A).[2] As in BrS, mutations of potassium channels are associated with a gain-of-function effect, whereas loss of function is observed in calcium and sodium channel mutations. Of note, few mutations have been functionally characterized, and currently, the mechanism or mechanisms through which mutations in the same genes leading to BrS or ERS phenotypes are obscure. Importantly, genetic mutations are identified in a small proportion of cases (<20%).

Despite the low rate of identified pathogenic mutations, there is a clear signal in the population suggesting that ERP is a heritable trait: offspring of ER-positive parents have a 2.5-fold increased risk of presenting with ERP on their ECG.[94,95] However, because, with few exceptions,[96] a Mendelian pattern of inheritance is not evident in most of cases,[97] an oligogenic inheritance can be hypothesized, but no data currently support this idea. In summary, it is clear that we have only started to scratch the surface of ERP genetic background, and therefore, genetic testing has currently a marginal role in the clinical management of ERP/ERS.

Clinical management and risk stratification

Many studies in the last decade have contributed to an understanding of the pathophysiology, the electrocardiographic definition, and the clinical manifestation of ERP. Still, there is a remarkable knowledge gap in the definition of a clear set of indications for the clinical management.[27] Even in the most recent experts' consensus document,[2] the only class I indication for ICD is for secondary prevention in ERP patients with a previous cardiac arrest. In these subjects, the use of quinidine could also have been considered to prevent recurrent ICD shocks. The use of ICD is also suggested (class IIb) for asymptomatic subjects with "strong" family history of SCD and "high-risk" ERP pattern. As mentioned earlier, the ECG features associated with higher risk of events are as follows: (1) the notching QRS morphology (as compared with the slurring morphology)[98]; (2) J-point elevation of more than 0.2 mV in the inferior leads[85]; (3) downsloping of ST segment.[85] However, there are still no data to quantify positive and negative predictive value, the number needed to treat, and the cost-effectiveness of ICD implantation for primary prevention of SCD in high-risk ERP patients. Thus, the clinical management remains ill defined, and the current recommendations are inadequately supported by the clinical evidence.

Early repolarization syndrome take-home messages and clinical implication

The key concepts emerging from the large body of clinical studies on ERP are as follows:

- ERP is frequently observed in young male subjects;
- Slurred or notched QRS in the inferior is more frequently present in patients with idiopathic VF than in controls;
- In the general population, ERP is associated with a detectable risk of SCD occurring in the structural normal heart, but most subjects with ERP appear to have a favorable outcome;
- When associated with one or more additional clinical features (history of arrhythmic events, short coupled PVCs, family history of SCD, family members with ERP pattern, a definitely pathogenic mutation), it is possible to define the presence of an ERS.
- The presence of ERP might be a risk factor for arrhythmic events in patients with coronary artery disease, LQTS, BrS, catecholaminergic polymorphic VT;
- ERP is a heritable trait, but only in a minority of cases can a Mendelian inheritance or single-gene mutations be detected;
- The indications for the use of ICD remain restricted to patients who already had an aborted cardiac death (those who have a class I indication independently from the

underlying disease); on the contrary, there are no robust guidelines for primary prevention of cardiac events in subjects with ERP.

Thus, although in some cases the detection of ERP is the only apparent cause of ventricular fibrillation or SCD in a family, the relatively high frequency of this ECG marker in the general population (with consequent low attributable risk) and the complex heritability support the idea that ERP is more often a disease-modifying factor and not a standalone disease. This view is supported by increasing clinical evidence. With the few exceptions of rare overt familial presentation of a malignant ERP phenotype, the current knowledge does not justify the systematic use of ICD for primary prevention. Future studies should aim at better delineating the role of ERP as a risk marker for arrhythmic cardiac events in cardiac disease.

REFERENCES

1. Osborn JJ. Experimental hypothermia; respiratory and blood pH changes in relation to cardiac function. Am J Physiol 1953;175(3):389–98.
2. Antzelevitch C, Yan GX, Ackerman MJ, et al. J-wave syndromes expert consensus conference report: emerging concepts and gaps in knowledge. Europace 2017;19(4):665–94.
3. Mazzanti A, Underwood K, Nevelev D, et al. The new kids on the block of arrhythmogenic disorders: short QT syndrome and early repolarization. J Cardiovasc Electrophysiol 2017;28(10):1226–36.
4. Antzelevitch C, Brugada P, Borggrefe M, et al. Brugada syndrome. Report of the second consensus conference. Endorsed by the Heart Rhythm Society and the European Heart Rhythm Association. Circulation 2005;111:659–70.
5. Priori SG, Napolitano C. Should patients with an asymptomatic Brugada electrocardiogram undergo pharmacological and electrophysiological testing? Circulation 2005;112(2):279–92.
6. Napolitano C, Bloise R, Monteforte N, et al. Sudden cardiac death and genetic ion channelopathies: long QT, Brugada, short QT, catecholaminergic polymorphic ventricular tachycardia, and idiopathic ventricular fibrillation. Circulation 2012;125(16):2027–34.
7. Litovsky SH, Antzelevitch C. Transient outward current prominent in canine ventricular epicardium but not endocardium. Circ Res 1988;62(1):116–26.
8. Yan GX, Antzelevitch C. Cellular basis for the electrocardiographic J wave. Circulation 1996;93(2):372–9.
9. Meijborg VM, Potse M, Conrath CE, et al. Reduced sodium current in the lateral ventricular wall induces inferolateral J-waves. Front Physiol 2016;7:365.
10. Medeiros-Domingo A, Tan BH, Crotti L, et al. Gain-of-function mutation S422L in the KCNJ8-encoded cardiac K(ATP) channel Kir6.1 as a pathogenic substrate for J-wave syndromes. Heart Rhythm 2010;7:1466–71.
11. Antzelevitch C, Yan GX. J wave syndromes. Heart Rhythm 2010;7(4):549–58.
12. Wilde AA, Postema PG, Di Diego JM, et al. The pathophysiological mechanism underlying Brugada syndrome: depolarization versus repolarization. J Mol Cell Cardiol 2010;49(4):543–53.
13. Zhang J, Sacher F, Hoffmayer K, et al. Cardiac electrophysiologic substrate underlying the ECG phenotype and electrogram abnormalities in Brugada syndrome patients. Circulation 2015;131:1950–9.
14. Abe A, Ikeda T, Tsukada T, et al. Circadian variation of late potentials in idiopathic ventricular fibrillation associated with J waves: insights into alternative pathophysiology and risk stratification. Heart Rhythm 2010;7(5):675–82.
15. Latcu DG, Bun SS, Zarqane N, et al. Ablation of left ventricular substrate in early repolarization syndrome. J Cardiovasc Electrophysiol 2016;27(4):490–1.
16. Koncz I, Gurabi Z, Patocskai B, et al. Mechanisms underlying the development of the electrocardiographic and arrhythmic manifestations of early repolarization syndrome. J Mol Cell Cardiol 2014;68:20–8.
17. Yan GX, Antzelevitch C. Cellular basis for the Brugada syndrome and other mechanisms of arrhythmogenesis associated with ST-segment elevation. Circulation 1999;100(15):1660–6.
18. Kimura M, Kobayashi T, Owada S, et al. Mechanism of ST elevation and ventricular arrhythmias in an experimental Brugada syndrome model. Circulation 2004;109(1):125–31.
19. Di Diego JM, Antzelevitch C. Pinacidil-induced electrical heterogeneity and extrasystolic activity in canine ventricular tissues. Does activation of ATP-regulated potassium current promote phase 2 reentry? Circulation 1993;88(3):1177–89.
20. Bloch Thomsen PE, Joergensen RM, Kanters JK, et al. Phase 2 reentry in man. Heart Rhythm 2005;2(8):797–803.
21. Miyazaki T, Mitamura H, Miyoshi S, et al. Autonomic and antiarrhythmic drug modulation of ST segment elevation in patients with Brugada syndrome. J Am Coll Cardiol 1996;27(5):1061–70.
22. Makimoto H, Nakagawa E, Takaki H, et al. Augmented ST-segment elevation during recovery from exercise predicts cardiac events in patients with Brugada syndrome. J Am Coll Cardiol 2010;56(19):1576–84.
23. Kasanuki H, Ohnishi S, Ohtuka M, et al. Idiopathic ventricular fibrillation induced with vagal activity in

patients without obvious heart disease. Circulation 1997;95(9):2277–85.

24. Mizumaki K, Nishida K, Iwamoto J, et al. Vagal activity modulates spontaneous augmentation of J-wave elevation in patients with idiopathic ventricular fibrillation. Heart Rhythm 2012;9(2):249–55.

25. Shinohara T, Kondo H, Otsubo T, et al. Exaggerated reactivity of parasympathetic nerves is involved in ventricular fibrillation in J-wave syndrome. J Cardiovasc Electrophysiol 2017;28(3):321–6.

26. Patocskai B, Barajas-Martinez H, Hu D, et al. Cellular and ionic mechanisms underlying the effects of cilostazol, milrinone, and isoproterenol to suppress arrhythmogenesis in an experimental model of early repolarization syndrome. Heart Rhythm 2016;13(6):1326–34.

27. Priori SG, Blomstrom-Lundqvist C, Mazzanti A, et al. 2015 ESC guidelines for the management of patients with ventricular arrhythmias and the prevention of sudden cardiac death: the task force for the management of patients with ventricular arrhythmias and the prevention of sudden cardiac death of the European Society of Cardiology (ESC). Endorsed by: Association for European Paediatric and Congenital Cardiology (AEPC). Eur Heart J 2015; 36(41):2793–867.

28. Brugada P, Brugada J. Right bundle branch block, persistent ST segment elevation and sudden cardiac death: a distinct clinical and electrocardiographic syndrome. A multicenter report. J Am Coll Cardiol 1992;20(6):1391–6.

29. Priori SG, Wilde AA, Horie M, et al. HRS/EHRA/APHRS expert consensus statement on the diagnosis and management of patients with inherited primary arrhythmia syndromes: document endorsed by HRS, EHRA, and APHRS in May 2013 and by ACCF, AHA, PACES, and AEPC in June 2013. Heart Rhythm 2013;10(12):1932–63.

30. Antzelevitch C, Yan GX. J-wave syndromes: Brugada and early repolarization syndromes. Heart Rhythm 2015;12(8):1852–66.

31. Ten Sande JN, Coronel R, Conrath CE, et al. ST-segment elevation and fractionated electrograms in Brugada syndrome patients arise from the same structurally abnormal subepicardial RVOT area but have a different mechanism. Circ Arrhythm Electrophysiol 2015;8(6):1382–92.

32. Veltmann C, Papavassiliu T, Konrad T, et al. Insights into the location of type I ECG in patients with Brugada syndrome: correlation of ECG and cardiovascular magnetic resonance imaging. Heart Rhythm 2012;9(3):414–21.

33. Nademanee K, Veerakul G, Chandanamattha P, et al. Prevention of ventricular fibrillation episodes in Brugada syndrome by catheter ablation over the anterior right ventricular outflow tract epicardium. Circulation 2011;123(12):1270–9.

34. Morita H, Zipes DP, Fukushima-Kusano K, et al. Repolarization heterogeneity in the right ventricular outflow tract: correlation with ventricular arrhythmias in Brugada patients and in an in vitro canine Brugada model. Heart Rhythm 2008;5(5):725–33.

35. Lambiase PD, Ahmed AK, Ciaccio EJ, et al. High-density substrate mapping in Brugada syndrome: combined role of conduction and repolarization heterogeneities in arrhythmogenesis. Circulation 2009; 120(2):106–17, 101–4.

36. Sunsaneewitayakul B, Yao Y, Thamaree S, et al. Endocardial mapping and catheter ablation for ventricular fibrillation prevention in Brugada syndrome. J Cardiovasc Electrophysiol 2012;23(Suppl 1): S10–6.

37. Pappone C, Brugada J, Vicedomini G, et al. Electrical substrate elimination in 135 consecutive patients with brugada syndrome. Circ Arrhythm Electrophysiol 2017;10:e005053.

38. Priori SG, Napolitano C. Sudden cardiac death syndromes in structurally normal hearts. ACCSAP version 9: adult clinical cardiology self-assessment program. Washington, DC: American College of Cardiology Foundation; 2016.

39. Priori SG, Napolitano C. Genetics of channelopathies and clinical implications. In: Fuster V, Harrington RA, Narula J, et al, editors. Hurst' the heart. 14th edition. New York: McGraw-Hill; 2017. p. 1910–23.

40. Priori SG, Gasparini M, Napolitano C, et al. Risk stratification in Brugada syndrome: results of the PRELUDE (PRogrammed ELectrical stimUlation preDictive valuE) registry. J Am Coll Cardiol 2012;59(1): 37–45.

41. Curcio A, Mazzanti A, Bloise R, et al. Clinical presentation and outcome of Brugada syndrome diagnosed with the new 2013 criteria. J Cardiovasc Electrophysiol 2016;27:937–43.

42. de Asmundis C, Mugnai G, Chierchia GB, et al. Long-term follow-up of probands with Brugada syndrome. Am J Cardiol 2017;119(9):1392–400.

43. Brugada J, Brugada R, Antzelevitch C, et al. Long-term follow-up of individuals with the electrocardiographic pattern of right bundle-branch block and ST-segment elevation in precordial leads V1 to V3. Circulation 2002;105(1):73–8.

44. Brugada P, Geelen P, Brugada R, et al. Prognostic value of electrophysiologic investigations in Brugada syndrome. J Cardiovasc Electrophysiol 2001; 12(9):1004–7.

45. Brugada J, Brugada P. Further characterization of the syndrome of right bundle branch block, ST segment elevation, and sudden cardiac death. J Cardiovasc Electrophysiol 1997;8(3):325–31.

46. Chen Q, Kirsch GE, Zhang D, et al. Genetic basis and molecular mechanism for idiopathic ventricular fibrillation. Nature 1998;392:293–6.

47. Mademont-Soler I, Pinsach-Abuin ML, Riuro H, et al. Large genomic imbalances in Brugada syndrome. PLoS One 2016;11:e0163514.

48. Li A, Saba MM, Behr ER. Genetic biomarkers in Brugada syndrome. Biomark Med 2013;7(4):535–46.

49. Holst AG, Saber S, Houshmand M, et al. Sodium current and potassium transient outward current genes in Brugada syndrome: screening and bioinformatics. Can J Cardiol 2012;28(2):196–200.

50. Marangoni S, Di Resta C, Rocchetti M, et al. A Brugada syndrome mutation (p.S216L) and its modulation by p.H558R polymorphism: standard and dynamic characterization. Cardiovasc Res 2011;91(4):606–16.

51. Tan BH, Valdivia CR, Song C, et al. Partial expression defect for the SCN5A missense mutation G1406R depends on splice variant background Q1077 and rescue by mexiletine. Am J Physiol Heart Circ Physiol 2006;291(4):H1822–8.

52. Bezzina CR, Barc J, Mizusawa Y, et al. Common variants at SCN5A-SCN10A and HEY2 are associated with Brugada syndrome, a rare disease with high risk of sudden cardiac death. Nat Genet 2013; 45(9):1044–9.

53. Priori SG, Napolitano C, Gasparini M, et al. Natural history of Brugada syndrome: insights for risk stratification and management. Circulation 2002;105(11):1342–7.

54. Mazzanti A, Maragna R, Priori SG. Genetic causes of sudden cardiac death in the young. Curr Opin Cardiol 2017;32:253–61.

55. Sroubek J, Probst V, Mazzanti A, et al. Programmed ventricular stimulation for risk stratification in the Brugada syndrome: a pooled analysis. Circulation 2016;133(7):622–30.

56. Morita H, Kusano KF, Miura D, et al. Fragmented QRS as a marker of conduction abnormality and a predictor of prognosis of Brugada syndrome. Circulation 2008;118(17):1697–704.

57. Sieira J, Conte G, Ciconte G, et al. A score model to predict risk of events in patients with Brugada syndrome. Eur Heart J 2017;38(22):1756–63.

58. Wu W, Tian L, Ke J, et al. Risk factors for cardiac events in patients with Brugada syndrome: a PRISMA-compliant meta-analysis and systematic review. Medicine (Baltimore) 2016;95(30):e4214.

59. Nakano M, Fukuda K, Kondo M, et al. Prognostic significance of late potentials in outpatients with type 2 Brugada electrocardiogram. Tohoku J Exp Med 2016;240(3):191–8.

60. Kawazoe H, Nakano Y, Ochi H, et al. Risk stratification of ventricular fibrillation in Brugada syndrome using noninvasive scoring methods. Heart Rhythm 2016;13(10):1947–54.

61. Sakamoto S, Takagi M, Kakihara J, et al. The utility of T-wave alternans during the morning in the summer for the risk stratification of patients with Brugada syndrome. Heart Vessels 2017;32(3):341–51.

62. Gray B, Kirby A, Kabunga P, et al. Twelve-lead ambulatory electrocardiographic monitoring in Brugada syndrome: potential diagnostic and prognostic implications. Heart Rhythm 2017;14(6):866–74.

63. Calvo M, Gomis P, Romero D, et al. Heart rate complexity analysis in Brugada syndrome during physical stress testing. Physiol Meas 2017;38(2): 387–96.

64. Behar N, Petit B, Probst V, et al. Heart rate variability and repolarization characteristics in symptomatic and asymptomatic Brugada syndrome. Europace 2017;19:1730–6.

65. Mazzanti A, Priori SG. Brugada syndrome: the endless conundrum. J Am Coll Cardiol 2016;68(6): 624–5.

66. Belhassen B, Rahkovich M, Michowitz Y, et al. Management of Brugada syndrome: thirty-three-year experience using electrophysiologically guided therapy with class 1A antiarrhythmic drugs. Circ Arrhythm Electrophysiol 2015;8(6):1393–402.

67. Anguera I, Garcia-Alberola A, Dallaglio P, et al. Shock reduction with long-term quinidine in patients with Brugada syndrome and malignant ventricular arrhythmia episodes. J Am Coll Cardiol 2016; 67(13):1653–4.

68. Wasserburger RH, Alt WJ. The normal RS-T segment elevation variant. Am J Cardiol 1961;8:184–92.

69. Shipley AM. Suppurative pericarditis: late results and methods of drainage. Ann Surg 1936;103(5): 698–705.

70. Rautaharju PM, Surawicz B, Gettes LS, et al. AHA/ ACCF/HRS recommendations for the standardization and interpretation of the electrocardiogram: part IV: the ST segment, T and U waves, and the QT interval: a scientific statement from the American Heart Association Electrocardiography and Arrhythmias Committee, Council on Clinical Cardiology; the American College of Cardiology Foundation; and the Heart Rhythm Society. Endorsed by the International Society for Computerized Electrocardiology. J Am Coll Cardiol 2009;53(11):982–91.

71. Macfarlane PW, Antzelevitch C, Haissaguerre M, et al. The early repolarization pattern: a consensus paper. J Am Coll Cardiol 2015;66(4):470–7.

72. Patton KK, Ellinor PT, Ezekowitz M, et al. Electrocardiographic early repolarization: a scientific statement from the American Heart Association. Circulation 2016;133(15):1520–9.

73. Goldman MJ. RS-T segment elevation in mid- and left precordial leads as a normal variant. Am Heart J 1953;46(6):817–20.

74. Klatsky AL, Oehm R, Cooper RA, et al. The early repolarization normal variant electrocardiogram: correlates and consequences. Am J Med 2003;115(3): 171–7.

75. Tikkanen JT, Anttonen O, Junttila MJ, et al. Long-term outcome associated with early repolarization

on electrocardiography. N Engl J Med 2009;361(26): 2529–37.

76. Ezaki K, Nakagawa M, Taniguchi Y, et al. Gender differences in the ST segment: effect of androgen-deprivation therapy and possible role of testosterone. Circ J 2010;74(11):2448–54.

77. Haïssaguerre M, Derval N, Sacher F, et al. Sudden cardiac arrest associated with early repolarization. N Engl J Med 2008;358(19):2016–23.

78. Nam GB, Kim YH, Antzelevitch C. Augmentation of J waves and electrical storms in patients with early repolarization. N Engl J Med 2008;358(19):2078–9.

79. Rosso R, Kogan E, Belhassen B, et al. J-point elevation in survivors of primary ventricular fibrillation and matched control subjects: incidence and clinical significance. J Am Coll Cardiol 2008;52(15):1231–8.

80. Krahn AD, Healey JS, Chauhan V, et al. Systematic assessment of patients with unexplained cardiac arrest: cardiac arrest survivors with preserved ejection fraction registry (CASPER). Circulation 2009;120(4): 278–85.

81. Siebermair J, Sinner MF, Beckmann BM, et al. Early repolarization pattern is the strongest predictor of arrhythmia recurrence in patients with idiopathic ventricular fibrillation: results from a single centre long-term follow-up over 20 years. Europace 2016; 18(5):718–25.

82. Sinner MF, Reinhard W, Muller M, et al. Association of early repolarization pattern on ECG with risk of cardiac and all-cause mortality: a population-based prospective cohort study (MONICA/KORA). PLoS Med 2010;7(7):e1000314.

83. Tikkanen JT, Junttila MJ, Anttonen O, et al. Early repolarization: electrocardiographic phenotypes associated with favorable long-term outcome. Circulation 2011;123(23):2666–73.

84. Olson KA, Viera AJ, Soliman EZ, et al. Long-term prognosis associated with J-point elevation in a large middle-aged biracial cohort: the ARIC study. Eur Heart J 2011;32(24):3098–106.

85. Cheng YJ, Lin XX, Ji CC, et al. Role of early repolarization pattern in increasing risk of death. J Am Heart Assoc 2016;5 [pii:e003375].

86. Naruse Y, Tada H, Harimura Y, et al. Early repolarization is an independent predictor of occurrences of ventricular fibrillation in the very early phase of acute myocardial infarction. Circ Arrhythm Electrophysiol 2012;5(3):506–13.

87. Rudic B, Veltmann C, Kuntz E, et al. Early repolarization pattern is associated with ventricular fibrillation in patients with acute myocardial infarction. Heart Rhythm 2012;9(8):1295–300.

88. Tikkanen JT, Wichmann V, Junttila MJ, et al. Association of early repolarization and sudden cardiac death during an acute coronary event. Circ Arrhythm Electrophysiol 2012;5(4):714–8.

89. Cheng YJ, Li ZY, Yao FJ, et al. Early repolarization is associated with a significantly increased risk of ventricular arrhythmias and sudden cardiac death in patients with structural heart diseases. Heart Rhythm 2017;14(8):1157–64.

90. Laksman ZW, Gula LJ, Saklani P, et al. Early repolarization is associated with symptoms in patients with type 1 and type 2 long QT syndrome. Heart Rhythm 2014;11(9):1632–8.

91. Tülümen E, Schulze-Bahr E, Zumhagen S, et al. Early repolarization pattern: a marker of increased risk in patients with catecholaminergic polymorphic ventricular tachycardia. Europace 2016;18(10): 1587–92.

92. Georgopoulos S, Letsas KP, Liu T, et al. A meta-analysis on the prognostic significance of inferolateral early repolarization pattern in Brugada syndrome. Europace 2018;20:134–9.

93. Watanabe H, Makiyama T, Koyama T, et al. High prevalence of early repolarization in short QT syndrome. Heart Rhythm 2010;7(5):647–52.

94. Reinhard W, Kaess BM, Debiec R, et al. Heritability of early repolarization: a population-based study. Circ Cardiovasc Genet 2011;4(2):134–8.

95. Noseworthy PA, Tikkanen JT, Porthan K, et al. The early repolarization pattern in the general population: clinical correlates and heritability. J Am Coll Cardiol 2011;57(22):2284–9.

96. Gourraud JB, Le Scouarnec S, Sacher F, et al. Identification of large families in early repolarization syndrome. J Am Coll Cardiol 2013;61(2): 164–72.

97. Ajijola OA, Sun AY. The genetics of the J wave patterns. J Electrocardiol 2013;46(5):395–8.

98. Zhang Z, Letsas KP, Yang Y, et al. Notching early repolarization pattern in inferior leads increases risk of ventricular tachyarrhythmias in patients with acute myocardial infarction: a meta-analysis. Sci Rep 2015;5:15845.

Syncope
Electrocardiographic and Clinical Correlation

Andrea Ungar, MD, PhD, FESC*, Martina Rafanelli, MD

KEYWORDS

- Syncope • Electrocardiogram • Arrhythmias

KEY POINTS

- Syncope is a frequent condition, owing to a transient global cerebral hypoperfusion, that may depend on a reduction of vascular total peripheral resistance and/or cardiac output.
- Cardiac syncope doubled the risk of death from any cause and increased the risk of nonfatal and fatal cardiovascular events.
- Arrhythmias are the most common cardiac causes of syncope. Both bradyarrhythmias and tachyarrhythmias may predispose to syncope.
- The first line evaluation relies on clinical history, physical examination, active standing test, 12-lead echocardiogram.
- The diagnostic yield of electrophysiological study in detecting the cause of syncope depends highly on the pretest probability.

EPIDEMIOLOGY

Syncope is a transient loss of consciousness owing to a transient global cerebral hypoperfusion and is characterized by a rapid onset, a short duration, and a spontaneous and complete recovery.[1] This condition is extremely common in the general population.[2] In the latest report of the Framingham Offspring study, 10% of the 7814 participants (mean age, 51 years; range, 20–96 years) reported at least 1 syncope. The prevalence of syncope is very high in patients between the age of 10 and 30 years, uncommon in adults with an average age of 40 years, and peaks again above the age of 65 years.[3]

CLASSIFICATION AND PATHOPHYSIOLOGY OF SYNCOPE

Box 1 provides a classification of the principal causes of syncope. The global cerebral hypoperfusion is responsible for an inadequate supply of oxygen and metabolic substrates to the brain[4] and is what differentiates syncope from other transient losses of consciousness without underlying cerebral hypoperfusion, such as epilepsy, hypoglycemia, and episodes of only apparent loss of consciousness, such as falls.[1]

Cerebral autoregulation maintains a constant blood flow within a wide range of pressures (systolic blood pressure between 60 and 190 mm Hg). When the systolic blood pressure decreases below this threshold, brain perfusion decreases slowly and progressively and, if this hemodynamic status lasts for 8 to 15 seconds, ischemia and ultimately loss of consciousness will follow.[5] Therefore, the main mechanism is a decrease in the systemic blood pressure (BP), which may depend on a reduction of vascular total peripheral resistance and/or cardiac output (CO).[1]

Syncope Unit, Geriatrics and Intensive Care Unit, University of Florence, Azienda Ospedaliero Universitaria Careggi, Viale Pieraccini 6, Florence 50139, Italy
* Corresponding author.
E-mail address: aungar@unifi.it

Card Electrophysiol Clin 10 (2018) 371–386
https://doi.org/10.1016/j.ccep.2018.02.007
1877-9182/18/© 2018 Elsevier Inc. All rights reserved.

Box 1
Classification of syncope

Reflex (neurally mediated) syncope

Vasovagal

  Orthostatic vasovagal: standing, or less common sitting

  Emotional: fear, pain, instrumentation, blood phobia

  Pain triggers: peripheral or visceral

Situational

  Micturition

  Gastrointestinal stimulation (swallow, defecation)

  Cough, sneeze

  Others (eg, laughing, brass instrument playing, weight lifting, after exercise)

Carotid sinus syncope

Syncope owing to orthostatic hypotension

Drug-induced orthostatic hypotension (eg, vasodilators, diuretics, phenothiazine, antidepressants)

Volume depletion (eg, hemorrhage, diarrhea, vomiting)

Primary autonomic failure (pure autonomic failure, multiple system atrophy, Parkinson's disease, dementia with Lewy bodies)

Secondary autonomic failure (diabetes, amyloidosis, spinal cord injuries, autoimmune autonomic neuropathy, paraneoplastic autonomic neuropathy, kidney failure)

Cardiac syncope

Arrhythmia as primary cause

  Bradycardia

  • Sinus node dysfunction (including bradycardia/tachycardia syndrome)

  • Atrioventricular conduction system disease

  • Implanted device malfunction

  Tachycardia

  • Supraventricular

  • Ventricular (idiopathic, secondary to structural heart disease or to channelopathies)

Structural disease

  Cardiac: Cardiac valvular disease, acute myocardial infarction/ischemia, hypertrophic cardiomyopathy, cardiac masses (atrial myxoma, tumors, etc)

  Pericardial disease/tamponade, congenital anomalies of coronary arteries, prosthetic valves dysfunction

Cardiopulmonary and great vessels

Pulmonary embolus, acute aortic dissection, pulmonary hypertension

Adapted from Moya A, Sutton R, Ammirati F, et al. Guidelines for the diagnosis and management of syncope (version 2009): the task force for the diagnosis and management of syncope of the European Society of Cardiology (ESC). Eur Heart J 2009;30:2636; with permission.

Vascular total peripheral resistance may be decreased by an inappropriate reflex activity causing vasodilatation through withdrawal of sympathetic vasoconstriction (vasodepressor reflex syncope) or by functional and structural impairment of the autonomic nervous system.[1] A decrease in CO may be caused by reflex bradycardia (cardioinhibitory reflex syncope), cardiovascular causes (arrhythmia, structural disease including pulmonary embolism and pulmonary hypertension), inadequate

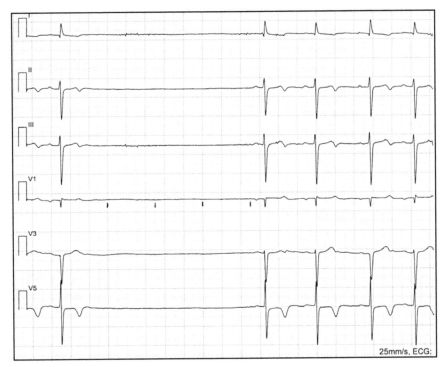

Fig. 1. Sinus arrest.

venous return owing to volume depletion or venous pooling, and chronotropic and inotropic incompetence through autonomic failure.[1] An interaction between different mechanisms is also possible; thus, a low total peripheral resistance may cause venous pooling of blood in the abdomen and lower limbs, in turn decreasing venous return and consequently CO.[1]

There is emerging evidence that low adenosine levels may be related to a sudden-onset syncope, without prodromes in patients with normal heart and normal electrocardiogram (ECG),[6] who frequently experience a long asystolic pause owing to paroxysmal atrioventricular (AV) block or sinus arrest.[7]

The prevalence of the causes of syncope differs depending on the age: reflex syncope is the most frequent cause at all ages,[2] cardiac syncope is the second most common cause,[8] and orthostatic hypotension is a frequent cause of syncope in very old patients. In the elderly, multiple causes are often present.[9]

CARDIAC SYNCOPE

Cardiac causes of syncope are highly represented in the older population.[10] In the Framingham study, cardiac syncope doubled the risk of death from any cause and increased the risk of nonfatal and fatal cardiovascular events, compared with those without syncope.[3]

Short-lived syncope of abrupt onset and recovery, supine, during (rather than after) exercise, or associated with palpitations or chest pain should be considered cardiac until proven otherwise. A history of heart disease is an independent predictor of cardiac syncope with a sensitivity of 95% and specificity of 45%.[11]

Cardiac syncope must be excluded in patients with known or suspected left ventricular systolic dysfunction, valvular disease, left ventricular outflow tract obstruction, in those with an abnormal surface ECG, and where the clinical context and concomitant investigations suggest pulmonary embolism. Neurally mediated cause

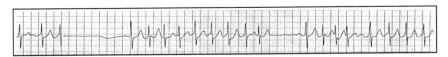

Fig. 2. Brady-tachy syndrome.

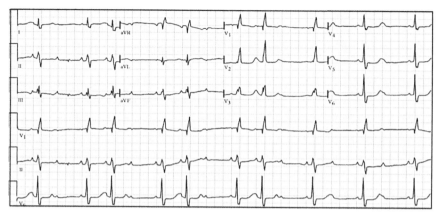

Fig. 3. Type II atrioventricular block.

of symptoms must not be assumed in any patient with these clinical and diagnostic features until a cardiac cause has been effectively excluded.

The Evaluation of Guidelines in Syncope Study score is a diagnostic score to identify cardiac syncope. Abnormal ECG and/or heart disease, palpitations before syncope, syncope during effort or in a supine position, absence of autonomic prodromes, and absence of predisposing and/or precipitating factors were found to be predictors of cardiac syncope. To each variable, a score from +4 to −1 was assigned according to the magnitude of regression coefficient. A score of greater than 3 identified cardiac syncope with a sensitivity of 95%/92% and a specificity of 61%/69%.[12]

Recently, the Canadian Syncope Arrhythmia Risk Score was developed to predict the 30-day risk of arrhythmia or death after emergency department (ED) disposition among patients presenting with syncope. Abnormal ECG (QRS duration >130 ms and QTc interval >480 ms), heart disease, and an absence of precipitating factors were associated with arrhythmia or death. A score of 0 or less was associated with less than a 1% risk, scores of 1 to 3 were associated with a 1.9% to 7.5% risk, and scores of 4 to 8 were associated with a 14.3% to 22.2% risk of arrhythmia or death within 30 days of ED disposition.[13] Nonetheless, these and others risk stratification tools perform no better than clinician judgment at predicting short-term serious outcome.[14]

Arrhythmic Syncope

Arrhythmias are the most common cardiac causes of syncope. Guidelines[1] and clinical scoring systems[12,15,16] for identifying high-risk patients

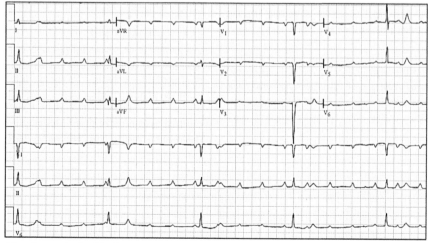

Fig. 4. Type III atrioventricular block.

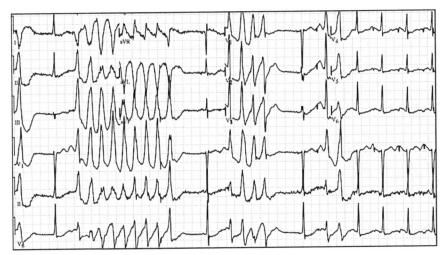

Fig. 5. Torsades de pointes.

include arrhythmias as a predictor of death and adverse events.

Brain hypoperfusion and syncope depend on a critical decrease in CO and contributory factors, such as the type of arrhythmia, the ventricular rate, the left ventricular function, the body position, and the adequacy of vascular compensation, which includes baroreceptor-mediated reflexes induced by a sudden hypotension.[17,18]

Both bradyarrhythmias and tachyarrhythmias may predispose to syncope.

The sick sinus syndrome is characterized by sinoatrial node dysfunction, either because of abnormal automaticity or sinoatrial conduction abnormalities. In this condition, syncope depends on long pauses owing to sinus arrest or sinoatrial block and a failure of escape mechanism and may also be reflex in origin (**Fig. 1**). These pauses are most frequently encountered when an atrial tachyarrhythmia suddenly stops (brady-tachy syndrome; **Fig. 2**).[17]

In case of severe forms of acquired AV block (Mobitz II block, 'high-grade,' and complete AV block), the cardiac rhythm may become dependent on subsidiary or escape pacemaker sites (**Figs. 3** and **4**). Syncope, which is closely related to these conditions, occurs because the delay before these pacemakers begin to 'fire' is long. Moreover, these subsidiary pacemaker sites typically have relatively slow rates (25–40 bpm).

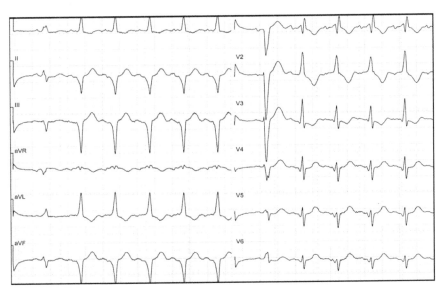

Fig. 6. Alternating left and right bundle branch block.

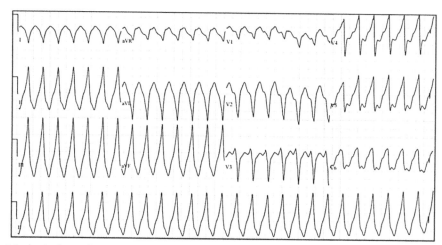

Fig. 7. Ventricular tachycardia.

Bradycardia also prolongs repolarization and predisposes to polymorphic ventricular tachycardia (VT), especially of the torsade de pointes type (**Fig. 5**).[1]

A sudden onset of paroxysmal tachycardia, both supraventricular or ventricular, may predispose to syncope or presyncope before vascular compensation development.[17,19] Unconsciousness may persist when the ventricular rate is high or ventricular activity is ineffective. Given that the recovery is not spontaneous, by definition the event is not a syncope, but a cardiac arrest.[1]

VT may be idiopathic, or secondary to structural heart disease or to channelopathies. In congenital long QT syndromes (LQTS), arrhythmias often follow a sudden adrenergic increase owing to exercise, arousal, and sudden auditory stimuli or an abrupt fright.[1] Brugada syndrome (BS) is a malignant arrhythmia syndrome manifesting as recurrent syncope or sudden cardiac death (SCD) owing to polymorphic VT or ventricular fibrillation (VF) in the absence of overt structural heart disease or myocardial ischemia.[18]

DIAGNOSTIC EVALUATION

The diagnostic protocol proposed by the European Society of Cardiology guidelines on syncope[1] is well enforceable at any age and, when applied, the rate of unexplained syncope decreases to 10.4%.[9] The first-line evaluation relies on clinical history, physical examination, active standing test, and 12-lead ECG.[1] The 12-lead ECG can be considered diagnostic, permits no further evaluation and institution of treatment, in cases of:

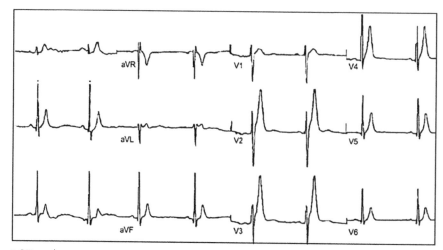

Fig. 8. Short QT syndrome.

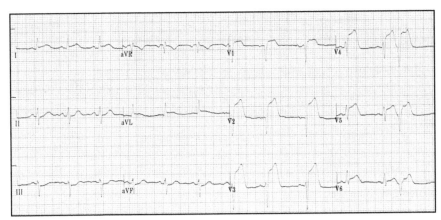

Fig. 9. ST segment elevation myocardial infarction.

- Persistent sinus bradycardia less than 40 bpm in awake or repetitive sinoatrial block or sinus pauses of greater than 3 s (see **Fig. 1**);
- Mobitz II second or third-degree AV block (see **Figs. 3** and **4**), alternating left and right bundle branch block (**Fig. 6**);

- VT (**Fig. 7**) or rapid paroxysmal supraventricular tachycardia (see **Fig. 2**);
- Nonsustained episodes of polymorphic VT (see **Fig. 5**) and long or short QT interval (**Fig. 8**); and
- Acute ischemia with or without myocardial infarction[1] (**Fig. 9**).

Box 2
Clinical features suggesting a diagnosis of cardiac syncope on initial evaluation

- During exertion or supine
- Presence of structural heart disease
  - Family history of unexplained sudden death at young age
  - Abnormal ECG
- Sudden-onset palpitation immediately followed by syncope
- ECG findings suggesting arrhythmic syncope:
  - Bifascicular block (defined as either LBBB or RBBB combined with left anterior or left posterior fascicular block)
  - Other intraventricular conduction abnormalities (QRS duration ≥0.12 s)
  - Mobitz II block, "high-grade" and complete AV block
  - Asymptomatic inappropriate sinus bradycardia (<50 bpm), sinoatrial block or sinus pause ≥3 s in the absence of negatively chronotropic medications
  - Nonsustained VT
  - Preexcited QRS complexes (see **Fig. 10**)
  - Long or short QT intervals
  - Early repolarization
  - RBBB pattern with ST elevation in leads V1-V3 (Brugada syndrome)
  - Negative T waves in right precordial leads, epsilon waves and ventricular late potentials suggestive of ARVC (see **Fig. 11**)
  - Q waves suggesting myocardial infarction.

Abbreviations: ARVC, arrhythmogenic right ventricular cardiomyopathy; AV, atrioventricular; ECG, electrocardiograph; LBBB, left bundle branch block; RBBB, right bundle branch block; VT, ventricular tachycardia.
  Data from Moya A, Sutton R, Ammirati F, et al. Guidelines for the diagnosis and management of syncope (version 2009): the task force for the diagnosis and management of syncope of the European Society of Cardiology (ESC). Eur Heart J 2009;30:2631–71.

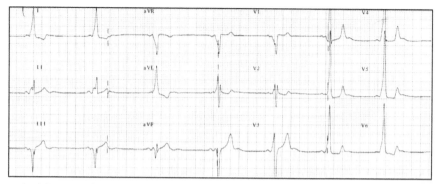

Fig. 10. Preexcited QRS complexes.

The initial evaluation may suggest a diagnosis of cardiac syncope, in case of specific clinical features (**Box 2**, **Figs. 10** and **11**).

When the cause of syncope remains uncertain after the initial evaluation, the next step is to assess the risk of major cardiovascular events or SCD.[1] Low-risk patients do not require further evaluation and can be discharged from the ED, whereas moderate-risk patients should undergo clinical and instrumental monitoring in observation units, inside the ED. High-risk patients should be monitored and treated properly in case of worsening.[20]

The evaluation of reflex, orthostatic, and structural cardiac syncope are not discussed in the present article.

Electrocardiographic Monitoring

ECG monitoring is aimed at diagnosing intermittent bradyarrhythmias and tachyarrhythmias, and is indicated when there is a high pretest probability of identifying an arrhythmia associated with syncope.[1]

Different systems of ECG ambulatory monitoring are available:

- In-hospital monitoring is indicated when the patient is at high risk of a life-threatening arrhythmia and, although the diagnostic yield varies from 1.9% to 16%, it is justified by the need to avoid immediate risk to the patient.[21,22]
- Holter ECG monitoring in syncope is of more value if the symptoms are very frequent, because daily episodes might increase the potential for a correlation between symptoms and ECG. However, in most patients, symptoms do not relapse during the monitoring period; therefore, the true yield of Holter ECG in syncope may be as low as 1% to 2%.[23]
- External or implantable loop recorders have a loop memory that continuously records and deletes ECG tracings. When activated by the patient, typically after a symptom has occurred, 5 to 15 minutes of preactivation ECG is stored and can be retrieved for

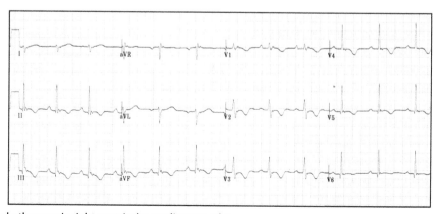

Fig. 11. Arrhythmogenic right ventricular cardiomyopathy.

analysis. External loop recorders can be useful for patients with relatively frequent syncope, when used early after the last episode.[1] A recent multicenter international registry showed a 24.5% diagnostic yield in patients with syncope.[24]

An implantable loop recorder is implanted subcutaneously, and has a battery life of more than 36 months. Last generation devices have a reduced size, with the same memory and battery, allowing a minimally invasive implantation and a daily wireless transmission to a service center with warning reports for predefined events.[25] An implantable loop recorder can be used either at the beginning or at the end of the diagnostic workup of the patients with syncope, because it has showed similar diagnostic yield.[26] Despite a high initial cost, the analysis of the cost per symptom–ECG yield has shown that implantable loop recorders may be more cost-effective than a strategy using conventional investigation.[1] An implantable loop recorder has been used also in patients with bundle branch block in whom paroxysmal AV block is likely despite negative complete electrophysiological evaluation.[27]

The gold standard for the diagnosis of arrhythmic syncope is the correlation between symptoms and ECG recording. The absence of an arrhythmia during a syncopal episode allows exclusion of an arrhythmia as the mechanism of the syncope (**Table 1**).[1]

Electrophysiologic Study

The diagnostic yield of electrophysiologic study (EPS) in detecting the cause of syncope depends greatly on the pretest probability and on the protocol applied, because positive results occur predominantly in patients with structural heart disease. Even if the development of noninvasive methods has decreased the use of EPS in the diagnostic workup of syncope, the test is useful in specific clinical situations.

- In patients with asymptomatic sinus bradycardia or sinoatrial block documented by 12-lead ECG or monitoring, there is a high pretest probability of bradycardia related syncope. An abnormal response is defined as 1.6 or greater or 2 s for sinus node recovery time or 525 ms or greater for a corrected sinus node recovery time.[1] Despite the prognostic value, a prolonged sinus node recovery time is not well-defined, patients with a corrected sinus node recovery time of 800 ms or greater showed an 8 times higher risk of syncope than

Table 1
Classification of electrocardiographic recordings

	Classification	Suggested Mechanism
Type 1, asystole (R-R pause ≥3 s)	Type 1A, sinus arrest: Progressive sinus bradycardia or initial sinus tachycardia followed by progressive sinus bradycardia until sinus arrest.	Probably reflex
	Type 1B, sinus bradycardia plus AV block: Progressive sinus bradycardia followed by AV block (and ventricular pause/s) with concomitant decrease in sinus rate sudden onset AV block (and ventricular pause/s with concomitant decrease in sinus rate)	Probably reflex
	Type 1C, AV block Sudden onset AV block (and ventricular pause/s) with concomitant increase in sinus rate	Probably intrinsic
Type 2, bradycardia	Decrease of heart rate >30% or <40 bpm for >10 s.	Probably reflex
Type 3, No or slight rhythm variations	Variations of heart rate <30% and heart rate >40 bpm.	Uncertain
Type 4, tachycardia: increase of heart rate >30% or >120 bpm	Type 4A, progressive sinus tachycardia	Uncertain
	Type 4B, atrial fibrillation	Cardiac arrhythmia
	Type 4C, supraventricular tachycardia (except sinus)	Cardiac arrhythmia
	Type 4D, ventricular tachycardia	Cardiac arrhythmia

Abbreviation: AV, atrioventricular; P intrinsic, probably intrinsic; P reflex, probably reflex.
Data from Brignole M, Moya A, Menozzi C, et al. Proposed electrocardiographic classification of spontaneous syncope documented by an implantable loop recorder. Europace 2005;7:14–8.

those with a corrected sinus node recovery time of less than this value.[28]

- In patients with bundle branch block, the risk of developing AV block increased from 2% in those without syncope to 17% in patients with syncope during follow-up.[29] EPS measures the His-ventricular interval at baseline, during incremental atrial pacing, and pharmacologic provocation with ajmaline, procainamide, or disopyramide. The more prolonged the His-ventricular interval is (<55 ms normal, ≥70 ms and ≥100 ms), the greater the progression rate to AV block over time.[30] The development of intra- or infra-His block during EPS predicts the development of spontaneous AV block with greater sensitivity.[31] Patients with positive EPS treated with a pacemaker showed a significant decrease in syncopal relapses, compared with untreated ones with negative EPS or to those who received an empiric pacemaker.[32] Nonetheless, about one-third of patients with negative EPS, who underwent implantable loop recorder implantation, developed intermittent or permanent AV block on follow-up.[27] Thus, EPS has a low negative predictive accuracy, and the absence of abnormal findings does not exclude the development of AV block.[1]

- The presence of palpitations before the development of syncope may suggest an SVT or VT, and EPS may be indicated in these patients. In case of previous myocardial infarction and preserved left ventricular ejection fraction, the induction of sustained monomorphic VT is strongly predictive of the cause of syncope,[33] whereas the induction of VF is considered a

Type 1 pattern in leads V1 and V2

Fig. 12. Type patterns 1 and 2.

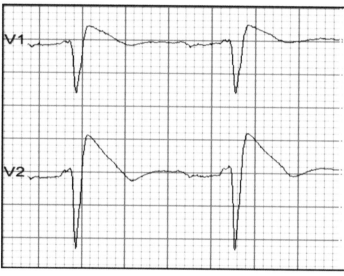

Type 2 pattern in lead V3

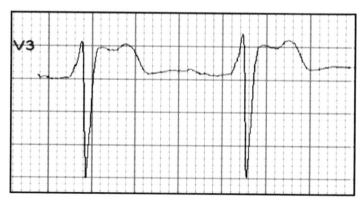

nonspecific finding.[34] The absence of induction of ventricular arrhythmias identifies a group of patients at a lower risk of arrhythmic syncope.[35]

THE BRUGADA SYNDROME

The BS is a genetic disorder with autosomal-dominant inheritance and variable phenotype, related to mutations affecting the sodium, potassium, or calcium ion channels in the cardiac cell membrane, characterized by abnormalities in the ECG (pseudo-right bundle branch block and persistent "coved type" ST-segment elevation in the leads V1–V2 or, rarely, in the inferior leads of ≥2 mm [≥0.2 mV]; **Figs. 12** and **13**) and increased risk of VT and SCD in apparently healthy individuals.

Asymptomatic typical ECG abnormalities, called the "Brugada pattern," were reported in 0.01% to 1.00% of adults.[36] The prevalence of patients with typical ECG features who experienced sustained VT or SCD, or "true BS," among individuals with the Brugada pattern is less well-studied. A metaanalysis of 30 studies revealed a 10% event rate over 2.5 years of follow-up in patients with the Brugada pattern.[37] Indeed, although most patients (64%) are diagnosed incidentally with the Brugada pattern and remain asymptomatic for their lifetime,[38] the BS is reportedly responsible for 4% to 12% of all SCDs and approximately 20% of SCDs in patients with structurally normal hearts.[39] The ECG often may shows dynamic fluctuations between normal,

Fig. 13. Type patterns 2 and 3.

Type 2 pattern lead V2

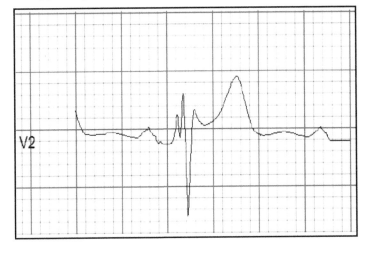

Type 3 pattern lead V1

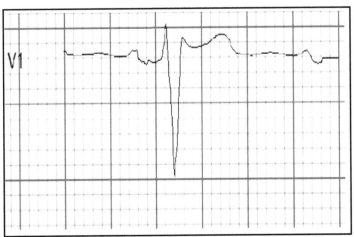

nondiagnostic and diagnostic ST segment patterns, thus hindering the diagnosis.[40]

The first presentation may be SCD. In successfully resuscitated patients, the precipitating arrhythmia is usually a polymorphic VT, or VF, often triggered by a ventricular premature beat. Other symptoms of BS include syncope, nocturnal agonal respiration (presumably caused by self-terminating VT/VF), palpitations, or chest discomfort. Symptoms tend to occur with increased vagal tone, usually at rest, during sleep, and after large meals, triggered by vagotonia-mediated aggravation of the putative electrophysiologic abnormalities.[40]

Fever has been also reported to unmask type 1 ECG and may trigger VT/VF. Fever could accelerate inactivation of the mutant Na^+ channels, or cause other alterations in cardiac electrophysiology, thus temporarily increasing the arrhythmic propensity in BS.[41]

Syncope is common in BS, occurring in 30% of patients. Both arrhythmic and reflex syncope are observed with different prognostic implications. Although arrhythmic syncope is an ominous sign, precipitated by runs of self-terminating VT with increased risk of SCD, reflex syncope with distinct clinical presentation does not impart an adverse prognosis.[37]

The diagnosis of BS requires:

- Documentation of the type 1 ECG (see **Fig. 12**), characterized by the "coved-type" ST segment elevation of 2 mm or more in leads V1 and/or V2, positioned in the second, third, or fourth intercostal space, occurring either spontaneously or after pharmacologic challenge. Superior positioning of the leads V1 and V2 up to the second intercostal space increases the sensitivity for the detection of a type 1 ECG (**Fig. 14**).
- In patients with nondiagnostic type 2 or type 3 ECG (see **Figs. 12** and **13**), the diagnosis can be made only if type 1 ECG is documented either spontaneously or with pharmacologic challenge.

Pharmacologic testing using intravenous class IA (eg, ajmaline, procainamide) or class IC (eg, flecainide, propafenone) antiarrhythmic drugs is indicated in case of strong clinical suspicion of BS in the absence of spontaneous type 1 ECG on serial recordings. The challenge does not contribute to risk stratification for SCD; thus, it should not be performed in subjects with a spontaneous type 1 ECG. The test is considered positive if the type 1 ST-segment elevation is unmasked, and should be terminated if frequent ventricular premature beats or other arrhythmias occur, or if the QRS

widens to greater than 130% of the baseline.[39] Ajmaline and flecainide are the two most frequently used medications in Europe for BS challenge. Ajmaline combines the advantages of higher sensitivity and a shorter half-life compared with flecainide, and is the preferred agent for pharmacologic testing.[42]

Table 2 provides the current treatment options for patients with BS, as suggested by the European Society of Cardiology guidelines.[43]

THE LONG QT SYNDROME

LQTS is a cardiac condition that displays an autosomal-dominant Mendelian inheritance with variable penetrance, rarely inherited in a recessive fashion associated with sensorineural deafness. The syndrome has a prevalence in the range of 1 in 2000 to 2500.[44] It is caused by genetically encoded abnormalities in cardiac ion channels:

- Potassium channel proteins KvLQT1 (*KCNQ1*) and HERG (*KCNH2*) mutations, leading to a reduction of net potassium current and delayed repolarization, are the basis for LQT types 1 and 2.
- Sodium channel protein NaV1.5 (*SCN5A*) mutation, leading to a gain of function in sodium channel and a persistent late, slow sodium influx, is the basis for LQT type 3.
- Potassium channel mutations can delay repolarization and lead to Andersen-Tawil syndrome (ATS1 or LQT type 7);
- Abnormal changes in intracellular Ca^{2+} handling can cause LQTS type 8.[45]

Although the current classifications of LQTS are genetically based, the most important clinical characteristic remains QT-interval prolongation, which may establish the prognosis of patients with LQTS, especially those with LQTS type 1 and 2. Differences in the mutations and electrophysiological mechanisms among the LQTS subtypes tend to produce distinctive differences in the T waves: LQTS type 1 has a broad-based T wave, LQTS type 2 has a low-amplitude and notched T wave, LQTS type 3 has a late-appearing T wave, and LQTS type 7 has a mild QT prolongation with a prominent U wave (**Fig. 15**). Severe sinus bradycardia has been reported in children with LQTS type1, and adults with LQTS type 1 can have normal resting heart rates but attenuated exercise rate responses. LQTS is also associated with increased QT dispersion, defined as the difference between the minimum and maximum QT intervals in the 12-lead ECG, which indicates ventricular

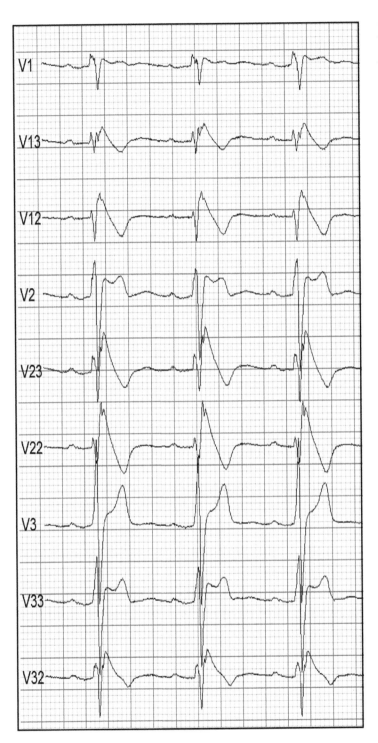

Fig. 14. Revealing type pattern 1 with simultaneous recording of leads V1 and V2 from the fourth, third, and second intercostal spaces.

repolarization heterogeneity. Prominent U waves and T-U complexes are also frequently seen. Standard ECG, but mostly ambulatory ECG, can show T-wave alternans, which is a beat-to-beat alternation in T-wave morphology, amplitude, QT interval, and polarity without concomitant QRS changes.[45]

LQTS is characterized clinically by palpitations, syncope, and SCD. Clinical events may be precipitated by specific triggers, such as exercise and

Table 2
Treatment options for patients with Brugada syndrome

Brugada Syndrome Therapy	Class of Recommendation	Level of Evidence
ICD implantation		
ICD is recommended in patients who a. are survivors of an aborted cardiac arrest, And/or b. Have spontaneous sustained VT.	I	C
ICD should be considered in patients with spontaneous type 1 ECG a history of syncope	IIa	C
S-ICD should be considered as an alternative to transvenous ICD in patients with an indication for ICD when antibradycardia and/or antitachycardia pacing, or cardiac resynchronization therapy is not needed.	IIa	C
S-ICD may be considered as an alternative to transvenous ICD when venous access is difficult, after the removal of a transvenous ICD for infections or in young patients with a long-term need for ICD therapy.	IIa	C
ICD may be considered in patients who develop VF during programmed ventricular pacing with 2 or 3 extra stimuli at 2 sites.	IIb	C
Pharmacologic therapy		
Quinidine or isoproterenol should be considered to treat electrical storms.	IIa	C
Quinidine should be considered in patients with an indication for ICD when the device is unavailable or contraindicated, and for the management of supraventricular arrhythmias.	IIa	C
Catheter ablation		
Catheter ablation may be considered in patients with a history of electrical storms or repeated appropriate ICD shocks.	IIa	C

Abbreviations: ECG, electrocardiograph; ICD, implantable cardiac defibrillator; S-ICD, subcutaneous implantable cardiac defibrillator; VT, ventricular tachycardia.

From Priori SG, Blomstrom-Lundqvist C, Mazzanti A, et al. 2015 ESC guidelines for the management of patients with ventricular arrhythmias and the prevention of sudden cardiac death. Eur Heart J 2015;36:2836; with permission.

specifically swimming in LQTS type 1, emotion and auditory stimulation especially on waking in LQTS type 2, and rest in LQTS type 3.[46] Because seizure activity attributable to cerebral anoxia during ventricular arrhythmias is relatively common, LQTS continues to be misdiagnosed as epilepsy.[47] The risk of adverse cardiac events relates to factors that facilitate the risk stratification, such as the length of the QT interval, childhood, male sex, genotype (LQTS types 2 and 3), and recurrent syncope.[46]

Torsades de pointes is a polymorphic VT with beat-by-beat changes in the QRS complex, which occurs frequently in LQTS (see **Fig. 5**). Although torsades de pointes usually terminates within seconds, it can recur repeatedly, cause faintness or syncope, and degenerate into VF, resulting in sudden death.[48,49]

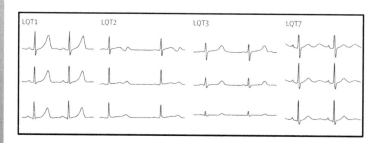

Fig. 15. Long QT syndrome subtypes.

Therapeutic options for patients with LQTS are β-adrenergic blockers, implantable cardioverter defibrillators, and left cardiac sympathetic denervation.[45,48]

REFERENCES

1. Moya A, Sutton R, Ammirati F, et al. Guidelines for the diagnosis and management of syncope (version 2009): the task force for the diagnosis and management of syncope of the European Society of Cardiology (ESC). Eur Heart J 2009;30:2631–71.

2. Olde Nordkamp LAR, van Dijk N, Ganzeboom KS, et al. Syncope prevalence in the ED compared to that in the general practice and population: a strong selection process. Am J Emerg Med 2009; 27:271–9.

3. Soteriades ES, Evans JC, Larson MG, et al. Incidence and prognosis of syncope. N Engl J Med 2002;347:878–85.

4. Van Lieshout JJ, Wieling W, Karemaker JM, et al. Syncope, cerebral perfusion, and oxygenation. J Appl Physiol 2003;94:833–48.

5. Wieling W, Thijs RD, van Dijk N, et al. Symptoms and signs of syncope: a review of the link between physiology and clinical clues. Brain 2009;132:2630–42.

6. Deharo JC, Guieu R, Mechulan A, et al. Syncope without prodromes in patients with normal heart and normal electrocardiogram: a distinct entity. J Am Coll Cardiol 2013;62:1075–80.

7. Brignole M, Guieu R, Tomaino M, et al. The mechanism of syncope without prodromes with normal heart and normal electrocardiogram. Heart Rhythm 2017;14:234–9.

8. Del Rosso A, Alboni P, Brignole M, et al. Relation of clinical presentation of syncope to the age of patients. Am J Cardiol 2005;96:1431–5.

9. Ungar A, Mussi C, Del Rosso A, et al. Diagnosis and characteristics of syncope in older patients referred to geriatric departments. J Am Geriatr Soc 2006;54:1531–6.

10. Brignole M, Menozzi C, Bartoletti A, et al. A new management of syncope: prospective systematic guideline-based evaluation of patients referred urgently to general hospitals. Eur Heart J 2006;27:76–82.

11. Alboni P, Brignole M, Menozzi C, et al. Diagnostic value of history in patients with syncope with or without heart disease. J Am Coll Cardiol 2001;37:1921–8.

12. Del Rosso A, Ungar A, Maggi R, et al. Clinical predictors of cardiac syncope at initial evaluation in patients referred urgently to general hospital: the EGSYS score. Heart 2008;94:1620–6.

13. Thiruganasambandamoorthy V, Stiell IG, Sivilotti MLA, et al. Predicting short-term risk of arrhythmia among patients with syncope: the Canadian syncope arrhythmia risk score. Acad Emerg Med 2017. https://doi.org/10.1111/acem.13275.

14. Costantino G, Casazza G, Reed M, et al. Syncope risk stratification tools vs clinical judgment: an individual patient data meta-analysis. Am J Med 2014; 127. 1126.e13–25.

15. Colivicchi F, Ammirati F, Melina D, et al. OESIL (Osservatorio Epidemiologico sulla Sincope nel Lazio) study investigators. Development and prospective validation of a risk stratification system for patients with syncope in the emergency department: the OESIL risk score. Eur Heart J 2003;24:811–9.

16. Quinn J, McDermott D, Stiell I, et al. Prospective validation of the San Francisco syncope rule to predict patients with serious outcomes. Ann Emerg Med 2006;47:448–54.

17. Brignole M, Gianfranchi L, Menozzi C, et al. Role of autonomic reflexes in syncope associated with paroxysmal atrial fibrillation. J Am Coll Cardiol 1993;22:1123–9.

18. Naseef A, Behr ER, Batchvarov VN. Electrocardiographic methods for diagnosis and risk stratification in the Brugada Syndrome. J Saudi Heart Assoc 2015;27:96–108.

19. Leitch JW, Klein GJ, Yee R, et al. Syncope associated with supraventricular tachycardia: an expression of tachycardia or vasomotor response? Circulation 1992;85:1064–71.

20. Casagranda I, Brignole M, Cencetti S, et al. Management of transient loss of consciousness of suspected syncopal cause, after the initial evaluation in the Emergency Department. Emergency Care Journal 2016;12:6046.

21. Chiu DT, Shapiro NI, Sun BC, et al. Are echocardiography, telemetry, ambulatory electrocardiography monitoring, and cardiac enzymes in emergency department patients presenting with syncope useful tests? A preliminary investigation. J Emerg Med 2014;47:113–8.

22. Benezet-Mazuecos J, Ibanez B, Rubio JM, et al. Utility of in-hospital cardiac remote telemetry in patients with unexplained syncope. Europace 2007;9:1196–201.

23. Bass EB, Curtiss EI, Arena VC, et al. The duration of Holter monitoring in patients with syncope. Is 24 hours enough? Arch Intern Med 1990;150:1073–8.

24. Locati ET, Moya A, Oliveira M, et al. External prolonged electrocardiogram monitoring in unexplained syncope and palpitations: results of the SYNARR-Flash study. Europace 2016;18:1265–72.

25. Pürerfellner H, Sanders P, Pokushalov E, et al. Miniaturized reveal LINQ insertable cardiac monitoring system: first-in-human experience. Heart Rhythm 2015;12:1113–9.

26. Brignole M, Vardas P, Hoffman E, et al. Indications for the use of diagnostic implantable and external ECG loop recorders. Europace 2009;11:671–6.

27. Brignole M, Menozzi C, Moya A, et al. Mechanism of syncope in patients with bundle branch block and negative electrophysiological test. Circulation 2001; 104:2045–50.

28. Menozzi C, Brignole M, Alboni P, et al. The natural course of untreated sick sinus syndrome and identification of the variables predictive of unfavorable outcome. Am J Cardiol 1998;82:1205–9.

29. McAnulty JH, Rahimtoola SH, Murphy E, et al. Natural history of 'high risk' bundle branch block. Final report of a prospective study. N Engl J Med 1982; 307:137–43.

30. Scheinman MM, Peters RW, Suave MJ, et al. Value of the H-Q interval in patients with bundle branch block and the role of prophylactic permanent pacing. Am J Cardiol 1982;50:1316–22.

31. Kaul U, Dev V, Narula J, et al. Evaluation of patients with bundle branch block and "unexplained" syncope: a study based on comprehensive electrophysiologic testing and ajmaline stress. Pacing Clin Electrophysiol 1988;11:289–97.

32. Moya A, Garcia-Civera R, Croci F, et al. Diagnosis, management, and outcomes of patients with syncope and bundle branch block. Eur Heart J 2011; 32:1535–41.

33. Olshansky B, Hahn EA, Hartz VL, et al. Clinical significance of syncope in the electrophysiologic study versus electrocardiographic monitoring (ESVEM) trial. The ESVEM Investigators. Am Heart J 1999; 137:878–86.

34. Mittal S, Hao SC, Iwai S, et al. Significance of inducible ventricular fibrillation in patients with coronary artery disease and unexplained syncope. J Am Coll Cardiol 2001;38:371–6.

35. Link MS, Kim KM, Homoud MK, et al. Long-term outcome of patients with syncope associated with coronary artery disease and a non diagnostic electrophysiological evaluation. Am J Cardiol 1999;83: 1334–7.

36. Gallagher MM, Forleo GB, Behr ER, et al. Prevalence and significance of Brugada-type ECG in 12,012 apparently healthy European subjects. Int J Cardiol 2008;130:44–8.

37. Probst V, Veltmann C, Eckardt L, et al. Long-term prognosis of patients diagnosed with Brugada

syndrome: results from the FINGER Brugada Syndrome Registry. Circulation 2010;121:635–43.

38. Juang JM, Huang SK. Brugada syndrome—an under-recognized electrical disease in patients with sudden cardiac death. Cardiology 2004;101: 157–69.

39. Priori SG, Wilde AA, Horie M, et al. HRS/EHRA/ APHRS expert consensus statement on the diagnosis and management of patients with inherited primary arrhythmia syndromes. Heart Rhythm 2013;10: 1932–63.

40. Veltmann C, Schimpf R, Echternach C, et al. A prospective study on spontaneous fluctuations between diagnostic and non-diagnostic ECGs in Brugada syndrome: implications for correct phenotyping and risk stratification. Eur Heart J 2006;27: 2544–52.

41. Adler A, Topaz G, Heller K, et al. Fever-induced Brugada pattern: how common is it and what does it mean? Heart Rhythm 2013;10:1375–82.

42. Vohra J, Rajagopalan S. Update on the diagnosis and management of Brugada syndrome. Heart Lung Circ 2015;24:1141–8.

43. Priori SG, Blomstrom-Lundqvist C, Mazzanti A, et al. 2015 ESC Guidelines for the management of patients with ventricular arrhythmias and the prevention of sudden cardiac death. Eur Heart J 2015;36: 2793–867.

44. Schwartz PJ, Stramba-Badiale M, Crotti L, et al. Prevalence of the congenital long-QT syndrome. Circulation 2009;120:1761–7.

45. Morita H, Wu J, Zipes DP. The QT syndromes: long and short. Lancet 2008;372:750–63.

46. Abrams DJ, MacRae CA. Long QT syndrome. Circulation 2014;129:1524–9.

47. MacCormick JM, McAlister H, Crawford J, et al. Misdiagnosis of long QT syndrome as epilepsy at first presentation. Ann Emerg Med 2009;54:26–32.

48. El-Sherif N, Turitto G. Torsade de pointes. In: Zipes DP, Jalife J, editors. Cardiac electrophysiology from cell to bedside. 4th edition. Philadelphia: WB Saunders; 1994. p. 687–99.

49. Zareba W, Moss AJ, Daubert JP, et al. Implantable cardioverter defibrillator in high-risk long QT syndrome patients. J Cardiovasc Electrophysiol 2003; 14:337–41.

Clinical Approach to Patients with Palpitations

Franco Giada, MD[a],*, Antonio Raviele, MD, FEHRA, FESC, FHRS[b]

KEYWORDS

- Palpitations • Diagnosis • Prognosis • Ambulatory ECG monitoring • Electrophysiological study

KEY POINTS

- Palpitations are among the most common symptoms that prompt patients to consult their general practitioner, cardiologist, or emergency health care services.
- The current management of patients with palpitations, despite extensive, costly, and time-consuming investigations, sometimes fails to establish a diagnosis.
- Prolonged ambulatory electrocardiogram monitoring serves to document the cardiac rhythm during palpitations when symptoms are paroxysmal and short lasting.
- Patients with palpitations rarely need to be hospitalized for exclusively diagnostic purposes, because invasive investigations, such as electrophysiological study and hemodynamic study, are rarely necessary.

INTRODUCTION

Palpitations are among the most common symptoms that prompt patients to consult their general practitioner, cardiologist, or emergency health care services. Very often, however, the diagnostic and therapeutic management of this symptom proves to be poorly efficacious and somewhat frustrating for both the patient and the physician. Indeed, in many cases a definitive, or at least probable, diagnosis of the cause of the palpitations is not reached, and no specific therapy is initiated. Therefore, many patients continue to suffer recurrences of their symptoms, which impair their quality of life and mental balance, leading to the potential risk of adverse clinical events and prompt continual recourse to health care facilities.

These difficulties stem from the fact that the palpitations are generally a transitory symptom. Indeed, at the moment of clinical evaluation, the patient is almost always asymptomatic and the diagnostic evaluation is based only on the search for pathologic conditions that may be responsible for the symptom.

DEFINITION AND PHYSIOPATHOLOGY

Palpitations are defined as an unpleasant perception of the heartbeat and are described by patients as a disagreeable sensation of throbbing or movement in the chest and/or adjacent areas. Indeed, in normal resting conditions, the activity of the heart is not generally perceived by the individual. However, during intense physical activity or emotional stress, it may be quite normal to become aware of one's own cardiac activity for brief periods; these sensations are regarded as physiologic palpitations, in that they represent the normal subjective perception of an increase in the frequency and strength of the contraction of the heart. Outside of such situations, instead, palpitations are considered to be pathologic.[1–5]

The mechanisms underlying palpitations are somewhat heterogeneous: contractions of the

Disclosure Statement: The authors have nothing to disclose.
[a] Sports Medicine and Cardiovascular Rehabilitation Unit, Cardiovascular Department, PF Calvi Hospital, Via Largo San Giorgio 3, Noale, Venice 30033, Italy; [b] Dell'Angelo Hospital, via Torre Belfredo 44, Mestre, Venice 30174, Italy
* Corresponding author.
E-mail address: francogiada@hotmail.com

heart that are too rapid, irregular, or particularly slow, as in cardiac rhythm disorders or in sinus tachycardia secondary to mental disturbance, systemic diseases, or the use of pharmaceutical drugs; very intense contractions and anomalous movements of the heart in the chest, as in the case of some structural heart diseases associated with cardiomegaly and/or increased stroke volume; and anomalies in the subjective perception of the heartbeat, whereby a sinus rhythm, sinus tachycardia, or minimal irregularities in the cardiac rhythm are felt by the patient and are poorly tolerated, as in the case of some psychiatric disorders.[1–7]

Clinical Presentation

Duration and frequency of palpitations

With regard to duration, palpitations may be either paroxysmal or persistent. In paroxysmal forms, the symptom terminates spontaneously within a period of time ranging from a few seconds to several hours. In persistent forms, the palpitations are ongoing and terminate only after adequate medical treatment. With regard to frequency, palpitations may occur daily, weekly, or monthly.

Types of palpitations

Patients use a wide range of sensations to describe their symptoms. The most common descriptions, and those most useful in clinical practice in differential diagnoses among the various causes of palpitations, enable palpitations to be classified according to the following main categories[1–5,8–21]: extrasystolic palpitations, tachycardiac palpitations, throbbing palpitations, and anxiety-related palpitations (**Table 1**).

Classification

From the etiologic point of view, the causes of palpitations can be subdivided into 5 main groups (**Box 1**): arrhythmic causes, structural cardiac causes, psychiatric causes, systemic causes, and the use of drugs or illicit substances.[1–5,8,9] It is not uncommon, however, for the patient to simultaneously manifest more than one potential cause of palpitations, or palpitations of different origins. Electrocardiographic documentation of a rhythm disorder during spontaneous symptoms provides the strongest evidence of causality; whenever this proves possible, therefore, the palpitations are classified as being of arrhythmic origin. By contrast, they are considered to be of nonarrhythmic origin when the underlying heart rhythm exhibits sinus rhythm or sinus tachycardia. Thus, according to this etiologic hierarchy, nonarrhythmic causes of palpitations emerge as definitive diagnoses only in cases in which the symptom-electrocardiogram (ECG) correlation excludes the presence of rhythm disorders.[4] When it is not possible to document the cardiac rhythm during the palpitations, nonarrhythmic causes are regarded as probable.

EPIDEMIOLOGY

The epidemiology of palpitations is, as yet, little known. Nevertheless, there is evidence to suggest that palpitations are a very frequent symptom in the general population[22] and, in particular, in patients suffering from hypertension or heart disease.[1,2] Indeed, few people would claim never to have felt their heart beating abnormally at some time in their lives. Moreover, palpitations account

Table 1
Types of palpitations and their clinical presentations

Type of Palpitation	Subjective Description	Heartbeat	Onset and Termination	Trigger Situations	Associated Symptoms
Extrasystolic	"Skipping a beat," "heart sinking"	Irregular, interspersed with periods of normal heartbeat	Gradual	Rest	
Tachycardiac	"Beating wings" in the chest	Regular or irregular, markedly accelerated	Sudden	Physical effort, cooling down	Hemodynamic impairment
Anxiety related	Anxiety, agitation	Regular, slightly accelerated	Gradual	Stress, Anxiety attacks	Aspecific symptoms
Throbbing	Heart pounding	Regular, normal frequency			

Adapted from Raviele A, Giada F, Bergfeldt L, et al. Management of patients with palpitations: a position paper of European Heart Rhythm Association. Europace 2011;13:920–34; with permission.

Box 1
Etiologic classification of palpitations

Palpitations due to arrhythmic causes

- Supraventricular extrasystole
- Ventricular extrasystole
- Supraventricular tachycardia
- Ventricular tachycardia
- Bradyarrhythmias: severe sinus bradycardia, sinus arrest, second- and third-degree atrioventricular block
- Anomalies in the functioning and/or programming of pacemakers and ICD

Palpitations due to structural heart disease

- Severe mitral regurgitation
- Severe aortic regurgitation
- Congenital heart diseases with significant shunt
- Atrial myxoma
- Mechanical prosthetic valves
- Cardiomegaly and/or heart failure of various causes
- Mitral valve prolapse

Palpitations of psychiatric origin

- Anxiety, panic attacks
- Depression, somatization disorders

Palpitations due to systemic causes

- Metabolic disorders: hyperthyroidism, pheochromocytoma, hypoglycemia, mastocytosis, postmenopausal syndrome
- States involving elevated stroke volume: fever (>38°C), anemia (HB <10 mg/dL), pregnancy (>20th week), Paget disease, arteriovenous fistula, hypovolemia
- Intolerance to orthostatism and functional syndromes: orthostatic hypotension, POTS, inappropriate sinus tachycardia

Palpitations induced by drugs or illicit substances

- Sympathicomimetics, vasodilators, anticholinergics, hydralazine
- Recent suspension of β-blockers
- Alcohol, cocaine, heroin, amphetamines, caffeine, nicotine, cannabis, synthetic drugs

Adapted from Raviele A, Giada F, Bergfeldt L, et al. Management of patients with palpitations: a position paper of European Heart Rhythm Association. Europace 2011;13:920–34; with permission.

---

for 16% of the symptoms that prompt patients to visit their general practitioner[23,24] and are second only to chest pain as the cause of specialist cardiologic evaluation.[6]

PROGNOSIS

Palpitations display a low mortality: about 1% per year.[23] A retrospective American study that analyzed case records obtained from general practitioners found no difference in 5-year mortality or morbidity between patients with palpitations and a group of asymptomatic control subjects.[24] Even in the above-mentioned study by Weber and Kapoor,[25] despite the frequent presence of palpitations of cardiac origin, 1-year mortality was only 1.6%.

In patients with palpitations, the recurrence of symptoms is, however, very frequent. In the study by Weber and Kapoor,[25] 77% of patients experienced at least one recurrence of palpitations, and the effect on their quality of life was unfavorable. These findings are confirmed by a prospective study conducted by Barsky and colleagues[19] on 145 patients with palpitations, who were followed up for 6 months and compared with an asymptomatic control group. These investigators observed that the patients with palpitations, despite having a favorable prognosis quoad vitam, remained symptomatic and functionally impaired over time and exhibited a high incidence of panic attacks and psychological symptoms. Although palpitations are generally associated with low rates of mortality,[4] in patients with structural or arrhythmogenic heart disease or a family history of sudden death, or if the palpitations are associated with symptoms of hemodynamic impairment (dyspnea, syncope, presyncope, dizziness, asthenia, chest pain, neurovegetative symptoms), they can have a direct impact on the prognosis.[1] However, even in patients without severe heart disease, palpitations may be due to significant arrhythmias, such as atrial fibrillation, atrial flutter, or ventricular ectopic beats, all of which require adequate investigation and treatment.

DIAGNOSTIC STRATEGY

In patients with palpitations, it is essential, for both diagnostic and prognostic purposes, to distinguish the type of palpitation; to search for possible structural and/or arrhythmogenic heart diseases and systemic or psychiatric conditions able to cause palpitations; and to obtain an electrocardiographic recording during symptoms. All patients suffering from palpitations should therefore undergo an initial clinical evaluation comprising history, objective examination, standard 12-lead ECG. In selected cases, a psychiatric evaluation and certain specific instrumental and laboratory investigations must be considered[8] (Fig. 1).

The initial clinical evaluation leads to a definitive or probable diagnosis of the cause of the palpitations in about half of the patients, excludes with reasonable certainty the presence of causes that have an unfavorable prognosis, and will indicate which specific investigations, if any, are necessary.[25]

If the initial clinical evaluation proves completely negative, which is more frequent in paroxysmal, short-lasting palpitations, the palpitations are deemed to be of unknown origin. In subjects with palpitations of unknown origin who have low probability of an arrhythmic cause, that is, patients without significant heart disease and those with anxiety-related or extrasystolic palpitations (Box 2), further investigations are not normally required; the patient should be reassured and a follow-up clinical examination may be scheduled. By contrast, in subjects with palpitations of unknown origin who have high probability of an arrhythmic cause (see Box 2), second-level investigations should be considered; these include ambulatory ECG (AECG) monitoring and electrophysiologic study (EPS). Table 2 shows the reported clinical characteristics of tachycardiac palpitations. Finally, even in the absence of arrhythmic risk criteria, second-level investigations should also be carried out in patients with palpitations of unknown origin whose symptoms are frequent or associated with impaired of quality of life or states of anxiety (see Fig. 1).

Standard Electrocardiogram

In the diagnosis of palpitations, 12-lead electrocardiographic recording during spontaneous symptoms constitutes the gold standard. Indeed, this enables the physician to definitively determine whether the palpitations are of arrhythmic origin (and generally provides an accurate diagnosis of the type of arrhythmia) or of nonarrhythmic origin, a distinction that has important diagnostic, prognostic, and therapeutic implications.[1–5,25] In

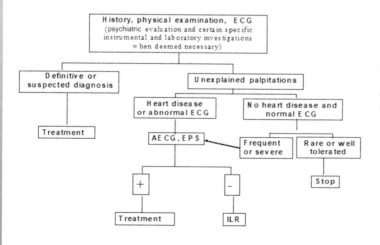

Fig. 1. Diagnostic flowchart of patients with palpitations. (Adapted from Raviele A, Giada F, Bergfeldt L, et al. Management of patients with palpitations: a position paper of European Heart Rhythm Association. Europace 2011;13:920–34; with permission.)

progress. This means that the palpitations must be of sufficiently long duration (generally at least an hour) and that they must not be accompanied by invalidating symptoms (syncope, presyncope, asthenia), which prevent the patient from reaching the emergency department.

AMBULATORY ELECTROCARDIOGRAM MONITORING

Prolonged AECG monitoring serves to document the cardiac rhythm during an episode of palpitations if this cannot be done by means of standard ECG, as in the case of paroxysmal and short-lasting symptoms.[26,27]

The devices currently used for AECG monitoring can be subdivided into 2 main categories: external and implantable. External devices comprise the Holter recorder, hospital telemetry (reserved for hospitalized patients at high risk of malignant arrhythmias), event recorders, external loop recorders and, very recently, mobile cardiac outpatient telemetry (MCOT). The implantable devices comprise pacemakers and implantable cardioverter-defibrillator (ICD) equipped with diagnostic features (used exclusively in patients requiring such devices for therapeutic purposes) and subcutaneous loop recorders (**Table 3**).

Holter

Although very widely used in everyday clinical practice, Holter monitoring has the following limitations: the period of monitoring is restricted to 24 to 48 hours or, in the latest devices, 7 days; the size of the device may prevent the patient

normal clinical practice, however, it is not always possible to record an ECG during spontaneous episodes of palpitations. Indeed, the patient must be able to reach the nearest emergency department while the palpitations are still in

---

Table 2
Clinical characteristics of tachycardiac palpitations

Type of Arrhythmia	Heart Beat	Trigger Situations	Associated Symptoms	Vagal Maneuvers
AVRT, AVNRT	Sudden onset regular with periods of elevated frequency	Physical effort, changes in posture	Polyuria, frog sign	Sudden interruption
Atrial fibrillation	Irregular with variable frequency	Physical effort, cooling down	Polyuria	Transitory reduction in heart rate
Tachycardia and atrial flutter	Regular (irregular if A-V conduction is variable) with elevated frequency			Transitory reduction in heart rate
Ventricular tachycardias	Regular with elevated frequency	Physical effort	Hemodynamic impairment	No effect

Abbreviations: A-V, atrioventricular; AVNRT, atrioventricular node reentrant tachycardia; AVRT, atrioventricular reentrant tachycardia.

Adapted from Raviele A, Giada F, Bergfeldt L, et al. Management of patients with palpitations: a position paper of European Heart Rhythm Association. Europace 2011;13:920–34; with permission.

Table 3
Recommendations for the use of ambulatory electrocardiogram monitoring techniques in patients with palpitations

	Holter Monitoring	Event Recorders	External Loop Recorders/MCOT	Implantable Loop Recorders
Advantages	Low cost; possibility of recording asymptomatic arrhythmias	Low cost; easy to use	Retrospective and prospective ECG records; possibility of recording asymptomatic arrhythmias automatically	Retrospective and prospective ECG records; quite good ECG records; monitoring capability up to 36 mo; possibility of record asymptomatic arrhythmias automatically
Limits	Monitoring limited to 24–48 h; size may prevent activities that may trigger the arrhythmias	Monitoring cannot be carried out for more than 3–4 wk; short-lasting arrhythmias are not recorded; arrhythmic triggers are not revealed; poor ECG records	Monitoring cannot be carried out for more than 3–4 wk; continual maintenance is required; devices are uncomfortable; quite poor ECG records	Invasiveness; risk of local complications at the implantation site
Indications	Daily palpitations; patients who are unable to activate a device for AECG monitoring	Compliant patients; infrequent and fairly long-lasting palpitations unaccompanied by hemodynamic impairment that is likely to hinder use of the device	Weekly short-lasting palpitations associated with hemodynamic impairment, in very compliant patients	Monthly palpitations associated with hemodynamic impairment; noncompliant patients; when all the other examinations prove inconclusive

Adapted from Raviele A, Giada F, Bergfeldt L, et al. Management of patients with palpitations: a position paper of European Heart Rhythm Association. Europace 2011;13:920–34; with permission.

from performing certain activities, such as physical exercise, which may be essential to triggering some arrhythmias; the correlation between the symptoms and the arrhythmias recorded is mainly based on the clinical diary, which the patient often fails to complete adequately.

Event Recorders

These small, easy-to-use, portable devices are applied to the patient's skin whenever symptoms are experienced. They provide prospective 1-lead electrocardiographic recording for a few seconds. The optimal duration of event recorder monitoring is generally 3 to 4 weeks.[28–30]

External Loop Recorders

These devices are connected continuously to the patient by means of skin electrodes. Equipped with a memory loop, they provide 1- to 3-lead electrocardiographic recording for a few minutes before and after activation by the patient when symptoms arise. The latest devices are also able to self-activate automatically when arrhythmic events occur. The optimal duration of external loop recorder monitoring is 2 to 4 weeks.[31–34]

Mobile Cardiac Outpatient Telemetry

This system is made up of an external recorder connected to the patient by means of skin electrodes and a portable receiver that is able to transmit an electrocardiographic trace to a remote operating center via the telephone. In this way, the patient's rhythm can be monitored in real time.

Implantable Loop Recorders

Similar in size to a pacemaker, implantable loop recorders (ILRs) are implanted beneath the skin through a small incision of about 2 cm in the left precordial region.[35] ILR are equipped with a memory loop and, once activated by the patient through an external activator at the moment when the symptoms arise, record a good-quality 1-lead electrocardiographic trace for several minutes before and after the event. They are also able to record any arrhythmic event automatically, that is, with no intervention by the patient. The duration of their monitoring capacity is limited only by the life of the internal battery, which can operate for up to 36 months.

Diagnostic Value

AECG monitoring is regarded as diagnostic only when it is possible to establish a certain correlation between the palpitations and an electrocardiographic recording.[26,27] In patients who do not develop symptoms during monitoring, therefore, this examination proves nondiagnostic.

Holter devices, external loop recorders, ILRs, and MCOT, which are able to record arrhythmic events automatically, without active intervention by the patient, are considered to be nondiagnostic with regard to the cause of palpitations even if the patient presents more or less significant, but asymptomatic, arrhythmias during the monitoring period. However, the presence of clinically significant arrhythmias that are asymptomatic, that is, not associated with palpitations, may suggest a probable diagnosis and/or guide the decision to undertake further investigations. In any case, the significance of these asymptomatic arrhythmias must be evaluated on the basis of their severity, prevalence in the age-group and population to which the patient belongs, and the presence of heart disease.

Whenever it is possible to establish a correlation between the patient's symptoms and an interpretable ECG recording, the specificity of AECG monitoring, at least in formulating a diagnosis of arrhythmic palpitations or nonarrhythmic palpitations, is 100%. The documentation of a normal sinus rhythm during clinical palpitations is therefore the quickest way to exclude an arrhythmic cause. By contrast, the sensitivity of AECG monitoring is extremely variable and depends on the following factors: the monitoring techniques used, the duration of monitoring, patient compliance, and the frequency of the symptoms.

In patients with palpitations of unknown origin, Holter has displayed a rather low diagnostic value (33%–35%).[36] In a meta-analysis of 7 studies conducted on patients with syncope and/or palpitations of unknown origin, Holter monitoring has been seen to display a diagnostic value of only 22%.[37] By contrast, in patients in whom the symptoms are quite frequent, that is, daily or weekly, external loop recorders and event recorders have shown both a higher diagnostic value (66%–83%) and a better cost-effectiveness ratio than Holter devices.[30,36] Finally, in patients with symptoms of possible arrhythmic origin, MCOT has been seen to exhibit a higher diagnostic value than the other external devices.[38–40]

ILRs have been successfully used to study syncope, in which they have shown a better cost-effectiveness ratio than the conventional tests,[35,41,42] and they could be useful also in the study of palpitations of unknown origin.[26,43,44] Indeed, the RUP (recurrent unexplained palpitations) study demonstrated the superiority of ILR over the conventional diagnostic strategy of Holter and event recorder monitoring and EPS in the evaluation of patients with infrequent palpitations, that is, monthly frequency, reporting both a higher diagnostic value (73% vs 21%) and a better cost-effectiveness ratio.[45]

Limits

AECG monitoring has some important limitations. Indeed, it is not always possible to formulate a precise diagnosis of the type of arrhythmia recorded, especially when single-lead ECG devices are used. The advantages and disadvantages of the individual devices used in AECG monitoring are reported in **Table 3**.

Indications

According to the American College of Cardiology/American Heart Association (ACC/AHA) guidelines for the use of AECG monitoring,[26,27] and European Heart Rhythm Association position paper,[46] recurrent palpitations of unknown origin constitute a class I indication. The recommendations regarding the choice of the AECG monitoring device most suited to the individual patient are reported in **Table 3**.

ELECTROPHYSIOLOGIC STUDY
Diagnostic Value

Unlike AECG monitoring, which records cardiac rhythm during spontaneous palpitations, EPS is a provocative test; EPS positivity therefore reveals only the presence of a pathologic substrate, which may (or may not) be responsible for the clinical symptoms. Few studies have used AECG monitoring to confirm the results of EPS in the diagnostic evaluation of patients with palpitations of unknown origin; the true diagnostic value of EPS in this context is therefore only partially known.[9,47,48] EPS is regarded as diagnostic when the induction of arrhythmias is accompanied by reproduction of the spontaneous symptoms, or when, even in the absence of symptoms, a sustained (>1 minute) supraventricular tachycardia or a sustained (>30 seconds, or necessitating urgent interruption) ventricular tachycardia is induced. When no arrhythmias with the above characteristics are induced, it is regarded as negative.

The diagnostic value of EPS depends heavily on the stimulation protocol used; aggressive protocols increase the sensitivity of the examination at the expense of its specificity and vice versa. EPS shows greater sensitivity in patients with structural or arrhythmogenic heart disease than in those without heart disease. Moreover, the sensitivity of EPS also seems to depend on the type of palpitation under investigation, being higher in tachycardiac palpitations than in extrasystolic or anxiety-related palpitations (see **Table 2**). By contrast, the specificity of EPS depends heavily on the type of arrhythmia induced. It is high (about 100%) when the induced arrhythmia is an atrioventricular nodal reentrant tachycardia, an atrioventricular reentrant tachycardia, or a monomorphic sustained ventricular tachycardia.[49,50] On the other hand, it is somewhat variable, especially in patients with structural heart disease, when an atrial fibrillation, an atrial flutter, a nonsustained ventricular tachycardia, a polymorphic ventricular tachycardia, or a ventricular fibrillation is induced.[51–56]

Limitations

Endocavitary EPS is costly, is invasive, requires hospitalization, and involves a risk of complications, albeit low. By contrast, transesophageal EPS is more economical, is semi-invasive, does not require hospitalization, and, although not always well tolerated by patients, rarely gives rise to complications. However, unlike endocavitary EPS, it does not enable the Hisian conduction system or ventricular vulnerability to be studied, nor does it allow ablative therapy for the induced arrhythmias to be performed during the same session.

Indications

According to the ACC/AHA guidelines,[47] "Long-term ambulatory recording is the most useful means of documenting the cardiac rhythm associated with palpitations" and "EPS is used if recording is unable to provide an answer." EPS is a class I indication in patients with palpitations of unknown origin during which an elevated heart rate is documented by a qualified person, and in patients with palpitations that precede syncope. EPS is a class II indication in patients with clinically significant palpitations suspected of being of cardiac origin in whom the symptoms are sporadic and cannot be documented. In patients with significant heart disease, endocavitary EPS is generally performed, whereas transesophageal EPS is preferred in patients without heart disease or with only mild heart disease.

EPS has some important advantages over AECG monitoring. First of all, it is able to correctly identify the type of arrhythmia responsible for the palpitations. Moreover, in the case of endocavitary EPS, it enables ablative therapy for the induced tachyarrhythmias to be performed during the same session in which the diagnosis is made. Finally, although EPS enables a diagnosis to be made and specific therapy to be initiated immediately, AECG monitoring requires the patient to experience a recurrence of symptoms. This delays the diagnosis and, should the palpitations be due to malignant arrhythmias, exposes the patient to the potential risk of adverse events. For this reason, in patients with significant heart disease and in those with palpitations that precede syncope, in whom the risk of adverse events is higher, EPS generally precedes the use of AECG monitoring. In all other cases, EPS normally follows AECG monitoring when this latter proves nondiagnostic.

THERAPY

Therapy for palpitations is of course directed toward the etiologic cause, whenever it can be determined. However, therapy must always be counterbalanced with the associated risks. For example, treating a benign arrhythmia, such as premature beats in the right ventricular outflow tract, with anti-arrhythmic drugs may induce proarrhythmia and result in secondary effects. After accurately identifying the cause of palpitations, a careful and balanced decision regarding therapy should be sought.

REFERENCES

1. Zimetbaum P, Josephson ME. Evaluation of patients with palpitations. N Engl J Med 1998;338: 1369–73.
2. Giada F, Raviele A. Diagnostic management of patients with palpitations of unknown origin. Ital Heart J 2004;5(8):581–6.
3. Pickett CC, Zimetbaum PJ. Palpitations: a proper evaluation and approach to effective medical therapy. Curr Cardiol Rep 2005;7:362–7.

4. Abbott AV. Diagnostic approach to palpitations. Am Fam Physician 2005;71:743–50.

5. Brugada P, Gursoy S, Brugada J, et al. Investigation of palpitations. Lancet 1993;341:1254–8.

6. Mayou R. Chest pain, palpitations and panic. J Psychosom Res 1998;44:53–70.

7. Flaker JC, Belew KRN, Beckman K, et al. Asymptomatic atrial fibrillation: demographic features and prognostic information from the Atrial Fibrillation Follow-up Investigation of Rhythm Management (AFFIRM) study. Am Heart J 2005;149:657–63.

8. Hlatky MA. Approach to the patient with palpitations. In: Goldman L, Braunwald E, editors. Primary cardiology. Philadelphia: WB Saunders; 1998. p. 122–8.

9. Zipes DP, Miles WM, Klein LS. Assessment of patients with cardiac arrhythmia. In: Zipes DP, Jalife J, editors. Cardiac electrophysiology: from cell to bedside. Philadelphia: WB Saunders; 1995. p. 1009–12.

10. Leitch J, Klein G, Yee R. Can patients discriminate between atrial fibrillation and regular supraventricular tachycardia? Am J Cardiol 1991;68:962–6.

11. Schwartz PJ, Locati EH, Napolitano C. The long QT syndrome. In: Zipes DP, Jalife J, editors. Cardiac electrophysiology: from cell to bedside. Philadelphia: WB Saunders; 1995. p. 788–811.

12. Gaita F, Giustetto C, Bianchi F. Short QT syndrome: a familial cause of sudden death. Circulation 2003; 108:965–70.

13. Lange R, Hillis D. Cardiovascular complications of cocaine use. N Engl J Med 2001;345:351–8.

14. Furlanello F, Vitali-Serdoz L, Cappato R, et al. Illicit drugs and cardiac arrhythmias in athletes. Eur J Cardiovasc Prev Rehabil 2007;14:487–94.

15. Chignon JM, Lepine JP, Ades J. Panic disorder in cardiac outpatients. Am J Psychiatry 1993;150: 780–5.

16. Barsky AJ, Cleary PD, Coeytaux RR, et al. Psychiatric disorders in medical outpatients complaining of palpitations. J Gen Intern Med 1994;9:306–13.

17. Barsky AJ, Cleary PD, Sarnie MK. Panic disorder, palpitations and awareness of cardiac activity. J Nerv Ment Dis 1994;182:63–71.

18. Jeejeebhoy FM, Dorian P, Newman DM. Panic disorder and the heart: a cardiology perspective. J Psychosom Res 2000;48:393–403.

19. Barsky AJ, Cleary PD, Coeytaux RR, et al. The clinical course of palpitations in medical outpatients. Arch Intern Med 1995;155:1782–8.

20. Tavazzi L, Zotti AM, Rondanelli R. The role of psychologic stress in the genesis of lethal arrhythmias in patients with coronary artery disease. Eur Heart J 1986;7(Suppl A):99–106.

21. Lessmeier TJ, Gamperling D, Johnson-Liddon V, et al. Unrecognized paroxysmal supraventricular tachycardia. Potential for misdiagnosis as panic disorder. Arch Intern Med 1997;157:537–43.

22. Messineo FC. Ventricular ectopic activity: prevalence and risk. Am J Cardiol 1989;64:53J–6J.

23. Kroenke K, Arrington ME, Mangelsdroff AD. The prevalence of symptoms in medical outpatients and the adequacy of therapy. Arch Intern Med 1990;150:1685–9.

24. Knudson MP. The natural history of palpitations in a family practice. J Fam Pract 1987;24:357–60.

25. Weber BE, Kapoor WH. Evaluations and outcomes of patients with palpitations. Am J Med 1996;100: 138–48.

26. Crawford MH, Bernstein SJ, Deedwania PC, et al. CC/AHA guidelines for ambulatory electrocardiography: executive summary and recommendations. A report of the American College of Cardiology/ American Heart Association task force on practice guidelines (committee to revise the guidelines for ambulatory electrocardiography). Circulation 1999; 100:886–9.

27. Kadish AH, Buxton AE, Kennedy HL, et al. ACC/AHA clinical competence statement on electrocardiography and ambulatory electrocardiography. A report of the ACC/AHA/ACP-ASIM task force on clinical competence (ACC/AHA Committee to Develop a Clinical Competence Statement on Electrocardiography and Ambulatory Electrocardiography). J Am Coll Cardiol 2001;38(7):2091–100.

28. Fogel RI, Evans JJ, Prystowsky EN. Utility and cost of event recorders in the diagnosis of palpitations, presyncope and syncope. Am J Cardiol 1997;79: 207–8.

29. Reiffel JA, Schulhof E, Joseph B. Optimum duration of transtelephonic ECG monitoring when used for transient symptomatic event detection. J Electrocardiol 1991;24:165–8.

30. Kinlay S, Leitch JW, Neil A. Cardiac event recorders yield more diagnoses and are more cost-effective than 48-hour Holter monitoring in patients with palpitations. Ann Intern Med 1996;124:16–20.

31. Zimetbaum PJ, Kim KY, Josephson ME, et al. Diagnostic yield and optimal duration of continuous-loop event monitoring for the diagnosis of palpitations. Ann Intern Med 1998;28:890–5.

32. Brown AP, Dawkins KD, Davies JG. Detection of arrhythmias: use of a patient-activated ambulatory electrocardiogram device with a solid-state memory loop. Br Heart J 1987;58:251–3.

33. Zimetbaum P, Kim KY, Ho KKL, et al. Utility of patient-activated cardiac event recorders in general clinical practice. Am J Cardiol 1997;79:371–2.

34. Antman EM, Ludmer PL, McGowan N, et al. Transtelephonic electrocardiographic transmission for management of cardiac arrhythmias. Am J Cardiol 1988; 58:1021–4.

35. Krahn AD, Klein GJ, Raymond Y, et al. Final results from a pilot study with an implantable loop recorder to determine the etiology of syncope in patients with

negative noninvasive and invasive testing. Am J Cardiol 1998;82:117–9.

36. Zimtbaum PJ, Josephson ME. The evolving role of ambulatory arrhythmia monitoring in general practice. Ann Intern Med 1999;150:848–56.

37. Di Marco JP, Philbrick JT. Use of ambulatory electrocardiographic (Holter) monitoring. Ann Intern Med 1990;113:53–68.

38. Joshi AK, Kowey PR, Prystowsky EN. First experience with a Mobile Cardiac Outpatient Telemetry (MCOT) system for the diagnosis and management of cardiac arrhythmias. Am J Cardiol 2005; 95:878–81.

39. Olson JA, Fouts AM, Padalinam BJ, et al. Utility of mobile outpatient telemetry for the diagnosis of palpitations, presyncope, syncope, and the assessment of therapy efficacy. J Cardiovasc Electrophysiol 2007;18(5):437–77.

40. Rothman SA, Laughlin JC, Seltzer J, et al. The diagnosis of cardiac arrhythmias: a prospective multi-center randomized study comparing mobile cardiac outpatient telemetry versus standard loop event monitoring. J Cardiovasc Electrophysiol 2007;18(3):248–9.

41. Krahn AD, Klein GJ, Yee R, et al. The high cost of syncope: cost implications of a new insertable loop recorder in the investigation of recurrent syncope. Am Heart J 1999;137:870–7.

42. Krahn AD, Klein GJ, Yee R, et al. Randomized assessment of syncope trial: conventional diagnostic testing versus a prolonged monitoring strategy. Circulation 2001;104(1):46–56.

43. Waktare JEP, Camm AJ. Holter and event recordings for arrhythmia detection. In: Zareba W, Maison-Blanche P, Locati EH, editors. Noninvasive electrocardiology in clinical practice. Armonk (NY): Futura Publishing Company; 2001. p. 3–30.

44. Paisey JR, Yue AM, Treacher K, et al. Implantable loop recorders detect tachyarrhythmias in symptomatic patients with negative electrophysiological studies. Int J Cardiol 2005;98:35–8.

45. Giada F, Gulizia M, Francese M, et al. Recurrent unexplained palpitations (RUP) study: comparison of implantable loop recorder versus conventional diagnostic strategy. J Am Coll Cardiol 2007;49(19): 1951–6.

46. Raviele A, Giada F, Bergfeldt L, et al. Management of patients with palpitations: a position paper of

European Heart Rhythm Association. Europace 2011;13:920–34.

47. Zipes DP, DiMarco JP, Gillette PC, et al. Guidelines for clinical intracardiac electrophysiological and catheter ablation procedures: a report of the American College of Cardiology/American Heart Association task force on practice guidelines (committee on clinical intracardiac electrophysiologic and catheter ablation procedures), developed in collaboration with the North American Society of Pacing and Electrophysiology. J Am Coll Cardiol 1995;26:555–73.

48. Bonso A, Delise P, Corò L. Palpitazioni d'origine sconosciuta: qual'è l'utilità della stimolazione atriale transesofagea?. In: Piccolo E, Raviele A, editors. Aritmie cardiache. Milan (Italy): Centro Scientifico Editore; 1991. p. 229–36.

49. Hyucke EC, Lai WT, Nguyen NX. Role of intravenous isoproterenol in electrophysiologic induction of atrioventricular node reentrant tachycardia in patients with dual atrioventricular node pathways. Am J Cardiol 1989;64:1131–7.

50. Morady F, Shapiro W, Shen E. Programmed ventricular stimulation in patients without spontaneous ventricular tachycardia. Am Heart J 1984;107:875–82.

51. Delise P, Bonso A, Allibardi PL. Clinical and prognostic value of atrial vulnerability. Evaluation using endocavitary and transesophageal electrophysiologic study. G Ital Cardiol 1990;20:533–42.

52. Brembilla-Perrot B, Spatz F, Khaldi E. Value of esophageal pacing in evaluation of supraventricular tachycardia. Am J Cardiol 1990;65:322–30.

53. Brembilla-Perrot B. Value of oesophageal pacing in evaluation of atrial arrhythmias. Eur Heart J 1994; 15:1085–8.

54. Delise P, Bonso A, Corò L. Endocavitary and transesophageal electrophysiology findings in idiopathic atrial fibrillation. G Ital Cardiol 1991;21:1093–9.

55. Fujimura O, Yee R, Klein G, et al. The diagnostic sensitivity of electrophysiologic testing in patients with syncope caused by transient bradycardia. N Engl J Med 1989;321:1701–7.

56. Brignole M, Menozzi C, Bottoni N. Mechanisms of syncope caused by transient bradycardia and the diagnostic value of electrophysiologic testing and cardiovascular reflexivity maneuvers. Am J Cardiol 1995;76:273–8.

Neonatal and Pediatric Arrhythmias
Clinical and Electrocardiographic Aspects

Fabrizio Drago, MD*, Irma Battipaglia, MD,
Corrado Di Mambro, MD

KEYWORDS

• Children • Neonates • Arrhythmias • ECG • Bradycardia • Tachycardia • Pediatric arrhythmias

KEY POINTS

- Correct interpretation of an electrocardiogram in children and neonates has different principles from adults; detailed knowledge of these age-dependent changes should be well-known to avoid misinterpretation.
- It is important to know that sinus arrhythmia, ectopic atrial rhythm, "wandering pacemaker," and functional rhythm can be normal characteristics in children.
- Treatment of tachyarrhythmias in children depends on natural history, and height and weight of the patient; in small children, medical treatment can postpone transcatheter ablation.
- Bradyarrhythmias can require pacemaker implantation in children.
- Endocardial or epicardial approach should be chosen depending on the weight and the height of the patient.

INTRODUCTION

Over the last years, arrhythmias have acquired a specific identity also in the field of pediatric cardiology. Pediatric electrophysiologists provide a better diagnostic and therapeutic process, but, for general pediatric cardiologists, it has always been difficult to recognize and treat even simple arrhythmias. This article aims to describe the electrocardiographic aspects of the pediatric electrocardiogram (ECG) and most frequent cardiac arrhythmias.

ELECTROCARDIOGRAPHY IN NEONATES AND CHILDREN: WHAT IS NOT PATHOLOGIC

The basic principles of ECG interpretation in children are identical to those applied in adults. However, progressive ECG changes in anatomy and physiology, taking place between birth and adolescence, result in some features that differ significantly from the normal adult pattern and vary according to the age of the child. Correct interpretation of the ECG is, therefore, potentially difficult, and a detailed knowledge of these age-dependent changes is critically important to avoiding misinterpretation and risky errors.[1]

For example, in pediatric patients, a positive T wave in V2 to V3 can have a "camel hump" aspect, that consists of a second peak starting on the first one-half of the descending part of the T wave. This configuration is due to the particular repolarization pattern in children, which describes a "figure-of-8" pattern rotating in a counterclockwise and then a clockwise direction. The "camel hump" T wave is absent in adults as the repolarization pattern modifies with the growth.

Disclosure Statement: The authors have nothing to disclose.
Paediatric Cardiology and Cardiac Arrhythmias Unit, Department of Paediatric Cardiology and Cardiac Surgery, Bambino Gesù Children's Hospital and Research Institute, Piazza Sant'Onofrio 4, Rome 00165, Italy
* Corresponding author.
E-mail address: fabrizio.drago@opbg.net

Card Electrophysiol Clin 10 (2018) 397–412
https://doi.org/10.1016/j.ccep.2018.02.008

Sinus arrhythmia, ectopic atrial rhythm, "wandering pacemaker," and junctional rhythm can be normal characteristics in children (15%–25% of healthy children can have these rhythms at the ECG).

Sinus Arrhythmia

According to several reported studies on 24-hour ECG Holter monitoring, all normal children and young adults have evidence of sinus arrhythmia, defined as spontaneous change in adjacent cycle lengths of 100% or more.[2–4] On the ECG, an irregular rhythm can be observed, with gradual variations in PP intervals, a sinus P wave that precedes each QRS, and rates varying with phase of breathing (increase with inspiration and decrease with expiration). During increased vagal tone, sinus pauses of various degree interrupted by escape beats and/or rhythms may be detected (escape beats may be of atrial, junctional, or ventricular origin).[5]

Wandering Pacemaker

This terminology is used when the ECG shows an irregular rhythm with ongoing changes in P wave morphology, with associated changes in PP interval during more than 2 beats, often appearing during period of low heart rates. Wandering atrial pacemaker rhythm is found in 25% of healthy newborn infants, 34% of healthy 10- to 13-year-old boys; 26% of 14- to 16-year-old boys; and 54% of medical students.[1–5] Atrial ectopic rhythm is distinguished from wandering atrial pacemaker rhythm by its unchanging P wave axis/morphology.

Junctional Rhythm

Junctional beats or rhythm can be found during phases of sinus arrhythmia and, for this reason, they are common in the pediatric population. On the ECG, we can observe (1) a regular rhythm with narrow QRS (or QRS resembling the patient's normal QRS), (2) heart rates between 40 and 100 bpm (according to the age), and (3) P waves dissociated from or after each QRS (retrograde conduction). The heart rate, relative to age and activity, is fundamental in deciding whether the junctional rhythm is normal and benign or junctional tachycardia should be considered.

In particular, junctional rhythm occurs in the age group of children with more vagotonia (13% of 10- to 13-year-old boys during sleep,[6] 45% of 7- to 10-year-old children,[1] and 19% of infants).[2] Endurance athletes have a 20% incidence of junctional rhythm, as well.[7]

PEDIATRIC ARRHYTHMIAS
Physiopathology

Cardiac arrhythmias are determined by a disorder in the generation or conduction of the electrical impulse. As for adult patients, also in pediatric patients (neonates, children, and adolescents) tachyarrhythmias are caused by enhanced automaticity, triggered activity or reentry mechanism, whereas bradyarrhythmias derive from missing generation of the impulse, or a slow or blocked conduction through the specific conduction system of the heart.[8–11]

Terminology and Classification

In pediatric patients, a diagnosis of bradycardia depends on the age.[12,13] In general, bradycardia is defined, at rest and awake, as a heart rate of less than 100 bpm in children up to 3 years old, less than 60 bpm in patients 3 to 9 years old, less than 50 bpm in patients 9 to 16 years old, and less than 40 bpm for patients older than 16 years. During sleep, these cutoffs are reduced by 15% to 20%.

A first-degree atrioventricular (AV) block is diagnosed when the PQ interval is longer than the maximum limit for age (140 ms in a child <1 year old, 150 ms in 1- to 5-year-old children, 160 ms in 5- to 10-year-old children, and 200 ms in older children).

Tachycardia is defined as a sequence of 3 or more beats at a rate that is more than 25% of the sinus rate at the onset of the arrhythmia (usually 120 bpm). Tachycardia can be sustained or not sustained (lasting >30 seconds or <30 seconds), paroxysmal (sudden onset and termination), or permanent/incessant (it is present for >20% of the time in 24 hours). A tachycardia is considered supraventricular if it originates from atria and the AV junction, and ventricular if it originates below the His bifurcation.

TACHYARRHYTHMIAS
Premature Supraventricular Beats

Generally, premature supraventricular beats are an idiopathic and clinically silent cardiac arrhythmia. Premature supraventricular beats originate from the atria or the AV junction and are diagnosed occasionally (sometimes during fetal life). Supraventricular extra beats, in neonates, can determine the so-called pseudo-bradycardia, when conduction to the ventricles is blocked, and usually disappears during the first year of life. This arrhythmia does not need to be treated.

Premature Ventricular Beats

Premature ventricular beats are usually idiopathic and not associated with symptoms. However, when they are documented, a cardiac disease or arrhythmias that are more complex must be excluded. Premature ventricular beats can be considered benign when they occur in normal heart as isolated beats, with 1 morphology, and are suppressed by exercise. In this case, they do not need any treatment and disappear spontaneously as the patients grows (**Fig. 1**).

Paroxysmal Supraventricular Reentry Tachycardia

Paroxysmal supraventricular reentry tachycardia is the most common arrhythmia in pediatric patients (82%). Its exact incidence is unknown, but it has been estimated from 1 in 250 to 1 in 1000, with a peak during the neonatal and prepubescent ages. Often, preschool children can describe palpitations as "precordial pain"; when the SVT is fast and not hemodynamically tolerated, weakness, dizziness, and syncope may occur. Reentry tachyarrhythmias can have a heart rate from 180 to 340 bpm.

- SVTs owing to accessory pathways is defined as AV reentry tachycardia and is the most

common form of tachycardia in pediatric patients (with an incidence increasing from 60% to 80% going from childhood into adolescence). These tachycardias have 2 peaks of incidence: the first year of life and ages 8 to 12. Accessory pathways, when they are capable of anterograde conduction, show ventricular preexcitation on the ECG (the association of ventricular preexcitation and symptoms related to the occurrence of SVT is called Wolff–Parkinson–White syndrome). Usually, this arrhythmia occurs in children with a structurally normal heart but, sometimes, it can be associated with an Ebstein anomaly, mitral valve prolapse, ventricular septal defect, and congenitally corrected transposition of the great arteries.[14–17] In neonates, SVT can be frequent because it is initiated by atrial extra beats, or only by the rapid acceleration of sinus rhythm during feeding or crying. After the first year of life, the frequency of recurrences tends to decrease because of a decrease in the number of atrial extra beats, and a better sympathovagal balance. Transesophageal pacing shows a disappearance of the reentry circuit in 50% of cases at 1 year of age[18] (**Fig. 2**).

- A paroxysmal SVT owing to a reentry in the AV node is defined as AV nodal reentry

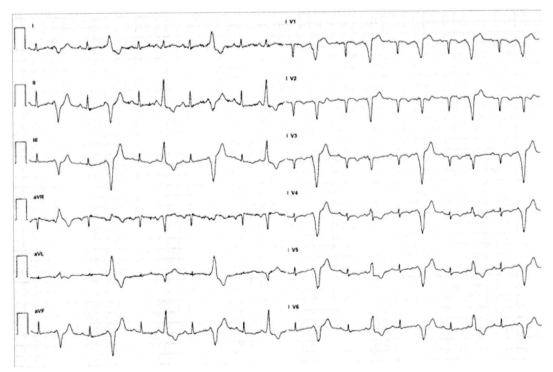

Fig. 1. Ectopic ventricular beats.

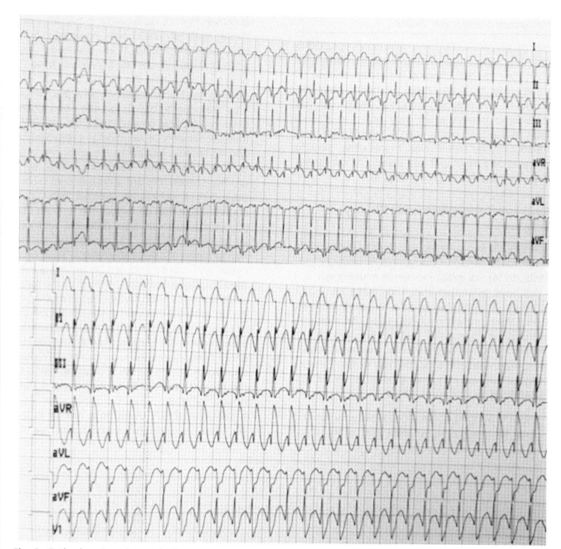

Fig. 2. Orthodromic atrioventricular reentry tachycardia with and without right bundle branch aberrancy.

tachycardia and it is rather rare in pediatric age (13%–16% of all SVTs). AV nodal reentry tachycardia is caused by a reentry through 2 different pathways, the slow pathway and the fast pathway. However, only 30% to 40% of children with this tachycardia show a double nodal conduction at the electrophysiologic study. Interestingly, AV nodal reentry tachycardia with 2:1 transient AV conduction block is present in 17% of children during electrophysiologic study, a much greater proportion than seen in adults (9%). Clinical manifestations of this tachycardia are variable and usually females are more symptomatic than male.[19] About its prognosis, AV nodal reentry tachycardia is a benign tachyarrhythmia and, nowadays, very safe. Effective ablation techniques exist for its treatment (such as

cryoablation with 3-dimensional mapping system guide)[20–27] (**Figs. 3** and **4**).

- Among the pediatric SVTs, there is a particular type of AV reentry tachycardia called permanent junctional reentry tachycardia. It represents 4% of all pediatric SVTs and it is due to the presence of an accessory pathway (usually on the right side of the heart, around the tricuspid annulus) capable of decremental retrograde conduction. In general, this is an incessant form of tachycardia very often responsible for left ventricular dysfunction. ECG tracings of this SVT are characterized by negative P wave in inferior leads and an RP interval that is longer than the PR interval.[28] Usually, permanent junctional reentry tachycardia onset is caused by an increase in sinus

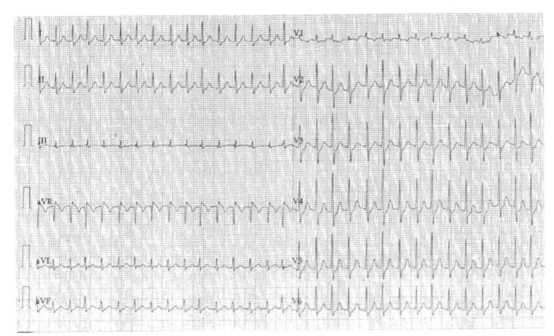

Fig. 3. Typical atrioventricular nodal reentry tachycardia.

rate. Permanent junctional reentry tachy-cardia is often resistant to drug therapy and, for this reason, the only treatment may be transcatheter ablation (recurrence rate of 20%). Nevertheless, spontaneous resolution has been described as well[29] (**Fig. 5**).

Therapy
Vagal maneuvers are effective in 70% of cases (diving reflex, Valsalva maneuver, carotid sinus massage, squatting position). When the SVT does not stop, antiarrhythmic drugs can be administered.

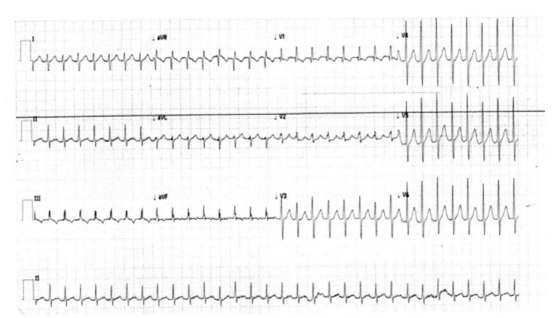

Fig. 4. Orthodromic atrioventricular reentry tachycardia in a patient with a right posteroseptal accessory pathway.

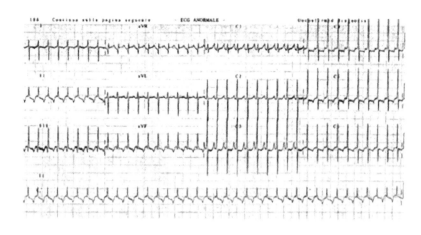

s/p Krenosin

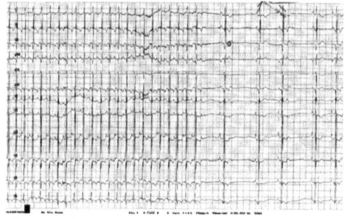

Fig. 5. Neonatal permanent junctional reentry tachycardia.

When the hemodynamic condition is stable, the first choice drug is adenosine fast bolus intravenously (IV). It can be repeated 3 times (100 μg/kg the first 2 times and then a double dose as a last attempt). If adenosine is unsuccessful, 1C class drugs are recommended (flecainide 1.5–2 mg/kg in 3–5 minutes, propafenone 1.5 mg/kg in 3–5 minutes). Amiodarone is used only in refractory cases or in patients with a reduced ejection fraction (5 mg/kg in 20 minutes followed by infusion of 10 mg/kg in 24 hours).

In cases of severe heart failure or cardiogenic shock, synchronized external electric cardioversion (0.5–1.5 J/kg) or transesophageal atrial pacing should be used.

In all forms of paroxysmal SVTs, antiarrhythmic prophylaxis should be started to avoid recurrences, using flecainide (2–7 mg/kg/d in 3 doses), propafenone (10–15 mg/kg/d in 3 doses), amiodarone (loading dose of 10–20 mg/kg/d in 1–2 administrations for 7–10 days; maintenance dose of 3–7 mg/kg/d in 1–2 administrations), or sotalol (2–8 mg/kg/d in 2–3 administrations). Class 1C drugs and amiodarone can be associated with beta-blockers (propranolol 1–3 mg/kg/d in 3–4 doses, nadolol 1–2 mg/kg/d in 1–2 doses, metoprolol 2–2.5 mg/kg/d in 2 administrations).

Transesophageal atrial pacing, especially in neonates, can test the efficacy of the medical treatment. Transcatheter ablation can be used any time in case of drug refractoriness or electively when the child weighs more than 20 to 25 kg.

Atrial Flutter

Atrial flutter is an intraatrial macroreentry tachycardia that can involve the whole atrium or just a part of it. The ECG is quite typical, with characteristic saw-tooth P waves. In pediatric patients, it has very fast atrial rate (275–580 bpm) but functional block in the AV junction (more often 2:1) slows down the ventricular rate.

Neonatal atrial flutter is rare (0.03% of neonates) and usually idiopathic.[30] In 12% to 33% of cases, it is associated with the presence of accessory pathways. In contrast, atrial flutter is common in patients with congenital heart disease, in particular when right atrial hypertrophy or dilation is present. Electrophysiologic study is useful to understand the arrhythmia mechanism and the existence of SVTs (AV reentry tachycardia, AV nodal reentry tachycardia) degenerating in atrial flutter (**Figs. 6** and **7**).

Therapy

In neonates, if well-tolerated, cardioversion can be delayed because sometimes the arrhythmia terminates spontaneously after 24 to 48 hours (26% of cases). For a persistent atrial flutter, electric or pharmacologic cardioversion using amiodarone (5 mg/kg in 20 minutes) can be practiced. In cases of hemodynamic intolerance, the electric cardioversion is the first-line therapy. In general, in neonates with no other arrhythmic substrate (eg, accessory pathways) there are no recurrences. Instead, in older patients a prophylactic therapy is needed: 1C antiarrhythmic drugs associated with beta-blockers or, as an alternative, amiodarone. In patients weighing more than 30 kg, transcatheter ablation can be considered.

Automatic Supraventricular Tachycardias

These tachyarrhythmias are generally owing to enhanced phase 4 automaticity, with "warm up/ cool down" behavior, often with wide fluctuations in the atrial rate secondary to the autonomic tone. They can be paroxysmal or permanent, and isolated or associated with structural heart disease. AV conduction can be variable. Automatic tachycardias are often associated with a heart rate only slightly higher than normal sinus rhythm, causing persistent weakness and reduced exercise tolerance.

However, after a while, it can provoke heart failure. A characteristic clinical scenario can be "tachycardiomyopathy," which can regress through an effective rate control. An IV bolus of adenosine can cause persistence of atrial tachycardia with complete or incomplete AV block. That tool can be useful in making the differential diagnosis and to evaluate the morphology and axis of ectopic P waves.

Ectopic atrial tachycardia

Ectopic atrial tachycardia is a rare tachycardia in pediatric patients (14% of all SVTs). It is more often due to an increased automaticity of myocardial cells, but triggered activity cannot be excluded. The most common ectopic foci are localized in the right appendage, in the crista terminalis, around the pulmonary veins, but a focus can exist at any place in the right or left atrium. On the ECG, the P wave can be visible and different from the sinus rhythm. Atrial rate during tachycardia ranges from 130 to 300 bpm, and it is influenced by autonomic tone variations. First- and second-degree AV blocks can be present (**Figs. 8** and **9**).

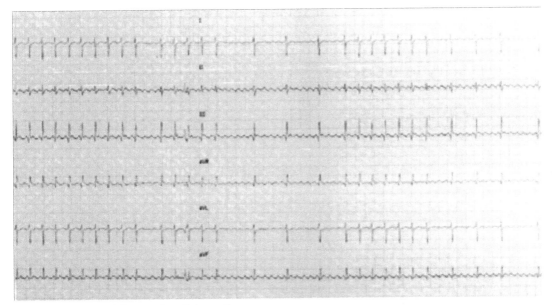

Fig. 6. Neonatal atrial flutter after diving reflex.

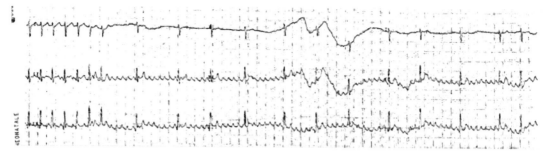

Fig. 7. Neonatal atrial flutter after subministration of Krenosin.

Multifocal atrial tachycardia

Multifocal atrial tachycardia is more common in neonates and in males. It is usually idiopathic, although it can be associated with syncytial respiratory virus infection. Multifocal atrial tachycardia is characterized by 3 or more different P wave morphologies and it is often incessant. First- and second-degree AV blocks cause variable PR and RR interval, and a relatively slow heart rate rarely driving to heart failure (**Figs. 10** and **11**).

Junctional ectopic tachycardia

Junctional ectopic tachycardia is distinguished in 2 forms: congenital junctional ectopic tachycardia, which is quite rare, and postoperative junctional ectopic tachycardia, which occurs after surgery for a congenital heart defect involving the AV junction (tetralogy of Fallot, ventricular septal defect, AV canal, truncus arteriosus, etc).[31–33]

Junctional ectopic tachycardia is due to automatic foci inside the AV junction (from the AV node to the His bundle). Both forms are associated with high mortality and morbidity. Idiopathic junctional ectopic tachycardia is often congenital and familiar in 50% of cases. It is usually incessant and this can cause heart failure and even sudden death owing to paroxysmal AV block (as a consequence of fibrosis of the AV junction owing to autoimmune mechanisms responsible for the tachycardia).

On the ECG, AV dissociation is generally present, as with ventricular tachycardia, but with a narrow QRS. However, in neonates and infants, a 1:1 ventriculoatrial retroconduction with negative P waves in inferior leads can be possible

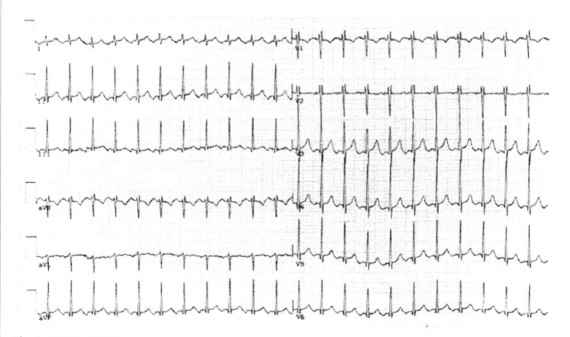

Fig. 8. Ectopic atrial tachycardia.

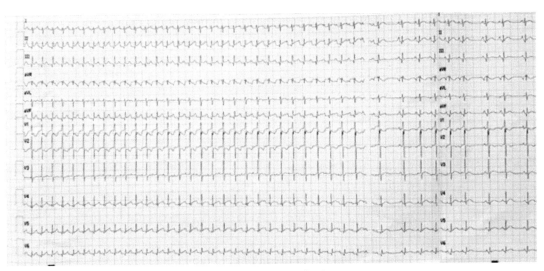

Fig. 9. Ectopic atrial tachycardia multiple atrioventricular conduction.

owing to a lower effective refractory period of AV node in this particular patients. The heart rate is between 140 and 370 bpm, and it can change with autonomic changes and body temperature (**Fig. 12**).

Therapy

Automatic tachycardias owing to an enhanced automatic activity cannot be terminate by pacing maneuvers. Pharmacologic therapy is usually effective, with the exception of idiopathic junctional ectopic tachycardia, which can be resistant to many drugs, and sometimes rate control is the only possible target to reach. In case of a stable hemodynamic state, first choice drug are beta-blockers (propranolol, nadolol, metoprolol); as an alternative class 1C antiarrhythmic drugs can be used (flecainide, propafenone). In cases of reduced ejection fraction or resistance to other antiarrhythmic drugs, the use of amiodarone is suggested.

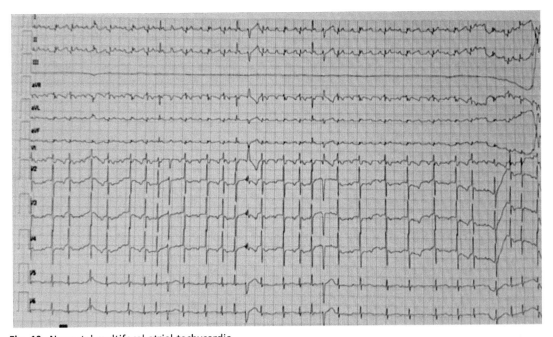

Fig. 10. Neonatal multifocal atrial tachycardia.

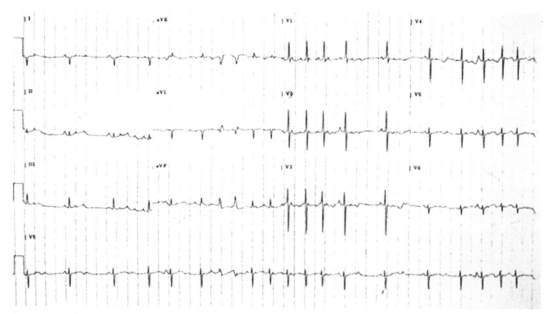

Fig. 11. Multifocal atrial tachycardia.

Transcatheter ablation can be effective in 80% to 85% of the cases and can be performed at any age when necessary or, electively, when the patient weights more than 20 kg. Cryoablation is suggested as a first-line strategy for junctional ectopic tachycardia, because radiofrequency transcatheter ablation can determine more easily damage to the His bundle with consequent need of PMK implant.

Ventricular Tachycardia

VT is rare in pediatric patients (5%–10% of all tachyarrhythmias). It can be idiopathic or an expression of a structural heart disease such as cardiomyopathy, myocarditis, cardiac tumor, electrolytes disorder, or a channelopathy. Secondary forms are more frequent than idiopathic ones. Idiopathic VTs include VT originating from the right ventricular outflow tract (58%), fascicular VT (23%), and polymorphic VT (19%). Idiopathic ventricular tachycardias are generally associated with a benign prognosis. In contrast, for VTs that are an expression of a structural disease, the prognosis depends on the primary disease.

The ECG shows typical signs of ventricular tachycardias: a large QRS, QRS axis different from the sinus rhythm, AV dissociation, fusion, and capture beats. An echocardiogram, Holter monitoring, exercise stress testing, and serum

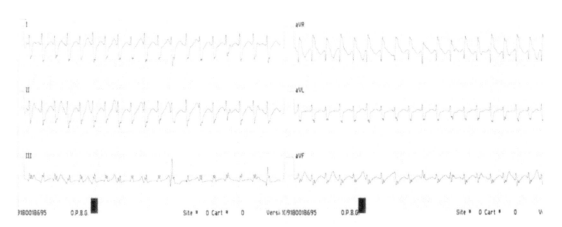

Fig. 12. Junctional ectopic tachycardia.

electrolytes check are indicated for all patients. In some cases, electrophysiologic study and more advanced imaging techniques are needed.

Therapy

If symptoms are severe or in cases of heart failure, synchronized electric cardioversion (or a DC shock for ventricular fibrillation) must be delivered (3–7 J/kg). Then, pharmacologic therapy to prevent recurrences can be started: lidocaine (1 mg/kg in bolus to repeat if necessary every 5 minutes, followed by infusion of 20–50 μg/kg/min), magnesium sulfate (30–50 mg/kg in bolus), and/or amiodarone. When the tachycardia is hemodynamically well-tolerated, amiodarone is the drug of choice in case of a reduction in ejection fraction. If the ejection fraction is preserved, propafenone, flecainide, sotalol, propranolol, nadolol, and metoprolol can be used alone or concomitantly. VTs can be treated by transcatheter ablation in case of refractoriness to drug therapy or in older patients (weight >30 kg or in patients after puberty; **Fig. 13**).

Neonatal ventricular tachycardia Neonatal VT is an incessant VT with a low heart rate that usually occurs in neonates with a normal structural heart. Usually, it does not require any treatment and it tends to disappear spontaneously after the first year of life. However, when VT is secondary to cardiac disease, it can be malignant, with a high and variable heart rate, and it can cause heart failure. Thus, it requires drug therapy, often combining

different drugs, or surgical or transcatheter treatment (**Figs. 14** and **15**).

Ventricular tachycardia originating from the right ventricle VT originating from the right ventricle is the most frequent type of VT. From a clinical point of view, these tachycardias can be or not be associated with symptoms (from palpitations to syncope). They are usually due to a triggered activity, but sometimes increased automaticity or reentry can be responsible for the cardiac arrhythmia. The ECG shows a left bundle branch block and inferior axis.[34] This VT can be paroxysmal (in this case, it is usually triggered by a physical activity), incessant, or iterative. The paroxysmal form is usually present in short runs of VT at 130 to 150 bpm, suppressed by an increase in sinus rhythm, not associated with symptoms, and carries a good prognosis. The incessant form causes longer runs of VT at heart rate greater than 150 bpm, which can cause heart failure. This form is treated by drugs (beta-blockers, class 1C, class III antiarrhythmic drugs) or by transcatheter ablation.

Fascicular ventricular tachycardia Fascicular VT originates from the inferior/septal wall of the left ventricle, sometimes from the inferior-posterior portion of the left bundle branch.[35] It shows right bundle branch block QRS complexes with superior axis (more rarely inferior axis) and a heart rate of 120 to 250 bpm. It usually occurs as a paroxysmal arrhythmia, during the second to fourth decades of life, and more frequently in

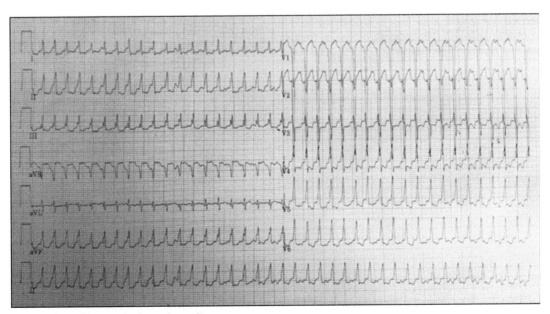

Fig. 13. Idiopathic ventricular tachycardia.

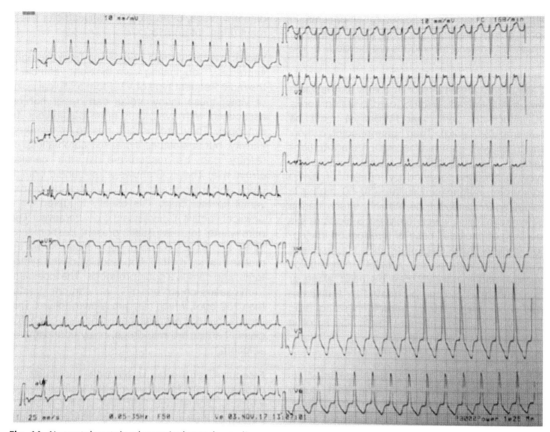

Fig. 14. Neonatal sustained ventricular tachycardia.

men. Often, fascicular tachycardia is triggered by physical activity or emotion. When it is not associated with symptoms, therapy is not necessary because the prognosis is good. When therapy is needed, verapamil is the first choice drug; beta-blockers, class 1C, 1B, class III drugs, or transcatheter ablation can be used.

BRADYARRHYTHMIAS
Atrioventricular Block

AV block is an arrhythmia owing to a disorder in AV conduction. First-degree AV block is characterized by a prolongation of the AV conduction (PR interval on ECG) over 17 to 20 ms, according to the

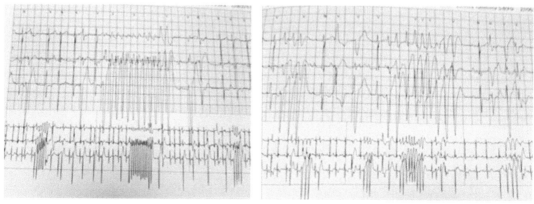

Fig. 15. Nonsustained ventricular tachycardia/ventricular flutter in patient with heart transplant (Holter electrocardiographic monitoring).

patient's age. Second-degree AV block (Mobitz 1) consists of a progressive prolongation of the PR interval until a P wave is blocked and not followed by a QRS. Second-degree AV block (Mobitz 2) is an intermittent and sudden block in the AV conduction (suddenly P waves are not followed by QRS). In third-degree AV block, there is a complete interruption of the AV conduction so that P waves are independent from QRS complexes, which derive from a junctional or ventricular escape rhythm.

AV block can be isolated or associated with a congenital heart disease (25%–50%). First-degree and second-degree Mobitz 1 AV block are clinically silent and are discovered occasionally. Second-degree Mobitz 2 and third-degree AV block can be asymptomatic, symptomatic (weakness, presyncope, or syncope), or associated with heart failure. Third-degree AV block can be congenital, and is sometimes associated with congenital heart disease (congenitally corrected transposition of the great arteries or univentricular heart). In 70% to 80% of congenital isolated AV block, maternal autoantibodies (SSA/Ro and SSB/La) cross the placenta between the 16th and 23rd weeks of gestation, damaging the fetal heart conduction system.[36,37]

Diagnosis is based on ECG, ECG Holter monitoring, event recorder devices, and implantable loop recorders. Echocardiography, exercise stress testing, and electrophysiologic study can complete the diagnostic process and prognostic stratification (**Figs. 16** and **17**).

Therapy

First-degree and second-degree AV block do not necessitate any therapy. Mobitz 2 and third-degree AV block require pacemaker implantation in the neonate if the heart rate is less than 55 bpm in a structurally normal heart or less than 70 bpm if a congenital heart disease is present. Pacemaker implantation is also recommended if a large QRS escape rhythm or ventricular dysfunction is present.

In neonates, the implant is epicardial. The preferred pacing site is the left ventricle apex and, if body dimension allows, dual-chamber pacing is preferred. In children weighing more than 20 kg, a transvenous implant can be performed, preferably choosing as pacing sites the right atrial appendage and the right ventricle septum.[38–42]

Sinus Atrial Node Dysfunction

Sinus atrial node dysfunction includes many different bradyarrhythmias, namely, sinus bradycardia, sinus pauses, and junctional bradycardia. ECG criteria for the diagnosis of sinus node dysfunction include sinus bradycardia, sinus pauses of greater than 3 seconds, and a slow escape rhythm. Some other arrhythmias may be wrongly interpreted as sinus node dysfunction include a second-degree AV block 2:1, bigeminal atrial extra beat blocked, and a complete AV block when atrial and ventricular rate seem synchronous.

Sinus atrial node dysfunction can be due to (1) noncardiac causes (neurologic or metabolic disorders) or (2) intrinsic anomalies of sinus node function. Sinus bradycardia, sinus pauses, and junctional escape beats can occur in 20% to 90% of normal neonates, and more often in preterm or low weight babies. In neonates, sinus pauses of 800 to 1000 ms can be present, but

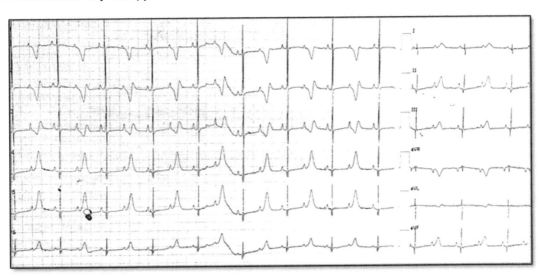

Fig. 16. Functional atrioventricular block 2:1 in long QT syndrome.

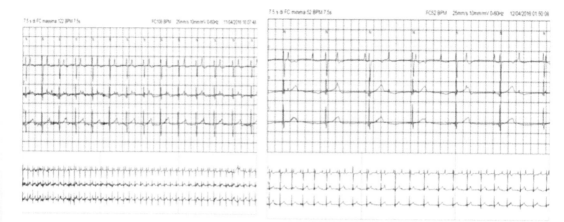

Fig. 17. Infant with first-degree atrioventricular block and complete atrioventricular block (electrocardiographic Holter monitoring).

pauses of longer than 2000 ms are considered pathologic. A junctional rhythm can be present in healthy neonates as well. Transient bradycardias and QT interval prolongation ($\leq$470 ms) can be the result of a stressful delivery, but usually these forms normalize in 48 to 72 hours.

A secondary sinus bradycardia in a neonate can be consequence of sepsis, central nervous system anomalies, hypothermia, hypopituitarism, intracranial hypertension, meningitis, maternal assumption of drugs, obstructive icterus, hypothyroidism, electrolytes or metabolic alterations, maternal autoimmune diseases. Sinus atrial node dysfunction can be associated with congenital heart disease in the natural history (eg, atrial septum defect, AV canal defect, Ebstein anomaly, and a single ventricle) or, more often, after heart surgery (eg, Fontan, Mustard, and Sening operations).

Patients with sinus atrial node dysfunction can be completely asymptomatic or may suffer from weakness, pallor, presyncope/syncope, or heart failure. Parents should be very careful to recognize symptoms that sometimes can be very sneaky.

If acute support is needed atropine (0.02–0.04 mg/kg IV), isoproterenol (0.02–0.05 μg/kg/min), adrenaline (0.01 mg/kg IV), or, if necessary, external transthoracic or transvenous pacing are suggested. When associated with symptoms, pacemaker implantation is among the class 1 indications.[43]

REFERENCES

1. Dickinson DF. The normal ECG in childhood and adolescence. Heart 2005;91:1626–30.
2. Southall DP, Richards J, Mitchell P, et al. Study of cardiac rhythm in healthy newborn infants. Br Heart J 1980;43:14–20.
3. Dickinson DF, Scott O. Ambulatory electrocardiographic monitoring in 100 healthy teenage boys. Br Heart J 1984;51:179–83.
4. Brodsky M, Wu D, Denes P, et al. Arrhythmias documented by 24 hour continuous electrocardiographic monitoring in 50 male medical students without apparent heart disease. Am J Cardiol 1977;39:390–5.
5. Randall WC, Wehrmacher WH, Jones SB. Hierarchy of supraventricular pacemakers. J Thorac Cardiovasc Surg 1981;82:797–800.
6. Scott O, Williams GJ, Fiddler GI. Results of 24 hour ambulatory monitoring of electrocardiogram in 131 healthy boys aged 10 to 13 years. Br Heart J 1980;44:304–8.
7. Viitasalo MT, Kala R, Eisalo A. Ambulatory electrocardiographic recording in endurance athletes. Br Heart J 1982;47:213–20.
8. Zipes DP, Jalife J, editors. Cardiac electrophysiology; from cell to bedside. 4th edition. Philadelphia: WB Saunders, Elsevier; 2004.
9. Wit AL, Rosen MR. Pathophysiologic mechanisms of cardiac arrhythmias. Am Heart J 1983;106:798.
10. Rosen MR. The links between basic and clinical cardiac electrophysiology. Circulation 1988;77:251.
11. Brugada J, Blom N, Sarquella-Brugada G, et al. Pharmacological and non-pharmacological therapy for arrhythmias in the pediatric population: EHRA and AEPC-Arrhythmia Working Group joint consensus statement. Europace 2013;15:1337–82.
12. Deal BJ, Wolff GS, Gelband H, editors. Current concepts in diagnosis and management of arrhythmias in infants and children. Armonk (NY): Futura; 1998.
13. Gillette PC, Garson A, editors. Clinical pediatric arrhythmias. 2nd edition. Philadelphia: WB Saunders; 1999.
14. Ko JK, Deal BJ, Strasburger JF, et al. Supraventricular tachycardia mechanism and their age

distribution in pediatric patients. Am J Cardiol 1992;69:1028–32.

15. Giardina AC, Ehlers KH, Engle MA. Wolff-Parkinson-White syndrome in infants and children. A longterm follow-up study. Br Heart J 1972;34:839–46.

16. Deal BJ, Keane JF, Gillette PC, et al. Wolff-Parkinson-White syndrome and supraventricular tachycardia during infancy: management and follow-up. J Am Coll Cardiol 1985;5:130–5.

17. Perry JC, Garson A. Supraventricular tachycardia due to WPW syndrome in children: early disappearance and late recurrence. J Am Coll Cardiol 1990; 16:1215–20.

18. Drago F, Silvetti MS, De Santis A, et al. Reciprocating supraventricular tachycardia in infants: electrophysiologically-guided medical treatment and long-term evolution of the reentry circuit. Europace 2008;10:629–35.

19. Drago F, Grutter G, Silvetti MS, et al. Atrioventricular nodal reentrant tachycardia in children. Pediatr Cardiol 2006;27:454–9.

20. Bauersfeld U, Pfammatter JP, Jaeggi E. Treatment of supraventricular tachycardias in the new millennium-drugs or radiofrequency catheter ablation? Eur J Pediatr 2001;160:1–9.

21. Van Hare GF, Javitz H, Carmelli D, et al. Prospective assessment after pediatric cardiac ablation: demographics, medical profiles, and initial outcomes. J Cardiovasc Electrophysiol 2004;15:759–70.

22. Drago F, Silvetti MS, Di Pino A, et al. Exclusion of fluoroscopy during ablation treatment of right accessory pathway in children. J Cardiovasc Electrophysiol 2002;13:778–82.

23. Miyazaki A, Blaufox AD, Fairbrother DL, et al. Cryoablation for septal tachycardia substrates in pediatric patients: mid-term results. J Am Coll Cardiol 2005;45:581–8.

24. Drago F, De Santis A, Grutter G, et al. Transvenous cryothermal catheter ablation of re-entry circuit located near the atrioventricular junction in pediatric patients: efficacy, safety, and midterm follow-up. J Am Coll Cardiol 2005;45:1096–103.

25. Drago F, Silvetti MS, De Santis A, et al. Lengthier cryoablation and a bonus cryoapplication is associated with improved efficacy for cryo catheter ablation of supraventricular tachycardias in children. J Interv Card Electrophysiol 2006;16: 191–8.

26. Drago F, Russo MS, Battipaglia I, et al. The need for a lengthier cryolesion can predict a worse outcome in 3D cryoablation of AV nodal slow pathway in children. Pacing Clin Electrophysiol 2016;39:1198–205.

27. Drago F, Battipaglia I, Russo MS, et al. Voltage gradient mapping and electrophysiologically guided cryoablation in children with AVNRT. Europace 2018; 20(4):665–72.

28. Drago F, Silvetti MS, Mazza A, et al. Permanent junctional reciprocating tachycardia in infants and children: effectiveness of medical and non-medical treatment. Ital Heart J 2001;2:456–61.

29. Lindinger A, Heisel A, Von Bernuth G, et al. Permanent junctional reentry tachycardia. A multicentre long-term follow up study in infants, children and young adults. Eur Heart J 1998;19: 936–42.

30. Texter KM, Kertesz NJ, Friedman RA, et al. Atrial flutter in infants. J Am Coll Cardiol 2006;48: 1040–6.

31. Villain E, Vetter VL, Garcia JM, et al. Evolving concepts in the management of junctional ectopic tachycardia. A multicentre study. Circulation 1990; 81:1544–9.

32. Sarubbi B, Musto B, Ducceschi V, et al. Congenital junctional ectopic tachycardia in children and adolescents: a 20 years experience based study. Heart 2002;88:188–90.

33. Dodge-Khatami A, Miller OI, Anderson RH, et al. Surgical substrates of postoperative junctional ectopic tachycardia in congenital heart defects. J Thorac Cardiovasc Surg 2002;123:624–30.

34. Vignati G, Drago F, Mauri L, et al. Idiopathic recurrent ventricular tachycardia in children: characteristics and long-term prognosis. G Ital Cardiol 1996;26: 747–55.

35. Ohe T, Aihara N, Kamakura S, et al. Long-term outcome of verapamil- sensitive sustained left ventricular tachycardia in patterns without structural heart disease. J Am Coll Cardiol 1995;25: 54–8.

36. Michealsson M, Engle M. Congenital complete heart block: an international study of the natural history. Cardiovasc Clin 1972;4(3):85–101.

37. Jaeggi ET, Hamilton RM, Silverman ED, et al. Outcome of children with fetal, neonatal or childhood diagnosis of isolated congenital atrioventricular block. A single institution experience of 30 years. J Am Coll Cardiol 2002;39:130–7.

38. Gillette PC, Zeigler VL, Winslow AT, et al. Cardiac pacing in neonates, infants and preschool children. Pacing Clin Electrophysiol 1992;15:2046–9.

39. Silvetti MS, Drago F, Grutter G, et al. Twenty years of cardiac pacing in paediatric age: 515 pacemakers and 480 leads implanted in 292 patients. Europace 2006;8:530–6.

40. Silvetti MS, Drago F, Marcora S, et al. Outcome of single-chamber, ventricular pacemakers with transvenous leads implanted in children. Europace 2007;9:894–9.

41. Drago F, Silvetti MS, De Santis A, et al. Closed loop stimulation improves ejection fraction in pediatric patients with pacemaker and ventricular dysfunction. Pacing Clin Electrophysiol 2007;30: 33–7.

42. Silvetti MS, Di Carlo D, Ammirati A, et al. Left ventricular pacing in neonates and infants with isolated congenital complete or advanced atrioventricular block: short-and medium-term outcome. Europace 2015;17:603–10.

43. Nof E, Luria D, Brass D, et al. Point mutation in the HCN4 cardiac ion channel pore affecting synthesis, trafficking, and functional expression is associated with familial asymptomatic sinus bradycardia. Circulation 2007;116:463–70.

Electrocardiogram and Imaging

An Integrated Approach to Arrhythmogenic Cardiomyopathies

Check for updates

Ketty Savino, MD[a],*, Giuseppe Bagliani, MD[b],
Federico Crusco, MD[c], Margherita Padeletti, MD[d],
Massimo Lombardi, MD, FESC[e]

KEYWORDS

- Electrocardiography • Cardiac imaging • Echocardiography • Cardiac magnetic resonance
- Arrhythmogenic cardiomyopathies • Arrhythmias

KEY POINTS

- Cardiovascular imaging has improved the management of patients with cardiac arrhythmias.
- Using echocardiography and magnetic resonance, the anatomic pattern of cardiomyopathies can be classified as hypertrophic, dilated, inflammatory, or right ventricular arrhythmogenic.
- A correct approach to the electrocardiogram (basal and during arrhythmias) should be used to identify the anatomic predictors of arrhythmias and sudden cardiac death by imaging techniques.

INTRODUCTION

Cardiovascular imaging radically changes the diagnosis of heart diseases. These tools accurately visualize heart morphology and function, study cardiac hemodynamics, stratify the cardiovascular risk, and address the most effective treatment.

Echocardiography is the most used imaging technique, because of its accuracy, availability, portability, safety, and cost. The transthoracic approach is the first diagnostic step: 2-dimensional (2D) and mono-dimensional (M-mode) examination provide qualitative and quantitative information about chambers size, volumes, and ventricular function. Pulsed, continuous, and color-Doppler studies allow an accurate analysis of cardiac hemodynamics. More recently, tissue Doppler imaging (TDI), speckle tracking, and 3-dimensional (3D) echocardiography have allowed the study of the earliest phases of systolic and diastolic ventricular dysfunction.

Cardiac magnetic resonance (CMR) is a gold-standard technique. Its strengths are the excellent image resolution, the intrinsic high contrast, absence of interference from lungs and bone, the 3D tomographic images, and multiple imaging techniques in a single system. Its disadvantages are the high cost, not widespread diffusion, long

Disclosure: No conflicts of interests.
[a] Cardiology and Cardiovascular Physiopathology, University of Perugia, Piazza Menghini, 1, Perugia 06129, Italy; [b] Arrhythmology Unit, Cardiology Department, Foligno General Hospital, Via Massimo Arcamone, Foligno 06034, Italy; [c] Radiology, Foligno Hospital, Via Massimo Arcamone, Foligno 06034, Italy; [d] Cardiology, Mugello Hospital, Viale della Resistenza, 60, 50032 Borgo San Lorenzo FI, Italy; [e] Multimodality Cardiac Imaging Section, Policlinico San Donato, San Donato Milanese, Piazza Edmondo Malan, 2, 20097 San Donato Milanese MI, Italy
* Correspondig author. Via Beata Chiara Luce Badano 4, Perugia 06125, Italy.
E-mail address: ketty.savino@unipg.it

acquisition time, and certain contraindications, such as claustrophobia and pacemakers.

Although imaging plays a key role in the setting of cardiomyopathies, it is "only" the integration with clinical history and electrocardiogram (ECG) that provides a comprehensive view of heart disease.

This article discusses the role of imaging in the diagnosis of heart disease that may cause arrhythmias and sudden cardiac death (SCD), integrated with the ECG.

In practical ways, some clinical cases are exposed and are analyzed for ECG and cardiovascular imaging.

From a practical point of view, the authors divided arrhythmogenic heart diseases into 4 groups:

- *Cardiomyopathies with hypertrophic pattern* (hypertrophic cardiomyopathy [HCM], restrictive cardiomyopathies, athlete's heart)
- *Cardiomyopathies with dilative pattern* (ischemic, nonischemic cardiopathy)
- *Inflammatory heart disease* (myocarditis)
- *Right ventricular diseases* (arrhythmogenic right ventricular cardiopathy) (**Table 1**).

Finally, the authors discuss predictors of arrhythmias and SCD, which are highlighted by cardiovascular imaging.

CARDIOMYOPATHIES WITH HYPERTROPHIC PATTERN

The hypertrophic pattern is present in many cardiopathies that have same phenotype but very different causes and physiopathologies.

Table 1
Different pattern in arrhythmogenic cardiomyopathies

Hypertrophic pattern	Hypertrophic cardiomyopathy Restrictive cardiomyopathy • Amyloidosis • Anderson-Fabry disease • Primitive restrictive cardiomyopathy • Sarcoidosis • Athlete's heart
Dilated pattern	Ischemic dilated cardiomyopathy Nonischemic dilated cardiomyopathy
Inflammatory heart disease	Myocarditis
Right ventricular disease	Arrhythmogenic right ventricular cardiomyopathy

Hypertrophic Cardiomyopathy

In HCM, the ECG has a wide spectrum of modifications ranging from normal or near normal to the most frequent changes in ST and T wave, and pathologic Q waves. These modifications can be isolated or combined.[1] In some cases, they are very suggestive of HCM, but they must be interpreted with an imaging tool for a definitive diagnosis.

Echocardiography is the crucial test for the definition of heart anatomy and function, offers a good prognostic stratification, and is recommended for the evaluation of patients with known or suspected HCM.[2] The transthoracic approach identifies the presence, location, and severity of ventricular hypertrophy; in most, the increased thickness is segmental and preferentially involves the basal interventricular septum, lateral wall, and apex, but it can be found at any location of the left ventricle (LV) and right ventricle (RV).[3] The increase of left ventricular mass depends on the extension of thickness segments. Other abnormalities are the systolic anterior movement (SAM) of the mitral valve, the left ventricular outflow tract obstruction (LVOTO), papillary muscles abnormalities, such as thickness, implant, muscle elongation, and accessory muscles. Color Doppler shows the presence and severity of mitral regurgitation; a midsystolic eccentric jet is suggestive of LVOTO.[4,5]

Atrial dilatation due to the increased left ventricular pressure and mitral regurgitation is important prognostic information.[6] Diastolic dysfunction aids in the understanding of symptoms and the stage of the disease.[7]

Generally, at the 2D echocardiography, radial contractile function is normal (normal ejection fraction [EF]), but left ventricular systolic function is reduced at global longitudinal strain.[8,9]

In most cases, echocardiography can correctly identify HCM diagnosis, all associated abnormalities (valvular regurgitation, presence, location, and grade of LVOTO), and studies of systolic and diastolic dysfunction. Hypertrophy severity, atrial enlargement, and diastolic dysfunction are good prognostic tools.

Unfortunately, there are some cases in which transthoracic echocardiography is limited from a suboptimal acoustic window and cannot accurately identify hypertrophy location or distribution; in these cases, other imaging tools can be useful.[2]

CMR is the gold-standard technique for providing information on ventricular function and morphology; it is particularly indicated for studying segmental thickness, ventricular function, left

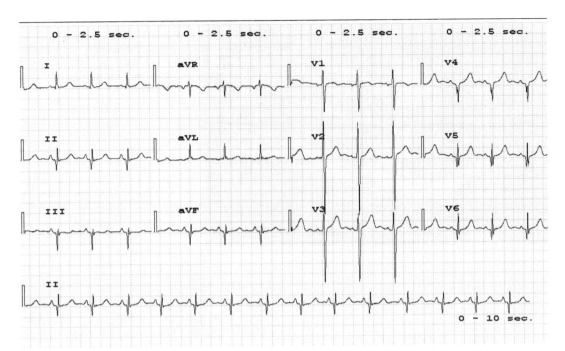

Fig. 1. Case 1 ECG: Q wave in inferior leads and pronounced R wave in leads V1, V2, and V3 as septal hypertrophy.

ventricular mass, LVOTO mechanism, and mitral kinesis and morphology.[10]

In addition to diagnostic capabilities, CMR can be applied for HCM prognostic stratification. Some recent meta-analyses showed significant associations between the presence of late gadolinium enhancement (LGE) and cardiovascular mortality, heart failure (HF), death, and all-cause mortality in HCM.[11,12] Furthermore, fibrosis (LGE) shows a trend toward an association between SDC or aborted SCD; indeed, extensive LGE seems a powerful risk marker for SDC, even after adjusting for baseline characteristics, including left ventricular EF. LGE of 20% of LV mass confers an almost 2-fold increase in SCD risk, and the risk appears to have a positive and continuous relationship with the extent of LGE.[12]

Therefore, despite that current European Society of Cardiology guidelines for management of HCM omit extensive LGE by quantitative contrast CMR in the HCM risk SCD score calculation, the extensive LGE may potentially be used as a prognostic marker to identify high-risk patients with HCM, who may be managed more aggressively, including more intensive medical treatment, surveillance, and device implantation.

The authors present 3 cases of HCM: the first with septal hypertrophy (**Figs. 1–4**), the second with diffuse left ventricular hypertrophy (**Figs. 5–7**), and the third with prevalent apical hypertrophy (**Figs. 8 and 9**).

Restrictive Cardiomyopathies

Restrictive cardiomyopathies are a heterogeneous group of cardiomyopathies, at least uncommon, with multiple causes and different morphologic characteristics.[13,14]

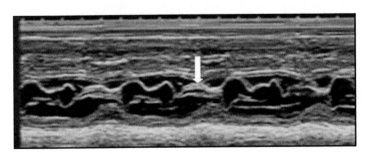

Fig. 2. Case 1: IVS hypertrophy reduces the outflow tract dimensions and causes SAM and LVOTO. At M-mode echocardiography, the anterior mitral leaflet moves toward the IVS (*arrow*). IVS, interventricular septum.

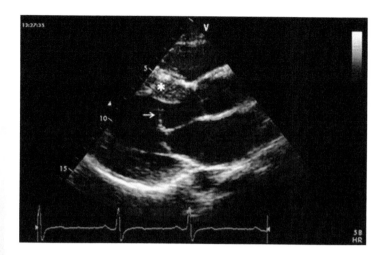

Fig. 3. Case 1: Parasternal long-axis view 2D echocardiography shows normal LV diameters, IVS hypertrophy (23 mm; *asterisk*) and SAM (*arrow*) as expression of LVOT obstruction.

They can be grouped into the following characteristics:

- Accumulation diseases with hypertrophic phenotype, such as the amyloidosis and Anderson-Fabry disease
- Endomyocardial forms, such as Loeffler disease and endomyocardial fibrosis
- Primitive restrictive cardiomyopathy characterized by an altered fibrous myocardial composition.

Although very different, they have in common the pathophysiologic mechanism with impaired ventricular relaxation, restriction filling, and high atrial pressures that occur with normal ventricular volumes, dilatation of both atria, normal or slightly reduced systolic function, a restrictive hemodynamic pattern, and caval veins dilated without excursion.

Echocardiography accurately detects morphology (chamber volumes, wall thicknesses, echogenicity) and function (EF, diastolic dysfunction, and restrictive hemodynamic pattern), but diagnosis is challenging. In these cases, CMR can be helpful for differential diagnosis.

Cardiac amyloidosis

The diagnosis of certainty regarding cardiac involvement is obtained with amyloid infiltration documentation by endomyocardial biopsy (EBM); however, ultrasounds can accurately diagnose the restrictive pattern and suspected disease. 2D echocardiography examination exhibits ventricular hypertrophy, wall thickness diffusely increased, echogenicity is like to "frosted glass", the interatrial septum and mitral and aortic leaflets are thickened and mild pericardial effusion is often present. Ventricular function is reduced. Diastolic pattern is restrictive (see later discussion).

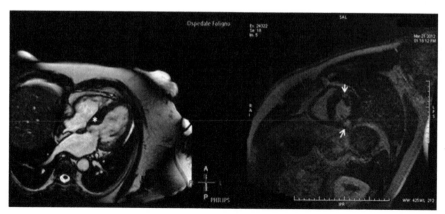

Fig. 4. Case 1: At CMR cine sequences, the basal IVS is hypertrophic (*asterisk*). At T1-weighted sequences LGE areas at the LV-RV junctions and in the inferior wall (*arrows*).

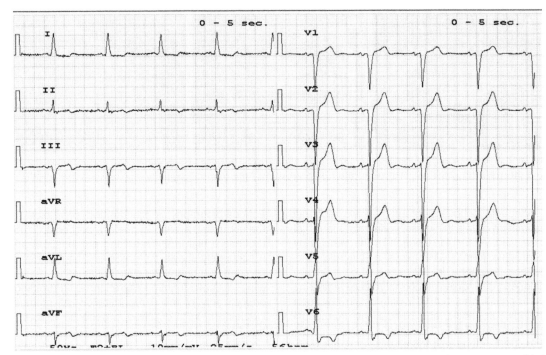

Fig. 5. Case 2: Typical ECG pattern for left ventricular hypertrophy: SV3 + RaVL greater than 2.5 mm and left ventricular overload. RaVL = R wave - aVL

At CMR, amyloidosis exhibits the same morphologic and functional modifications as described in the echocardiography section; however, it is gadolinium injection that has a peculiar signal: the blood pool is hyperintense to the T1-weighted sequences with a rapid washout with a low contrast between myocardium and blood.[15] In later discussion, the authors present 2 cases of amyloidosis, the first in low-voltage sinus rhythm and pseudo-infarct pattern (**Figs. 10–14**), and the second with atrial tachycardia and intraventricular conduction delay in a patient with amyloidosis (**Figs. 15–17**).

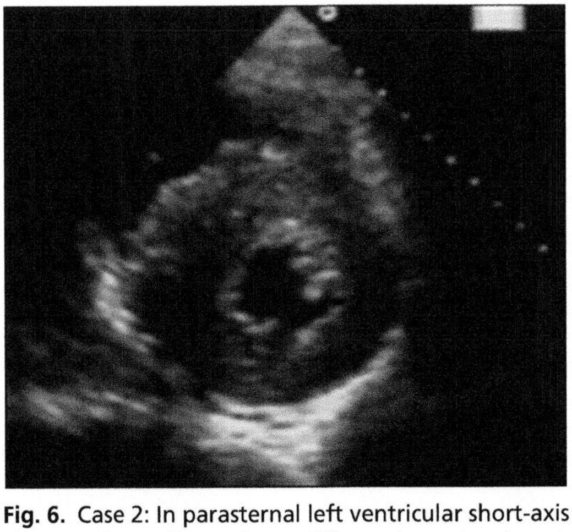

In Anderson-Fabry disease, the echocardiographic phenotype is hypertrophic, but classic restriction can also be present. In these cases CMR addresses the diagnostic suspicion (**Table 2**).

In sarcoidosis, heart involvement is rare but prognostically unfavorable. There are no typical echocardiographic features, but distortion of the myocardial wall and alterations of parietal kinetics, often with noncoronary distribution, may be present, as well as associated with diastolic and/or systolic function alterations, as shown in case 6 (**Figs. 18–21**).

Athlete's Heart

In the athlete's heart, echocardiography may show an increase in parietal thickness, slight left ventricular dilatation, and normal ventricular function. In some cases, differential diagnosis may be required with other hypertrophic cardiomyopathies (especially HCM). In these cases, CMR does not show myocardial fibrosis at LGE, which is, however, present in structural cardiopathy.

Fig. 6. Case 2: In parasternal left ventricular short-axis view echocardiography, diffuse hypertrophy is visualized.

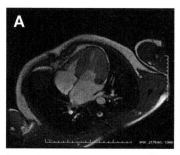 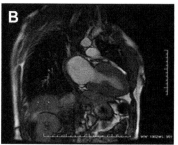 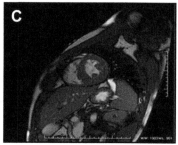

Fig. 7. Case 2: CMR in SSFP: Diffuse left ventricular hypertrophy in HCM in 4 chambers (*A*), vertical long-axis (*B*), and short-axis (*C*) planes. SSFP, steady-state free precession. Anterolateral papillary muscle is located apically.

Although echocardiography allows accurate estimation of wall thickness, ventricular mass, volume, and ventricular function in the various hypertrophic forms, CMR plays a key role when echocardiography is not responsive. It is also unique in distinguishing phenotypically similar hypertrophic forms, but very different in physiopathology, prognosis, and clinical and therapeutic management. **Table 2** lists the echocardiography and CMR criteria that identify the different forms of hypertrophic cardiopathies.

CARDIOMYOPATHIES WITH DILATED PATTERN

Ventricular dilatation and dysfunction are the ultimate means of both ischemic and nonischemic cardiomyopathy.

History, ECG, and echocardiography often lead to diagnosis. Cardiac imaging plays a central role in the diagnosis and in guiding treatment.[16]

Echocardiography is the method of choice for the accuracy, availability, safety, and cost.[16] This tool has a high diagnostic and prognostic value. It accurately shows the grade of chamber dilatation, left and right ventricular dysfunction, remodeling, diastolic function alterations, and presence and severity of mitral regurgitation. All of these indices are, in themselves, prognostic factors of the disease.[17]

CMR can complete the echocardiographic study in some cases; in fact, it is acknowledged as the gold standard for the measurements of volume, mass, and EF of both LVs and RVs. It is the best alternative modality for patients with nondiagnostic echocardiography and is the preferred imaging method to establish the cause of heart failure.[18] For example, CMR with LGE assesses myocardial fibrosis and allows the visualization of myocardial fibrosis/scars, differentiating between ischemic and nonischemic heart failure.[18]

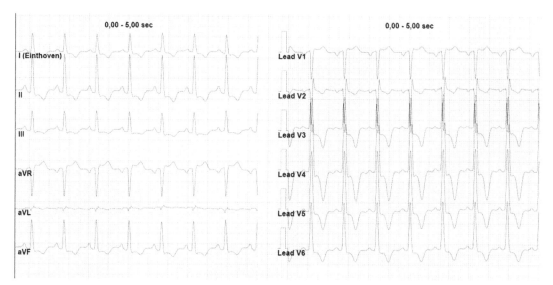

Fig. 8. Case 3 ECG: T-wave inversion, relative to apical hypertrophy, is present in D1, D2, D3, aVF, and from V3 to V6 leads. In these cases, additional imaging features of HCM are needed.

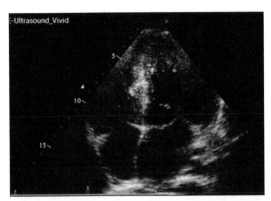

Fig. 9. Case 3: In 2D 4-chamber-view echocardiography, diffused left ventricular hypertrophy is visible and more evident at the apex.

INFLAMMATORY CARDIOPATHIES

The cause of myocarditis often remains undetermined, but a variety of infectious agents, systemic diseases, drugs, and toxins can cause the disease. Clinical presentation is variable, ranging from chest pain and palpitations with transient ECG changes to life-threatening cardiogenic shock and ventricular arrhythmias.[19] All ages are involved, although it is most frequent in young individuals. These different clinical scenarios imply that the diagnosis requires a high level of suspicion and the use of appropriate investigations to identify the cause and confirm the diagnosis.

ECG is usually abnormal, but signs are neither specific nor sensitive. However, some ECG changes are more suggestive of myocarditis than others (ST segment elevation is typically concave and diffuse without reciprocal changes, AV block, QRS prolongation, Q waves, and repolarization abnormalities).[20]

Echocardiography identifies an instrumental framework similar to ischemic heart disease (regional wall motion abnormalities) and/or congestive heart failure (global ventricular dysfunction with cardiac dilatation, sometimes complicated by mitral regurgitation and diastolic dysfunction).[21]

CMR provides noninvasive tissue characterization of the myocardium and can support the

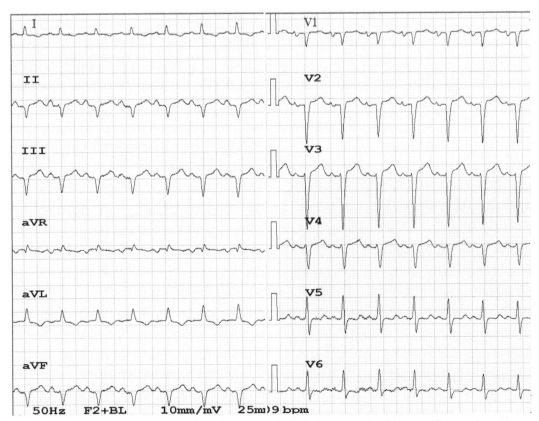

Fig. 10. Case 4 ECG: Low voltage on limb leads and pseudo-infarct pattern had high specificity and positive predictive value for the diagnosis of amyloidosis.

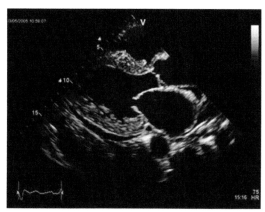

Fig. 11. Case 4: Parasternal long-axis view echocardiography: increased wall thickness (left ventricular hypertrophy), mitral and aortic leaflets thickening, hypermyocardial reflexion (frosted glass), pericardial effusion. Mitral leaflets have a reduced opening as a severe left ventricular dysfunction.

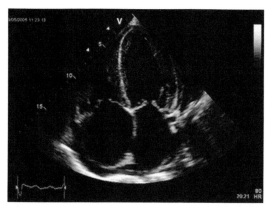

Fig. 13. Case 4: Apical 4 chambers: left and right atrium dilatation, normal ventricular volumes, increased wall thickness (left ventricular hypertrophy), mitral and tricuspidal leaflets thickening, myocardial hyperreflexion (frosted glass), pericardial effusion.

diagnosis of myocarditis. The timing of CMR is before EMB in stable patients.

Because the histopathologic features of this process are edema, hyperemia, and altered cellular homeostasis, CMR tissue characterization recognizes the presence and distribution of edema at T2-weighted sequences in the acute phase and LGE in the chronic phase as expression of intramyocardial fibrosis.[22]

The diagnosis of myocarditis, according to Lake Louise criteria, can be achieved if at least 2 criteria are positive (78% accuracy); however if the clinical suspect is high and the CMR identifies only one criterion or no one is reasonable to repeat the investigation 1 to 2 weeks later.[23]

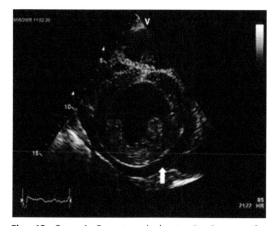

Fig. 12. Case 4: Parasternal short-axis view at the papillary muscle level: increased wall thickness (left ventricular hypertrophy), hypermyocardial reflexion (frosted glass), pericardial effusion (*arrow*).

In later discussion, the authors present a case of subendocardial myocarditis (**Figs. 22** and **23**) and epicardial myocarditis (**Figs. 24** and **25**).

RIGHT VENTRICULAR CARDIOMYOPATHIES
Arrhythmogenic Right Ventricular Cardiomyopathy

The arrhythmogenic right ventricular cardiomyopathy (ARVC) is a progressive hereditary cardiomyopathy with a higher risk of ventricular arrhythmias and SCD.[24] It is characterized histologically by fibrofatty replacement of myocardium with subsequent ventricular dilation and systolic dysfunction.[25] Ventricular fibrillation (VF) may occur during the process of cell death, whereas macro-reentry ventricular tachycardia (VT) is related to fibrofatty scars.[26]

ARVC diagnosis is challenging because most patients are asymptomatic, and sudden death is often the first manifestation of the disease.

Some phenotypic variants follow:

- The "classical" form that mainly involves the RV, whereas the LV is only affected in the late stages of the disease. In this case, diagnostic criteria of the disease are ventricular arrhythmias from macro-reentry that have a QRS morphology type of left bundle branch block.
- The "biventricular" variant in which the 2 ventricles are involved in parallel.
- The "left dominance" variant in which left ventricular involvement is dominant on the right.

Making a correct diagnosis is critically important and requires many diagnostic techniques.

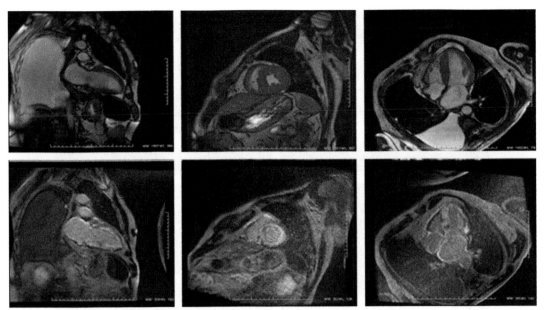

Fig. 14. Case 4: CMR in amyloidosis: cine sequences show diffuse hypertrophic pattern and dilated atrium. At LGE, T1-weighted sequences are shown with low interface between blood and myocardium global subendocardial enhancement typical for amyloidosis.

In current ARVC diagnostic criteria, the good diagnostic sensitivity is based, among others, on cardiovascular imaging.[27]

In the early stage of the classical form, with right involvement, morphofunctional localized abnormalities are present (dyssynergic areas or aneurysm); in the advanced phases, the disease evolves toward RV outflow dilatation, increased ventricular volumes (especially at the RV outflow tract), and reduced RV EF.

Echocardiography can show regional RV wall motion abnormality, increased RV dimension, and reduced RV EF, especially in advanced phases of disease. CMR plays a major role in diagnosing ARVC with fairly high sensitivity and specificity in recognizing the disease in the early stage.

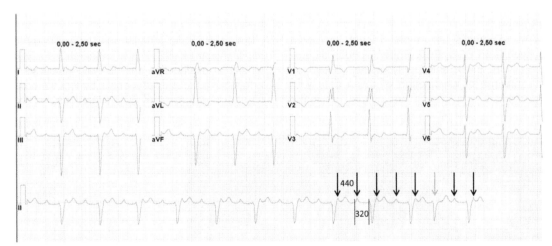

Fig. 15. Case 5 ECG: Atrial tachycardia and diffuse intraventricular conduction delay in a patient with amyloidosis. Atrial tachycardia (*arrows*), A-A interval 440 milliseconds, with 2:1 atrioventricular conduction is present. A complete right bundle branch block and left anterior fascicular block are present (bifascicular block); a long A-V interval should raise suspicion of a more advanced intraventricular block (trifascicular block). In these cases, suspected amyloidosis is very challenging, and cardiac imaging (echocardiography and CMR) is needed for diagnosis.

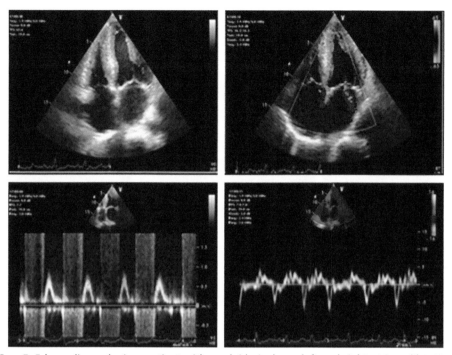

Fig. 16. Case 5: Echocardiography in a patient with amyloidosis shows left and right atrium dilatation, normal ventricular volumes, increased wall thickness (left and right ventricular hypertrophy), mitral and tricuspidal leaflets thickening, myocardial hyperreflexion (frosted glass) without pericardial effusion. At mitral flow and interventricular septal TDI, restrictive diastolic pattern is shown. At color Doppler, mild mitral and tricuspidal regurgitation is shown.

Although the criteria do not list tissue characterization, such as diagnostic parameters, many studies have demonstrated the additive value of both adipose infiltration and fibrosis. In particular, there seems to be an unfavorable outcome in subjects with right ventricular arrhythmias and tissue disorders.[28]

The diagnosis is made through a score derived from ECG, ECG-Holter, echocardiography, CMR, EMB, and family history. Based on the strength of association of these data with the disease, the criteria are defined as major or minor. Combining the major and minor criteria, it is possible to obtain a reliable diagnosis of ARVC (2 major criteria or 1 major criterion and 2 minor or 4 minor criteria), probable ARVC (1 major criterion and 1 minor or 3 minor criteria), or possible ARVC (1 major criterion or 2 minor).

In asymptomatic patients, nonsustained ventricular tachycardia (NSVT) and moderate to severe ventricular dysfunction are the main indicators of arrhythmic risk. Other prognostic factors are probing status, extension of ECG alterations, number

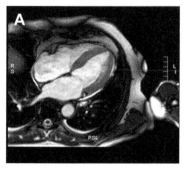
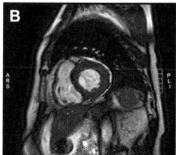
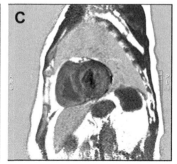

Fig. 17. Case 5: In the same patient in **Fig. 16**, CMR cine sequences show diffuse hypertrophy of both ventricles (*A*, *B*); at black blood T1-weighted sequences (*C*), low contrast between myocardium and blood is present.

Table 2
Morphologic parameters for diagnosis of cardiomyopathies with hypertrophic pattern

	HCM	Amyloidosis	Anderson-Fabry Disease	Athlete's Heart
Hypertrophic pattern	Asymmetric Symmetric Midventricular Apical	Symmetric	Symmetric	Symmetric
Increased LVM	+++	+++	+++	+
LVOT obstruction	Frequent	Very rare	Rare	Absent
LGE	Focal intramyocardial junction	Subendocardial Frosted glass Valves Atria Heterogeneous pattern	Inconstant Intramyocardial Inferolateral wall	Rare
Native T1 mapping	Increased	Greatly increased	Reduced	Normal
Myocardial annulment at LGE	Annulled	Not annulled	Annulled	Annulled
Δ T1 (myocardium/ blood) in LGE	High	Low	High	High
Other characteristics	SAM Accessory papillary muscles Apical aneurysms	IAS hypertrophy RV hypertrophy Valves leaflet thickening Pericardial effusion		Diastolic wall thickness to volume ratio <0.15 Normal LVM after deconditioning

Abbreviations: AS: atrial septum; L, left ventricular mass.

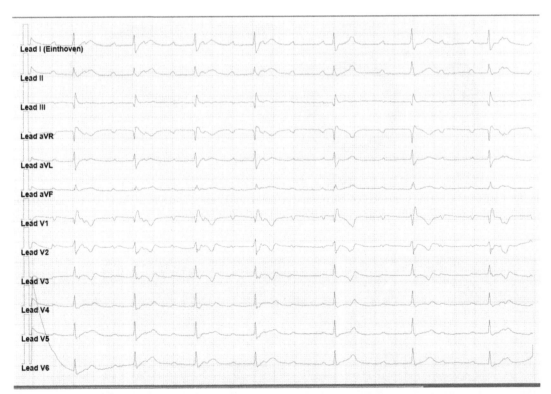

Fig. 18. Case 6 ECG: Sinus tachycardial rhythm with atrioventricular II degree 2:1 block (first 4 QRS), followed by paroxysmal complete atrioventricular block with junctional escape rhythm. Patient with right-septal cardiac sarcoidosis. Right bundle branch block is also present.

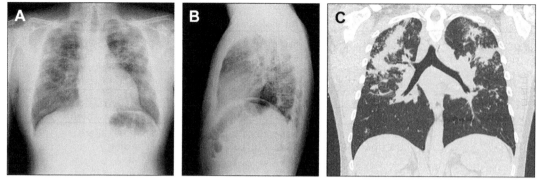

Fig. 19. Case 6: At chest radiograph (*A, B*) reticulonodular opacities with middle and upper zone distribution. At chest CT (*C*), irregular thickening of hilar interstitium in a perilymphatic distribution with peripheral large pulmonary opacities.

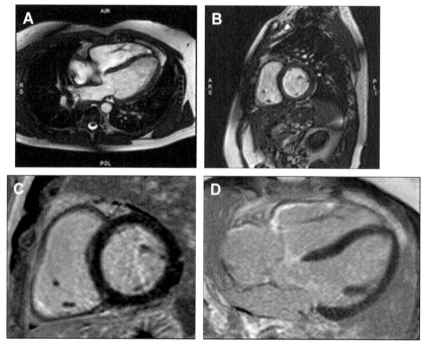

Fig. 20. Case 6 CMR: at cine sequences (*A, B*), normal volumes, thicknesses, and kinesis. At T1-weighted post-gadolinium sequences (*C, D*), faint subendocardial right wall, and right IVS LGE.

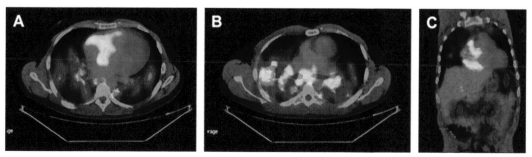

Fig. 21. Case 6: At PET-CT (*A–C*): PET avidity in perilymphatic interstitium and in right atrial, right ventricular, right atrioventricular cardiac walls.

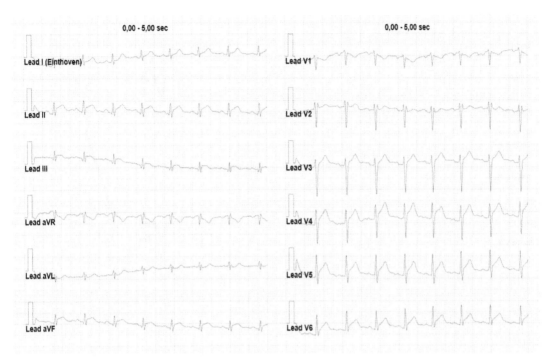

Fig. 22. Case 7: ECG of a patient with acute myocarditis: sinus tachycardia (100 bpm), normal atrioventricular conduction, low QRS voltage in limb leads, diffuse ST elevation.

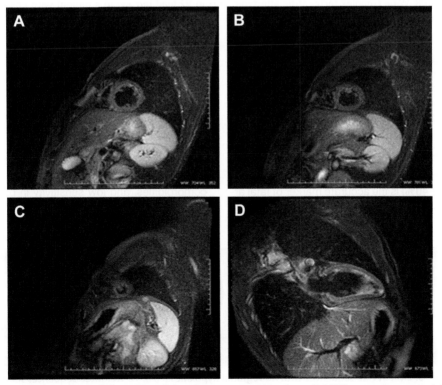

Fig. 23. Case 7 CMR in myocarditis: at T2-weighted sequences, subendocardial LV hyperenhancement from basal to apical segments in short-axis view (*A–C*) and longitudinal plane (*D*) are shown.

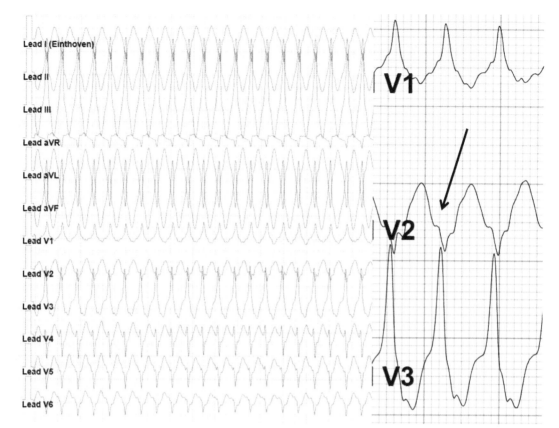

Fig. 24. Case 8: Wide complex tachycardia and typical QS in V2 lead (*arrow*) in a patient with epicardial septal myocarditis.

and complexity of ventricular premature beats at Holter, and VT/VF inducibility to programmed ventricular stimulation.

The last case concerns an advanced ARVC (**Figs. 26–28**).

PREDICTORS OF SUDDEN CARDIAC DEATH

Severe systolic left ventricular dysfunction (EF ≤35%–40%) is the accurate marker of fatal arrhythmias. For this population, implantable cardioverter-defibrillator (ICD) represents the optimal therapy for primary prevention of SCD, and current guidelines recommended its use in class IA.[29]

The extensive use of the device has shown treatment efficacy, but has highlighted some relevant limitations. EF, itself, has low specificity because it does not differentiate the risk of SCD from the death or congestive heart failure or comorbidities, and low sensitivity in patients with preserved or moderately reduced EF.[30] These

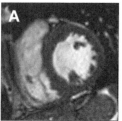
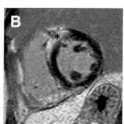
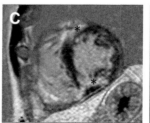
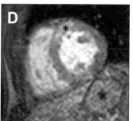

Fig. 25. Case 8: CMR at cine sequences with no regional hypokinesia (*A*); T2-weighted sequences show epicardial edema of the anteroseptal and inferior sub-epimesocardial LGE at T1-weighted post-gadolinium sequences (*asterisk* in *B* and *C*), with first-pass hyperemia in the same regions (*asterisk* in *D*).

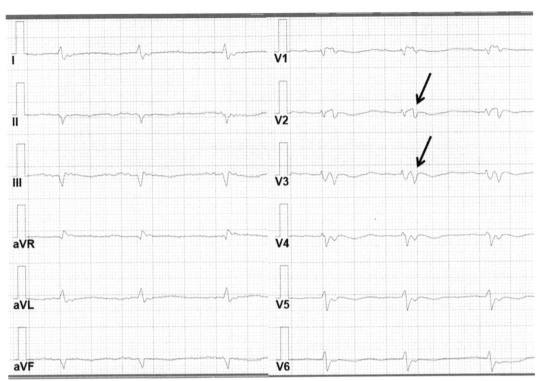

Fig. 26. Case 9 ECG: Sinus rhythm, very low P wave, and QRS voltages in a patient with ARVC. In right precordial leads, a wide epsilon wave is well evident (*arrow*).

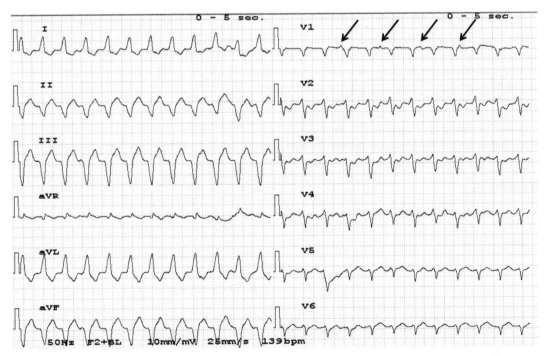

Fig. 27. Case 9: In the same patient as in **Fig. 26**, other ECG shows VT and atrioventricular dissociation (*arrows* on the P waves).

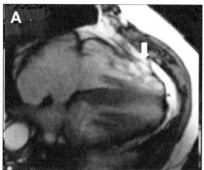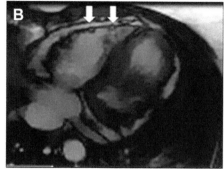

Fig. 28. Case 9: CRM in ARVC: In cine sequences (SSFP) RV dilatation, regional wall thinning (*arrow* in *A*), and 3 wall RV bulging (*arrows* in *B*) are visible.

data are supported by the evidence that more than one-third of ICDs do not have the appropriate interventions during the follow-up. Thus, a negligible proportion of patients do not have any benefit while are subjected to ICD side effects.

The limits of the SCD risk stratification are due to the following various factors[31,32]:

- 50% of SCDs occur in subjects without a known cardiopathy
- Approximately three-fourths of events are in subjects with EF greater than 40%
- Fatal arrhythmias are generated by dynamic electrophysiologic mechanisms
- EF represents the indicator of ICD implant indicator but does not consider the cause of left ventricular dysfunction, the evolution of the disease, and the phenotype.

Numerous recent CMR studies have shown solid evidence that the presence and extension of myocardial fibrosis/scar (LGE) are accurate predictors of major arrhythmias and improve the EF risk stratification.[33,34] Therefore, in the near future, CMR may become a useful tool for arrhythmic and SCD risk stratification "beyond EF" in different heart diseases and for decision making in ICD therapy device implantation.[35]

REFERENCES

1. McLeod CJ, Ackerman MJ, Nishimura RA, et al. Outcome of patients with hypertrophic cardiomyopathy and a normal electrocardiogram. J Am Coll Cardiol 2009;54:229–33.
2. Elliott PM, Anastasakis A, Borger MA, et al. 2014 ESC guidelines on diagnosis and management of hypertrophic cardiomyopathy: the task force for the diagnosis and management of hypertrophic cardiomyopathy of the European Society of Cardiology (ESC). Eur Heart J 2014;35:2733–79.
3. Klues HG, Schiffers A, Maron BJ. Phenotypic spectrum and patterns of left ventricular hypertrophy in hypertrophic cardiomyopathy: morphologic observations and significance as assessed by two-dimensional echocardiography in 600 patients. J Am Coll Cardiol 1995;26:1699–708.
4. Wigle ED, Sasson Z, Henderson MA, et al. Hypertrophic cardiomyopathy. The importance of the site and the extent of hypertrophy. A review. Prog Cardiovasc Dis 1985;28:1–83.
5. Maron MS, Olivotto I, Zenovich AG, et al. Hypertrophic cardiomyopathy is predominantly a disease of left ventricular outflow tract obstruction. Circulation 2006;114:2232–9.
6. O'Mahony C, Jichi F, Pavlou M, et al. A novel clinical risk prediction model for sudden cardiac death in hypertrophic cardiomyopathy (HCM Risk-SCD). Eur Heart J 2014;35:2010–20.
7. Nagueh SF, Appleton CP, Gillebert TC, et al. Recommendations for the evaluation of left ventricular diastolic function by echocardiography. Eur J Echocardiogr 2009;10:165–93.
8. Maciver DH. A new method for quantification of left ventricular systolic function using a corrected ejection fraction. Eur J Echocardiogr 2011;12:228–34.
9. Urbano-Moral JA, Rowin EJ, Maron MS, et al. Investigation of global and regional myocardial mechanics with 3-dimensional speckle tracking echocardiography and relations to hypertrophy and fibrosis in hypertrophic cardiomyopathy. Circ Cardiovasc Imaging 2014;7:11–9.
10. Puntmann VO, Gebker R, Duckett S, et al. Left ventricular chamber dimensions and wall thickness by cardiovascular magnetic resonance: comparison with transthoracic echocardiography. Eur Heart J Cardiovasc Imaging 2013;14:240–6.
11. Green JJ, Berger JS, Kramer CM, et al. Prognostic value of late gadolinium enhancement in clinical outcomes for hypertrophic cardiomyopathy. JACC Cardiovasc Imaging 2012;5:370–7.
12. Weng Z, Yao J, Chan RH, et al. Prognostic value of LGE-CMR in HCM. A meta-analysis. JACC Cardiovasc Imaging 2016;9:1392–402.

13. Angelini A, Calzolari V, Thiene G, et al. Morphologic spectrum of primary restrictive cardiomyopathy. Am J Cardiol 1997;80(8):1046.

14. Seward JB, Casaclang-Verzosa G. Infiltrative cardiovascular diseases: cardiomyopathies that look alike. J Am Coll Cardiol 2010;55:1769–74.

15. Di Bella G, Pizzino F, Minutoli F, et al. The mosaic of the cardiac amyloidosis diagnosis: role of imaging in subtypes and stages of the disease. Eur Heart J Cardiovasc Imaging 2014;15(12):1307–15.

16. Ponikowski P, Voors AA, Anker SD, et al. 2016 ESC guidelines for the diagnosis and treatment of acute and chronic heart failure. Eur Heart J 2016;37: 2129–200.

17. Lang RM, Badano LP, Mor-Avi V, et al. Recommendations for cardiac chamber quantification by echocardiography in adults: an update from the American Society of Echocardiography and the European Association of Cardiovascular Imaging. Eur Heart J Cardiovasc Imaging 2015;16:233–70.

18. Gonzalez JA, Kramer CM. Role of imaging techniques for diagnosis, prognosis and management of heart failure patients: cardiac magnetic resonance. Curr Heart Fail Rep 2015;12:276–83.

19. Moon JC, Messroghli DR, Kellman P, et al. Myocardial T1 mapping and extracellular volume quantification: a Society for Cardiovascular Magnetic Resonance (SCMR) and CMR Working Group of the European Society of Cardiology consensus statement. J Cardiovasc Magn Reson 2013;15:92.

20. Caforio ALP, Pankuweit S, Arbustini E, et al. Current state of knowledge on aetiology, diagnosis, management, and therapy of myocarditis: a position statement of the European Society of Cardiology Working Group on myocardial and pericardial diseases. Eur Heart J 2013;34:2636–48.

21. Ukena C, Mahfoud F, Kindermann I, et al. Prognostic electrocardiographic parameters in patients with suspected myocarditis. Eur J Heart Fail 2011;13: 398–405.

22. Pinamonti B, Alberti E, Cigalotto A, et al. Echocardiographic findings in myocarditis. Am J Cardiol 1988;62:285–91.

23. Friedric MG, Sechtem U, Schultz-Menger J, et al. International consensus group on cardiovascular magnetic resonance in myocarditis: a JACC white paper. J Am Coll Cardiol 2009;53:1475–87.

24. Basso C, Corrado D, Marcus F, et al. Arrhythmogenic right ventricular cardiomyopathy. Lancet 2009;373:1289–300.

25. Thiene G, Nava A, Corrado D, et al. Right ventricular cardiomyopathy and sudden death in young people. N Engl J Med 1988;318:129–33.

26. Sen-Chowdhry S, Syrris P, Prasad SK, et al. Left-dominant arrhythmogenic cardiomyopathy: an under-recognized clinical entity. J Am Coll Cardiol 2008;52:2175–87.

27. Marcus FI, McKenna WJ, Sherrill D, et al. Diagnosis of arrhythmogenic right ventricular cardiomyopathy/dysplasia proposed modification of the task force criteria. Circulation 2010;121:1533–41.

28. Aquaro GD, Pingitore A, Strata E, et al. Cardiac magnetic resonance predicts outcome in patients with premature ventricular complexes of left bundle branch block morphology. J Am Coll Cardiol 2010; 56(15):12435–43.

29. Silvia G, Priori SG, Blomstro-Lundqvist C, et al. 2015 ESC guidelines for the management of patients with ventricular arrhythmias and the prevention of sudden cardiac death. Eur Heart J 2015;36:2793–867.

30. Epstein AE, Di Marco JP, Ellenbogen KA, et al. 2012 ACCF/AHA/HRS focused update incorporated into the ACCF/AHA/HRS 2008 guidelines for device-based therapy of cardiac rhythm abnormalities. A report of the American College of Cardiology Foundation/American Heart Association task force on practice guidelines and the Heart Rhythm Society. Circulation 2013;127:e283–352.

31. Moss AJ, Zareba W, Hall WJ, et al, Multicenter Automatic Defibrillator Implantation Trial II Investigators. Prophylactic implantation of a defibrillator in patients with myocardial infarction and reduced ejection fraction. N Engl J Med 2002;346:877–83.

32. Weeke P, Johansen JB, Jorgensen OD, et al. Mortality and appropriate and inappropriate therapy in patients with ischaemic heart disease and implanted cardioverter defibrillators for primary prevention: data from the Danish ICD register. Europace 2013; 15:1150–7.

33. Klem I, Weinsaft JW, Bahnson TD, et al. Assessment of myocardial scarring improves risk stratification in patients evaluated for cardiac defibrillator implantation. J Am Coll Cardiol 2012;60:408–20.

34. Kuruvilla S, Adenaw N, Katwal AB, et al. Late gadolinium enhancement on CMR predicts adverse cardiovascular outcomes in non-ischemic cardiomyopathy: a systematic review and meta-analysis. Circ Cardiovasc Imaging 2014;7:250–8.

35. De Maria E, Aldrovandi A, Borghi A, et al. Cardiac magnetic resonance imaging: which information is useful for the arrhythmologist? World J Cardiol 2017;26:773–86.

Moving?

Make sure your subscription moves with you!

To notify us of your new address, find your **Clinics Account Number** (located on your mailing label above your name), and contact customer service at:

Email: journalscustomerservice-usa@elsevier.com

800-654-2452 (subscribers in the U.S. & Canada)
314-447-8871 (subscribers outside of the U.S. & Canada)

Fax number: 314-447-8029

Elsevier Health Sciences Division
Subscription Customer Service
3251 Riverport Lane
Maryland Heights, MO 63043

ELSEVIER

Printed and bound by CPI Group (UK) Ltd, Croydon, CR0 4YY

03/10/2024

01040383-0004